Textbook of Community Children's Nursing

Edited by

Anna Sidey RSCN RGN DN Cert

Independent Adviser, Community Children's Nursing, UK

David Widdas RSCN RGN Dip Community Health Nursing
Dip Health Promotion MSc

*Nurse Consultant for Children with Complex Care Needs, North and South Warwickshire,
Coventry and Rugby Primary Care Trusts, UK*

Foreword by

Elizabeth Fradd MSc RSCN SCM RN HVCert FRCN

Independent Health Service Adviser, UK

SECOND EDITION

ELSEVIER

EDINBURGH LONDON NEW YORK OXFORD PHILADELPHIA ST LOUIS SYDNEY TORONTO 2005

ELSEVIER

An imprint of Elsevier Limited

First edition 2000
Second edition 2005
  Reprinted 2005

ISBN 0 7020 2729 4

British Library Cataloguing in Publication Data
A catalogue record for this book is available from the British Library

Library of Congress Cataloguing in Publication Data
A catalogue record for this book is available from the Library of Congress

ELSEVIER your source for books, journals and multimedia in the health sciences

www.elsevierhealth.com

Working together to grow
libraries in developing countries

www.elsevier.com | www.bookaid.org | www.sabre.org

ELSEVIER   BOOK AID International   Sabre Foundation

The publisher's policy is to use paper manufactured from sustainable forests

Printed in China

Contents

Section Two

Philosophical Issues Underpinning the Delivery of Community Children's Nursing Practice

Section Three

Dimensions of Community Children's Nursing Practice

Section Four

Advancing Community Children's Nursing Practice

Contributors

Jackie Acornley RSCN RGN BA(Hons) Dip Nursing
Team Leader, Cambridge Community Children's Nursing Team, Cambridge, UK

Dorothy Bean RGN RSCN RHV BSc Med
Senior Lecturer Palliative Care, Oxford Brookes University, Oxford, UK

Michael Bland RGN RSCN DipHe BSc(Hons)
Senior Lecturer, Department of Nursing, Faculty of Health, University of Central Lancashire, Preston, UK

Sue Burr RSCN RGN RHV RNT MA OBE FRCN
Former Adviser in Children's Nursing, Royal College of Nursing, UK

Steve Campbell BNurs PhD RGN RSCN RHV NDN Cert FRSH
Head of Nursing Research and Development, Head of Research and Development, City Hospitals Sunderland NHS Trust, Professor of Nursing Practice, Northumbria University, UK

Linda Cancelliere RSCN RGN DipDN BA(Hons) CPT
Community Children's Nurse Manager, Telford and Wrekin Primary Care Trust, Shropshire, UK

Anne Casey RSCN MSc FRCN
Editor, Paediatric Nursing, Royal College of Nursing Publishing Company, Harrow, UK

Melanie Coombes RNMH Dip Community Nursing Studies
Consultant Nurse, North Warwickshire PCT, Nuneaton, UK

Tara Davis DipHE RN BSc(Hons) PGDip
Community Children's Nurse, Kensington and Chelsea Primary Care Trust, London, UK

Bridgit Dimond MA LLB DSA AHSM Barrister-at-Law
Emeritus Professor of University of Glamorgan, UK

Sue Dryden
RSCN RGN MA DN Cert
Assistant Director, Children's Services, Broxtowe and Hucknall Primary Care Trust, UK

Sue Facey
BSc(Hons) MSc RSCN RGN Dip N
Community Children's Nursing Sister, The Children's Unit, The Great Western Hospital, Swindon, UK

Julia Fearon
BSc(Hons) RGN RSCN
Laser Nurse Specialist, Department of Plastic Surgery, Birmingham Children's Hospital NHS Trust, Birmingham, UK

Caroline Fitzgerald
RGN RSCN DN BSc(Hons)
Community Children's Nurse Team Leader, Kensington and Chelsea Primary Care Trust, London, UK

Jo Holder
RNMH Dip Community Nursing Studies
Community Children's Nurse, Community Children's Team, Rugby, UK

Julie Hughes
RGN RSCN BSc(Hons) PGCEA MScEd
Learning Coordinator, London Region National Health Service University, UK

Mark Jones
MSc BSc(Hons) RN RHV
Director, Community Practitioners' and Health Visitors' Association, London, UK

Suzanne Jones
RGN RSCN ENB 988 MSc PGD Advanced Nursing Practice
Programme Development Manager, Children's Services, Birmingham and the Black Country Strategic Health Authority, UK

Paulajean Kelly
RGN RSCN MSc BSc PGCE
Lecturer in Child Health Nursing, Florence Nightingale School of Nursing and Midwifery, Research Fellow, Queen Mary's College, London, UK

Peter Kent
BA(Hons)
Independent Consultant, Helix Partners, London, UK

Sharon Linter
RGN RSCN BSc MA
Deputy Chief Nurse for Children's Services, Trust Headquarters, St James University Hospital, Leeds, UK

Lorly McClure
MSc PGCEA BA RGN DN RHV
Lecturer, School of Health and Social Care, The University of Reading, UK

Tracey Malkin
RGN RSCN BSc(Hons) RHV MSc ANP
Advanced Children's Nurse/Community Children's Team Leader, Cheadle Hospital, Cheadle, UK

Chris Middleton
RSCN RGN RNT Dip NEd MA Socio-Legal Studies (Children)
Senior Health Lecturer, University of Nottingham School of Nursing, UK

Sue Miller
RGN RSCN DN Cert Ed BSc(Hons) MSc
Senior Lecturer, Children's Nursing, School of Nursing and Midwifery, University of Hertfordshire, Hatfield, UK

Debbie Mills
NNEB HPS IIHT IAIM
Children's Palliative Care Community Play Specialist, Diana Community Children's Nursing Team, Leicester Frith Hospital, Leicester, UK

Sean Mountford

Sarah Neill
MSc PGDE BSc(Hons) RGN RSCN
Senior Lecturer in Children's Nursing, School of Health, University College Northampton, UK

Susan Procter
RGN BSc(Hons) PhD Cert Ed
Professor of Primary Health Care Research, St Bartholomew School of Nursing and Midwifery, London, UK

Phillippa Russell
OBE DSc(Soc) BA
Special Policy Adviser on Disability, National Children's Bureau, Disability Rights Commissioner, UK

Brian Samwell
MMedsci BA RGN RSCN PGCE
Clinical Service Manager, Borders General Hospital, Borders Health Board, UK

Anna Sidey
RSCN RGN DN Cert
Independent Adviser, Community Children's Nursing, Shropshire, UK

Maybelle Tatman
MB BS MSc FRCP FRCPCH
Consultant Community Paediatrician and Clinical Director, Child & Family Services, Coventry Teaching Primary Care Trust, Gulson Hospital, Coventry, UK

Saleha Uddin
Link Worker, Community Children's Nursing Service, Tower Hamlets Primary Care Trust, London, UK

Lisa Whiting
MSc BA (Hons) RN RSCN RNT LTCL
Senior Lecturer Children's Nursing, School of Nursing and Midwifery, University of Hertfordshire, Hatfield, UK

Mark Whiting
MSc BNursing RSCN RN DN Cert HV Cert PG Dip Ed RNT
Consultant Nurse, Children with Complex Health Needs, Hertfordshire Partnership NHS Trust

David Widdas
RSCN RGN Dip Community Health Nursing Dip Health Promotion MSc
Nurse Consultant for Children wih Complex Care Needs, North and South Warwickshire, Coventry and Rugby Primary Care Trusts, UK

Kath Williamson   RGN RSCN PG Cert
Clinical Nurse Specialist, Child and Adolescent Mental Health Service, Derbyshire Mental Health Services, NHS Trust, UK

Christine Wint   BSc(Hons) RSCN
Senior Lecturer Community Children's Nursing, University of Central England, Birmingham, UK

Lynn Young   RN DN CPT
Primary Health Care Adviser, Royal College of Nursing, London, UK

Foreword

When the first edition of this book was published in 2000, I predicted that it would become essential reading for nurses caring for sick children in the community. The fact that only five years later a second edition has been necessary, is testament both to its supreme value as a textbook, and to the many changes taking place in the field of children's services. In my view it is an excellent and important read for all children's healthcare professionals.

New chapters in this edition reflect the growing maturity of community children's nurses as well as their confidence to influence the future, although Acornley argues the case for greater corporate identity in the future in order to secure the best for children (Chapter 10). In addition, this new book reflects the changing political arena in which they work. For example Jones and Tatman explore strategic planning and commissioning of services (Chapter 15). The organic nature of nursing practice is reflected in new chapters about how the role of the community children's nurse has advanced (Chapter 30), as well as the difficult but important transition period into adult services (Chapter 32). However, alongside the sharing in many chapters of the exciting developments in practice, there is also the reality of what it is like to deliver complex care; for example the reflections of Widdas, Sidey and Dryden in Chapter 22 on the funding of care.

Perhaps the chapter which is the most striking for me, given what I know has been the relentless momentum of community children's nursing, is the one describing the evolution of the specialty. The story told by Whiting in Chapter 2 is complemented by the chapter that follows, describing recent changes within the NHS and how they affect children's services. It is historic reading and an important record of progress for future reference.

The book follows the same logical pathway as the first edition. The broad strategic and operational issues sensibly come first, along with the historical perspective. Recently there have been extraordinary moves to improve the quality of services for children, the like of which I have never seen, for example the raised profile of children on the political agenda, new indicators to assist in the determination of quality care, followed by inspection against standards. Philosophical issues are explored, and finally there are two sections about the practice of community children's nurses. Importantly the book covers many areas of care children's nurses in clinical practice may experience, including the acutely ill child, those with a mental health problem or a learning disability, those who are carers themselves, or those receiving palliative care.

Importantly, however, the book not only covers clinical care, but also includes a number of chapters that are fundamental to the safe and effective delivery of care; for example benchmarking, dependency scoring, information management and economic evaluation. These sections will be particularly informative for managers and service commissioners.

What is clear to me, from my first reading of the book, is that Whiting's observation is true. Services across the UK have indeed painstakingly sought out the right model of care for the children and families in their locality. I know this to be true from my work in the Commission for Health Improvement, when we inspected children's services. I believe this individualism has contributed to the richness of the services provided and therefore to the content of this book.

I particularly wish to thank the editors Anna Sidey and David Widdas for drawing together authors from such diverse backgrounds, resulting in the production of a comprehensive guide to community children's nursing. My final comment must, however, be about the children themselves. They are the inspiration for this book, and I hope that those involved in their care when they are at their most vulnerable will read it and gain inspiration from it. Importantly I hope they persist in listening to the children, so that care can continue to flourish and reflect what is in their best interest in the future.

Nottingham 2005   Elizabeth Fradd Msc RSCN SCM RN HVCert FRCN

Preface

'In the culture I grew up in you did your work and did not put your arm around it to stop other people from looking. You took the earliest opportunity to make knowledge available'.

James Black, December 1998
Winner of the Nobel Prize for Medicine

In the first edition of the first book devoted to community children's nursing contributors brought together historical, contemporary and future perspectives of this exciting discipline. It was impossible to cover all aspects of expanding service provision but it has nevertheless been very well received not only by Community Children's Nurses (CCNs) but also a surprising range of interested readers!

At the time of writing it remains the only textbook specifically addressing the speciality of community children's nursing. In the fast moving world of the NHS and community nursing this revision reflects the professional development and expanding dimensions of care for sick children and their families.

Within this second edition many of the original chapters have been extensively updated, expanded or rewritten to reflect the NHS reforms and the expansion of practice. Five chapters have been updated by new contributors. Particular thanks and appreciation are offered to Andrea Lambert (Chapter 23), Patricia Livsey (Chapter 9), Aidan Macfarlane (Chapter 3), Kirsty Read (Chapter 25) and Helen Shipton (Chapter 27) for their work for the first edition that has been extracted, edited and updated or rewritten. Julia Muir, the former co-editor, was unable to work on this edition but her influence is valued and evident within the new text. The second edition continues the aim to be a foundation text and we hope it will be extensively viewed and used as a signpost to further study. A challenging conclusion may provide some direction for this.

The title Community Children's Nurse was formalised in the early 1990s (see pp 31 and 97) and is used throughout this text to encourage its adoption as part of the drive towards a corporate identity for community children's nursing. While exploring and explaining developments in CCNs' practice the book seeks to rekindle debate about the need for and value of an identifiable national strategy and corporate identity for the profession (see Chapter 10). The term 'children' rather than 'paediatric' is used wherever possible to reflect the person-centred approach. In addition, when referring to 'child and young person' we intend it to reflect the National Service Framework (NSF) definition, i.e. from birth to nineteenth birthday. Some commonly accepted abbreviations are included and unqualified throughout: HM (Her Majesty), NHS (National Health Service), DoH (Department of Health) and UK (United Kingdom).

The emerging NSF is a constant theme in this second edition as it will be in children's services for some years to come. A key area of the NSF is transition and a new chapter explores the interface between children's and adult services (see Chapter 32).

In the first edition readers found the 'further reading' sections of each chapter useful but because of extensive duplication further reading is now at the end of the book together with chapter-specific and generic websites.

The size of the book, and, in some cases, shortage of information, prevented the inclusion of proposed topics. In particular this includes areas of specific practice that readers of the first edition urged the editors to include. The need for clear professional and practical guidance on the administration of medicines was one of the most requested. An expanding group of both formal and informal carers are now responsible for this increasingly complex area of practice in the range of settings recognised as 'the community'. We accept there is a dearth of literature to support this practice and acknowledge increasing concerns about what constitutes secure and 'required' administration of medicines.

Furthermore, our combined experience as CCNs leads us to promote a wider embracing of 'enabling and empowering' practice (see Chapter 11). Whilst many CCNs deliver care that reflects this approach we are also aware of situations where practice does not. As a consequence families may fail to develop the empowering control and broad ranging expertise that constitute the cornerstones of family care (p 354). Failure to empower can be disabling and we have endeavoured to weave the 'enabling and empowering' theme into each chapter.

With these issues in mind this second edition is prepared as a key resource for all existing and prospective CCNs and also for nurses, allied professionals, commissioners and providers of services who have direct or indirect contact with children and their families. This is a book 'from practice, for practice' and intended to inform, provide support, stimulate debate and promote community children's nursing. Knowledge combined with individual philosophies of care is a powerful advocate for sick children and their families. Chapter 1 refers to CCNs as 'practitioners of care' and 'taking the lead'. We believe the reader will find from within these pages the knowledge to increase their repertoire of skills to do just that.

Anna Sidey   David Widdas
Shropshire   Warwickshire
                                                          2005

Acknowledgements

To John for his unconditional help and patience throughout the project.

To Becky for her invaluable support and administrative skills.

Thank you to Dr Brian Silk and the spirit of Donna for their belief and confidence.

Thank you to Joan Finney and Margaret Hoskin for the inspiration of their nursing practice.

For Emily and Laura for tolerating and accepting every venture.

SECTION 1

Organisational Facets Influencing the Professional Development of Community Children's Nursing

SECTION CONTENTS

This first section considers the many facets that have preceded and influenced the professional development of community children's nursing, alongside the current issues that demand attention. It provides a historical context, outlining the development of nursing, professional bodies and community children's nursing in particular. The realisation of specialist practitioner education is presented through a 100-year account before exploring the current educational agenda. Contemporary issues are also examined, including the dynamic changes in the 'new NHS' and the need for community children's nurses to 'get political'. With the demands for collaborative practice, opportunities for working in partnership with other agencies are described. The intention here is to offer a foundation to the remaining text.

Chapter 1

A short journey down a long road: the emergence of professional bodies

Chris Middleton

> **KEY ISSUES**
> - The late nineteenth century saw nursing achieve respectability, although its definition as 'women's work' meant low status.
> - The first professional organisations in nursing disagreed over training, examination and registration of nurses, a split that was to deepen.
> - The unionisation of nursing was seen as unethical and contrary to the traditions of vocation and service.
> - The division between the unions and the professional bodies allowed others, outside nursing, to dictate policy and development.
> - The low status of nursing obstructs its recognition as a true profession.
> - By mirroring the development of medicine, nursing has adopted inappropriate medical models in approaches to care.
> - The re-emergence of primary healthcare and the rediscovery by community children's nursing of its roots have provided nursing with a new opportunity to raise its profile and status.
> - Recent government policies have recognised the value of nurses and nursing for the contribution they can make to the health of the population.
> - Different ways of working and new alliances offer nurses serious opportunities to lead, especially in the field of community care.

INTRODUCTION

Nursing is at once an ancient art and a modern science. Shaped over the last 100 years by external forces and internal weaknesses, nursing is now, as is healthcare, redefined and rediscovered and ready to take up its rightful place in the new NHS. This chapter, while charting the well-known waters of the development of nursing, does so with an eye to the parallels of the emerging status of women in society and developments in medicine.

The delivery of healthcare in the UK has come full circle, with the emphasis now on primary health and the delivery of healthcare in the community rather than secondary care based in hospital. Community children's nursing is, therefore, now ideally placed to, with others, lead the challenges of healthcare provision in this century.

DEVELOPMENT OF MODERN NURSING

The development of 'modern' nursing can be traced to the mid-nineteenth century, although the concept of nursing has much older roots, arising from the care offered to the sick by members of religious orders. Records dating back to 1095 note the practice of nursing as a public service throughout the monastic movement, a service staffed predominantly by men.

With the dissolution of the monasteries in this country in the sixteenth century, the references to nursing as an organised activity all but disappear from the records. It is not until the eighteenth century, with the development of the voluntary hospitals, that nursing starts to re-appear, with any significance, in the history books.

The provisions of the Poor Law Amendment Act 1834 (the 'New Poor Law') led to the establishment of workhouse infirmaries. The intent of the Act was to make life in the workhouse so unpleasant that paupers would rather work than rely on the guardians for support, thus reducing claimants and costs. But this was not to be the case when it was discovered that much poverty was due not to idleness but to illness. The building of the workhouse infirmaries and the consequent expansion of the Poor Law medical service led to a greater understanding of the sanitary conditions of the labouring classes and the social costs of sickness. This in turn led to the birth of public health legislation in this country.

Paradoxically the 1834 Act can also be seen to be the turning point for the development of nursing. New infirmaries were being built. In 1869 the first poor law school of nursing in London was established with the involvement of Florence Nightingale. It only lasted nine years but it set a precedent for the others that followed.

In the British Medical Journal in 1870 (p 415), Dr Dudfield, reporting on the reduction of mortality that using 'trained' poor law nurses had brought to St Margaret's Workhouse, Kensington, said: 'Much has been done by your board to ameliorate the condition of the sick, infirm and the aged, without in any way making the establishment attractive to that class of poor for whom the workhouses were originally intended'. The growth of the infirmaries and the recognition of the contribution of nurses led to the formation, by Louisa Twining, of the Workhouse Infirmary Nursing Association. The standards of nursing and medical care in the infirmaries continued to improve and by the late 1880s the infirmaries had become so specialised that many of them were becoming 'true' hospitals.

Around this time the winds of change were blowing for nursing in this country. This change movement was also catalysed to a large extent by the reforms being implemented by the religious nursing sisterhoods in Europe. In Britain, Florence Nightingale, who was strongly influenced by these sisters of charity, was recognised as an influential agent of nursing reform. In the latter half of the nineteenth century her work and ideas had quite a major impact on the future structure and philosophy of nursing.

Nursing history cannot be and should not be viewed in isolation from social history, and it is important to consider the development of the emerging profession in its social and political context. The end of the nineteenth and the beginning of the twentieth centuries saw huge strides being made in the women's suffrage movement. Victorian women were enjoying a previously unknown independence in society. However this newfound independence for women did not bring with it a newfound status. Victorian society was riven with wide social divisions. Importantly it was deeply patriarchal and as nursing became identified as primarily women's work it was inevitably seen as subordinate to that of the man/doctor. Any consideration of the development of and professionalisation of nursing in the UK must also, therefore, review the parallel emergence of the medical profession and the reasons for the dominance of the latter over the former.

Before the discovery of germ theory in the nineteenth century the role of doctors was largely ameliorative. It was the propagation of this theory that increased their prestige in the public's estimation and this, coupled with the reduction of deaths from infectious diseases at that time, assured their superior position. However, this acclaim is probably based on good 'PR' rather than fact. The reduction in the death rate was due to an understanding of the germ theory and of the cause and spread of disease and its practical application in the area of public health, not as a result of any advance in medical science. The public health model of illness at the time was based on the concept of 'bad air'. One of the most effective strategies to control or eliminate this bad air was the introduction of improved sanitation; it was this relatively simple measure that was actually responsible for the reduction in deaths from infectious diseases.

The medical profession, to protect its dominant status, needed to classify health problems in a way that indicated they were amenable to medical (doctor-led) intervention; the biomechanical model, in which healthcare interventions are based upon the diagnosis and treatment of a specific aetiology, suited the profession's needs perfectly. Medical practice became firmly rooted in 'centres of disease' hospitals. As hospitals developed, more nurses were needed to staff them, but the requirement was now not just for quantity of nurses but also for quality of nurses. Nightingale, and others of her social class at that time, had prompted an explosion of interest in nursing and had endowed it with an air of respectability:

'Nursing's values and culture were expropriated by women of a higher social status and greater wealth than the working-class women who had formed the bulk of the earliest nurses. Self sacrifice, loyalty, obedience and dedication were the key attributes to be instilled into educated young women of "good character".'

(Hart 1996 p 6)

These educated young women of good character were required to train as nurses to staff the rapidly developing voluntary hospitals. Unfortunately it is these very origins of modern nursing that determined it now as women's work, and in turn this laid the foundations for how nurses were, and to a large extent still are, treated as workers within a patriarchal society.

With the advent of training for nurses the battle lines were drawn for the next fight, which was to establish a register of nurses and also a national final examination at the end of any training course to provide a common benchmark of suitability for registration.

BIRTH OF THE PROFESSIONAL ORGANISATIONS

According to Abel-Smith (1960), the first professional organisation was the British Nurses Association. This group was led by Miss Ethel Manson, who later married Dr Bedford Fenwick. Mrs Bedford Fenwick believed that the only way to ensure the highest possible standard of nursing was to restrict entry to the profession to the daughters of the higher social classes. In 1887, Bedford Fenwick founded the British Nurses Association in direct opposition to the Hospitals' Association, founded by Henry Burdett, a hospital administrator, which had set up a nursing section with its own central registry. Bedford Fenwick's association also set up its own registration system while it pushed for an official national register of nurses.

However, Mrs Bedford Fenwick's idea for a register of nurses was strongly opposed by Florence Nightingale. Her main objection to the style of registration being proposed was the introduction of an examination to test knowledge. Nightingale herself placed more emphasis on the personal qualities of the person than her intellectual capacity. Other opposition came from Sydney Holland (Abel-Smith 1960 p 3) of the London Hospital where Mrs Bedford Fenwick had worked as a ward sister. He wrote: 'We want to stop nurses thinking themselves anything more than they are, namely, the faithful carriers out of the doctor's orders.'

In contrast to their opposition to nurse registration, the medical profession strongly supported the registration of midwives. Following the creation of the midwifery register under the provisions of the Midwives Act 1902, a select committee was appointed in 1904 to review the issue of registration for nurses. The outcome of their deliberations was in favour of registration. However, it would be some 15 years before Parliament acted on these findings. The requirement for nurses during the First World War brought further impetus for registration and a national standard in training. As a result the College of Nursing was founded. The intention was that the College should become the recognised body for determining the syllabus for nurse training and approving nurse-training institutions and also the registration body for qualified nurses. That was also the desire of the British Nurses Association. After three years of bitter wrangling between the two organisations Parliament decided that the way forward with nurse registration was to form its own General Nursing Council (GNC) with the Nurses' Registration Act 1919. The first state final examination was held in 1925 and the first nurses were admitted to the Register by examination.

The divisions in nursing revealed by the registration debate were mirrored in the attempts by nurses to unionise. Employers and the medical profession obstructed these moves until 1910 when the National Asylum Workers Union (NAWU) was formed. Their priorities were more pay and a shorter working week. The emphasis at the turn of the century on training and registration had produced a shortage of trained nurses. This was exacerbated by the First World War and by 1918 there was a major shortage of suitable women to train as nurses. According to Hart (1996 p 7) the extra burden this placed on existing staff 'had been justified by arguing that increased duties, longer hours and fewer days off were in the interests of good patient care'.

Discontent with pay and working conditions reached a peak in the mid 1930s when many nurses turned to the, by now, widely recognised trade unions for support. However, the College of Nursing, whose articles expressly forbade it becoming a trade union, continued to voice its opposition to the unionisation of nursing and condemned nurses who demanded better working conditions as being unethical, claiming that these demands 'had little in common with the ideals of service which must animate every nurse worthy of her name' (Hart 1996 p 8).

In 1939 the Government finally set up a committee to investigate nursing shortages. The committee's recommendation was to meet the unions' demands, an idea that was rejected by the Government at the time. It was not until the formation of the NHS in 1948 that the objectives of nationally negotiated pay and conditions of service were finally achieved.

Within the NHS, the pay and conditions of service of nurses and midwives was to be decided by the Whitley Council. The Council's staff side consisted of union and professional association representatives. The union representation was from the Confederation of Health Service Employees (COHSE), formed from the earlier merger of the National Union of County Officers (NUCO) and NAWU's successor, the Mental Hospital and Institutional Workers' Union. The Royal College of Nursing (RCN), as the College of Nursing had become, with the support of the other professional associations claimed the largest number of seats of any individual organisation on the Council. With their opposing political and philosophical views, this ensured that nursing was relatively powerless and split.

Twenty years of Whitley Council failure meant that by the 1970s health workers' salaries were out of step and depressed. Nurses, faced with cutbacks in services and resources, became more militant and both the RCN and COHSE responded to their concerns with pay campaigns. In 1979 the Conservative Government, with an anti-nationalised industries, public services and trades unions philosophy, took power. The next 10–15 years saw COHSE and the RCN becoming more and more similar in their demands for nurses' pay and conditions, but still maintaining a distance by disputing how these demands were to be met by the Government. Unfortunately this continued bickering and lack of unity, an echo from the days of the professionalisation debate, allowed the

Government to weaken further nursing's influence in healthcare provision by the introduction of general management.

> *'The division between nursing's trade unions and professional associations is almost unique in labour history, indicating nursing's positions somewhere between a skilled trade and a profession. It would be difficult to imagine, for example, doctors or dockers allowing themselves to be so thoroughly split and, consequently, weakened. The differences between them reflect the evolution of nursing's many strands and the people who became nurses.'*
>
> (Hart 1996 p 5)

Hart (1996) makes the very valid point that, although nurses are continually accused of failing to articulate their needs and act in their own best interests, this accusation fails to take account of the fact that they work in and are products of a professionalised service. This has traditionally worked against their interests, denying them choices and exercising power in such a way as to ensure that those issues are never adequately discussed, an opinion perhaps shared by Rafferty (1995) when she said: 'The history of nursing is rarely one of triumph in the face of adversity but of struggle and compromise and often defeat.'

PROFESSIONALISATION OF NURSING

The continuing struggle of nursing to establish itself as an important intellectual force in healthcare delivery and/or reform can be explained in part by its own enduring ability to stab itself in the back. Equally influential, though, are its close but subordinate relationships with medicine and a legacy of populist images, the angel, the battleaxe and the tart, that work to undermine public and professional confidence. To overcome these hurdles nursing needs firstly to define itself independently from medicine and secondly to provide with this definition information for itself and the public about its worth, value and status. In a climate of advancing technology in healthcare and a move from a disease focus to a health focus, nurses are in a prime position to establish themselves as a profession on an equal footing with their medical colleagues.

Professionalisation was (and still is) to prove as elusive a quarry as registration had been. Unsurprisingly the issues appear to be the same. Nursing opinion is split between declaring itself a profession by virtue of meeting the necessary criteria to do so, and endlessly debating whether to do so is advantageous. External opinion and activity may serve to hamper the process further. Crouch (1996 p 12) argues that weak governing frameworks and organisational marginality within health services hamper the acceptance of nursing as a profession. She goes on to say: 'Health services, professional and organisational bodies, government and in some cases nurses themselves, have allowed nursing to become marginalised, resulting in loss of power for nurses and an increase in bureaucracy.'

Carter (1994) argues that the professionalisation process and debate has been impeded by nursing's failure to confront patriarchal attitudes in the clinical context. The roots of this, Carter believes, lie with Florence Nightingale and her insistence that nurses ask permission from a doctor before carrying out even basic caring tasks, a demand which should not be considered out of the context of the prevailing social attitudes towards women at this time. The ethos of the Victorian age was characterised by an acceptance of male superiority over women.

This doctor–nurse tension is an important consideration in the profession debate. Nurses who perceive professional status as offering them independence, autonomy and empowerment, and therefore a 'way out' of the traditional subservience, see the doctors as an example of how professional status can benefit its members. 'Doctors have money, high social standing and autonomy so why shouldn't we?' (Salvage 1985). However, as Rafferty (1996) points out, the work of Witz (1992) and Davies (1995) suggests that professions are 'gendered institutions', organised around male patterns of career development and priorities. Nursing, as a female-dominated occupation, does not fit easily into the traditional mould within which the archetypal professions have been cast. If this situation is to change, it needs to be challenged by both men and women. It is necessary to pit the occupation of the dominant role by men against the hesitancy of women to challenge their own responsibility for maintaining it.

SPECIALISATION

Although specialisation in name can be traced back to the Nurses Registration Act 1919, Castledine (1998 p 3) argues that:

> 'If specialisation infers a narrowing of the range of work to be done, and an increase in depth of knowledge and skill, then we must take the setting up of the first training school in nursing after the Crimean War by Florence Nightingale as the starting point for specialisation and identification of clinical nursing in the United Kingdom.'

However, he then goes on to distinguish between 'specialisation **of** nursing', achieved by the introduction of registration and training, and 'specialisation **in** nursing', which is the issue of concern here. According to Scott (1998), the late 1950s and 1960s in the UK saw an increase of specialisation in nursing, particularly in the acute sector. The RCN (1977) saw that this was due in part to a parallel increase in specialisation in medicine; as medical science advances and specialisation increases, suitably prepared nurses must be available to identify the implications of these advances for nursing practice, to prescribe changes in nursing care and to advise on new techniques, in order that the nursing care of patients may reflect these advances.

Developments in the technology of medicine increased the cost of healthcare. To maintain the ideals of the NHS as a service 'free at the point of delivery', hospital administrators had to develop strategies for keeping down the cost of healthcare delivery. One approach was to cluster together high-tech/high-cost resources into regional centres. This led, naturally, to an increased demand for hospital nurses with specialist knowledge and skills. At this time there was no nationally recognised or regulated system of post-registration education. To meet the demand, therefore, many hospitals set up their own *ad hoc* clinical courses. The GNC was powerless to act to regulate these courses, and ensure standards were being maintained, as it had responsibility only for pre-registration education and training.

In 1970, in response to the profession's urgent demands, the Government set up the Joint Board of Clinical Nursing Studies (JBCNS) to monitor and set standards for post-basic courses. NHS re-organisation in the 10 years between the mid 1960s and the mid 1970s had a significant impact on the organisation of nursing. Important among these effects was the Salmon Report (1966) that reorganised the management of nursing, but in doing so, according to Castledine (1998), it also shifted attention from the clinical role of the nurse. The status of the patient care aspect of the nurses' role dropped even further.

The plethora of specialised advanced nursing courses that were produced under the JBCNS appeared to have, at their heart, an increasing emphasis on medical treatment. Castledine (1998) offers the opinion that this was due in part to the 'theory–practice divide' in nursing, leading to a confusion about which way practice should develop.

Specialisation in nursing was not a concept that was universally welcomed. In a report in 1980 (Department of Health and Social Security 1980), the Chief Nursing Officer stated that this would lead to fragmented patient care and would further disintegrate the nursing function. The favoured pathway at the time was that of the general or generalist nurse. This concept is significant as a comment on the internal politics of nursing; however, criticisms of specialisation in nursing are probably not without foundation as early attempts to create specialist nurse roles fell into the trap of following the medical biomechanical model too closely.

By the 1980s there was a backlash. The Merrison Report (1979) had commented on the situation in North America where it had investigated the creation of clinical nurse specialists, nurses whose area of specialisation was clinical nursing. They recognised that a similar model could work in the UK and made specific recommendations about appropriate remuneration for the acquisition and use of advanced nursing skills.

'RE-EMERGENCE' OF PRIMARY HEALTHCARE

The arena for the involvement of nurses in healthcare delivery has never been restricted to that of the acute, secondary sector, although the years since the inception of the NHS have probably focused on its profile in institutions. The existence of primary healthcare, more accurately for the time, public healthcare, can be recognised pre-Nightingale.

The time of the Industrial Revolution had changed the employment picture in Britain. From being a largely agricultural, rural-based community system, the new factories attracted people into the cities and towns in large numbers, which led to massive overcrowding and associated health problems. Wages were not high and many people lived in poverty in these conditions. During the latter half of the eighteenth century various groups were formed in an attempt to improve the sanitary conditions and teach the people about public health. Among these was the Ladies Sanitary Association (LSA) (1861), which was formed to teach mothers about health. However, according to Baly (1995), they were not very successful in achieving their aims so they employed 'a respectable woman to go from door to door giving advice and help as the opportunity offered'.

These women were originally called 'health missioners', but when the LSA changed its name to the Ladies Health Society, they became 'health visitors'. Eventually these 'health visitors' came under the direction of the Medical Officer of Health and were part paid by the Local Authority (Baly 1995). These early prototypes are not to be confused with the current version of health visitors. They were not nurses and they were not trained. In 1892 Florence Nightingale was influential in procuring some technical training for 'lady health visitors', but by the start of the twentieth century concerns about the health of children, increasing infant mortality and the maternal death rate created a new role for the health visitor. She moved from someone who worked by educating and persuading the whole family to a professional who worked to take on the health and welfare of the baby and mother from the midwife, now a trained and registered professional in her own right. Initially these new health visitors were required to have a medical degree or to have undergone a full nursing course (Baly 1995).

At the turn of the twentieth century Nightingale herself recognised the impact of a person's environment on their health status and much of her work was directed towards prevention. She also had a significant impact on William Rathbone when he was pioneering district nursing and health visiting services.

It is not until later in the twentieth century that we start to see primary healthcare being put back under the spotlight. Developments in the technology of medicine had increased the cost of healthcare. Consumers who had grown up with the NHS were becoming more aware of their own health needs and of the shortcomings of the service and were starting to make their voices heard through patient support groups. The Government set up Community Health Councils in 1974 to provide a consumer's voice in healthcare policy and practice.

During the 1980s surveys were reporting an increasing dissatisfaction among the public with regard to waiting lists, outpatients and the 'inpatient experience'. The Government's response to this was to introduce the ethos of the free market system into the structure and management of the NHS. This was a cost-driven exercise, but the secondary intention was to promote good practice in healthcare delivery at a local level.

In the late 1980s the growth of the primary care sector proceeded apace. Services that had traditionally been the exclusive domain of hospitals were being relocated into the community service, such as minor surgery and specialist outpatient services. Increasingly, what would once have been considered intensive and complex nursing care procedures are being carried out in the community setting; this, of course, has important, and often overlooked, implications for informal carers.

In part, these issues of spiralling acute care costs and growing public protest about the quality of secondary sector care helped to drive the shift of emphasis from institutional to community-based care. Other factors are demographic trends, changing patterns of illness and the development of less-invasive medical treatments. The UK was not alone in experiencing this push towards a greater focus on primary healthcare. In 1978 the World Health Organization (WHO) published 'Health for all by the year 2000', which requested states' parties to place primary care firmly at the centre of their health policies and systems (WHO 1978).

The emergence of community children's nursing as a speciality has slightly different roots. The negative impact of hospitalisation on children had been recognised for some time, and in the early 1950s the work of Bowlby (1965) had demonstrated that children were not just small adults: they reacted differently to stressful situations and had special emotional and physical needs that should be met by specialised services. In 1959 the Platt Report (Ministry of Health 1959) strongly recommended the provision of special nursing services for the home care of children, putting an emphasis on avoiding hospitalisation if at all possible and meeting children's health needs in the community. Unfortunately Platt was largely ignored and developments in community children's nursing were slow and sparse until the early 1990s. Why this should have been so is unclear but since the last decade of the twentieth century the growth of this service has outstripped its adult counterparts (Whiting 2003).

PRESSURES ON THE SYSTEM

In 1997 Bell wrote: 'Nurses in the primary health care setting are currently experiencing unprecedented change both from within their working environment and as members of a developing profession' (Bell 1997). According to Coote (1998) there has been expressed public anxiety about health risks, but any action is usually about concerns with the NHS, not health. 'This may be because people feel impotent about it. The links between cause and effect are unclear to them. They or we don't know who to blame, or what can be done to make things better' (Coote 1998 p 2).

There is a need to take collective action to improve public health. This is certainly not a new phenomenon, but it is clear that earlier strategies have not worked. For example, the Health of the Nation (HOTN) strategy, which from 1992 to 1997 was the central plank of health policy in England, represented the first explicit attempt by government to provide a strategic approach to improving the overall health of the population. In spite of being widely welcomed, it failed to realise its full potential. In 'The Health of the Nation – a policy assessed: the executive summary of two reports into the failings of the HOTN strategy', there were recommendations for future health policy initiatives. Prominent among these was the need to 'make public health part of the core business by embedding it in the organisational culture' (DoH 1998a). As Coote (1998 p 2) says: 'Most activity which makes a difference will come from the bottom up; it will depend on effective, inter-agency working at local level.'

In its White Paper 'The New NHS. Modern, dependable' (DoH 1997) the Government made a clear statement about the need to strengthen the contribution made by nursing. Additionally, the Health Services Circular (DoH 1998b) 'Better health and better health care' outlined a set of activities to ensure that staff at all levels were enabled to maximise their contribution to health and healthcare through the implementation of 'The new NHS. Modern, dependable' and 'Our healthier nation' (DoH 1998c).

Certainly the message that strikes out from 'Our healthier nation' is that everybody has a part to play in improving the health of the population. The Government was committed to producing a national contract for better health under which it would join in partnerships with local communities and individuals to improve health. Action was to be focused in four priority areas:

- coronary heart disease and stroke
- cancers
- accidents
- mental health

and the settings for these were determined as:

- healthy schools (focusing on children)
- workplaces (focusing on adults)
- neighbourhoods (focusing on older people).

However, in July 2000 the Government published the NHS Plan (DoH 2000) a radical action plan for 10 years that set out measures to put people and patients at the heart of the health service. It promised:

- more power and information for patients
- more hospitals and beds
- more doctors and nurses
- much shorter waiting times for hospital and doctor appointments
- cleaner wards, better food and facilities in hospital
- improved care for older people
- tougher standards for NHS organisations and better rewards for the best.

In order to achieve these major changes the Government decided it had to set priorities:

1. Target the diseases that are the biggest killers such as cancer and heart disease.
2. Pinpoint the changes that were most urgently needed to improve people's health and wellbeing and deliver the modern, fair and convenient services people want.

The Modernisation Board is leading the changes and ten Taskforces have been established to drive forward the improvements in:

- coronary heart disease
- cancer
- mental health
- older people
- children
- waiting times and access to services
- the NHS workforce
- quality
- reducing inequalities and promoting public health
- investment in facilities and information technology.

To help staff and organisations translate the NHS Plan into reality the Government also set up the Modernisation Agency.

What community children's nursing has to consider is where and how it fits into this strategy. As in 'Our Healthier Nation' there are some very encouraging messages for nurses and nursing within this strategy document. Health promotion is becoming a more integral part of healthcare provision than it has been in the past (see Chapter 13). Nurses are in a prime position to take this on board, and have the potential for significant influence in this area. According to 'Liberating the Talents' (DoH 2002a) this will mean:

- a service where patients and the public have a greater choice and a greater voice
- opportunities to provide more secondary care in community settings
- extending nursing roles including taking on some work currently undertaken by General Practitioners
- a key role in delivering 24-hour first-contact care across a range of settings
- a major role in delivering National Service Frameworks
- having a greater voice in decision making
- a focus on preventing and tackling inequalities
- greater skill mix and leadership opportunities.

Clearly the NHS Plan was not a strategy designed to be bolted on to existing structures. It brought with it a whole raft of changes to the structures for the delivery of healthcare. Importantly for primary care, the power for determining, and the resources for meeting, the healthcare needs of the community are shifted from the resource-hungry, but illness-focused, secondary care sector, to the primary sector. Ninety per cent of all patient journeys begin and end in primary care. For most people primary care is the NHS. The shifting of resources inevitably leads to the shifting of the power balance. This was set out in the document 'Shifting the Balance of Power' (DoH 2002b).

- **Primary Care Trusts** (PCTs) have become the lead NHS organisation in assessing need, planning and securing all health services and improving health. This is forging new partnerships with local communities and leading the NHS contribution to joint working with local government and other partners.
- **NHS Trusts** continue to provide services, working within delivery agreements with PCTs. Trusts will be expected to devolve greater responsibility to clinical teams and to foster and encourage the growth of clinical networks across NHS organisations. High-performing Trusts will earn greater freedoms and autonomy in recognition of their achievements.
- **Strategic Health Authorities** have replaced the previous Health Authorities. They lead the strategic development of the local health service and performance manage PCTs and NHS Trusts on the basis of local accountability agreements.

- The **Department of Health** is changing the way it relates to the NHS, focusing on supporting the delivery of the NHS Plan. The Department of Health Regional Offices have been abolished and four new Regional Directors of Health and Social Care oversee the development of the NHS and provide the link between NHS organisations and the central department. Modernisation Agency, Leadership Centre and the NHS University will support the development of frontline staff and services.

THE FUTURE

At the end of the last century Bell (1997) noted O'Keefe et al's earlier (1992) dire prediction of a pending health crisis which must be taken seriously by community nurses, together with the need for them to take full account of key factors that have the potential to underpin the predicament:

- shift in emphasis from biomedical, curative approaches to preventive approaches
- 'epidemiological transition' from childhood illnesses to chronic and degenerative disorders
- iceberg of sickness
- environmental pollution
- user dissatisfaction
- widening gap between demand and supply
- demographic time bomb.

We can predict that primary healthcare as a concept and in practice is at, and will remain at, the very heart of healthcare and health service development. This has been stated clearly by recent governmental and international health strategies, and is inevitable if healthcare costs are to be managed. Recent Government initiatives have made it clear that community nurses will be key workers in strategies for improving health.

'This Plan cannot be delivered without the support of nurses, midwives and health visitors. If patients and communities are to benefit from the investments in the NHS nurses in primary care will need to be at the forefront of change and innovation. The NHS Plan is an opportunity to turn rhetoric into reality'

(DoH 2002a)

CONCLUSION

In the late nineteenth century modern nursing was born into a deeply patriarchal and socially divided Victorian British society. At its beginning it had in its grasp what we now know to be the root of effective healthcare provision, public health and primary care. But, partly as a result of social gender values and partly as a result of its persistent inability to present a united front, nursing soon lost any lead it had to the male-dominated medical profession. In seeking to re-establish itself as a valid force for healthcare assessment and delivery nursing has faced many battles. Changes have been imposed from outside by forces that have recognised the inherent weakness of an internally divided group. In the face of such onslaught nursing has struggled to define itself and its role but most of the time its biggest enemy has probably been itself.

Fifty plus years after the creation of the NHS the social, political and economic wranglings, that have been a familiar characteristic of healthcare provision in the UK, have finally conspired to produce healthcare policies and strategies that rely on nurses to ensure their success. These, coupled with the establishment of primary care as the very heart of these policies, mean that community nurses with their special skills and understanding of communities can and must take up the challenge.

REFERENCES

Abel-Smith B 1960 A history of the nursing profession. Heinemann, London

Baly M E 1995 Nursing & Social Change. Routledge, London

Bell R 1997 Towards the next millennium. In: Burley S, Mitchell E E, Melling K, Smith M, Chilton S & Crumplin C (eds) Contemporary community nursing. Arnold, London, p 259

Bowlby J 1965 Child care and the growth of love. 2nd edn. Penguin, Harmondsworth

British Medical Journal 1870 Workhouse Reform. BMJ, London, p 415

Carter H 1994 Confronting patriarchal attitudes in the fight for professional recognition. Journal of Advanced Nursing 19(2):367–372

Castledine G 1998 In: Castledine G & McGee P (eds) Advanced and specialist nursing practice. Blackwell Science, Oxford, Ch. 1, p 3

Coote A 1998 Cited in: Expert analysis of the new health strategy. Department of Health, Target. Online. Available: www.dh.gov.uk 14 September 2004

Crouch S 1996 Professionals – myth or reality? Nursing Management 3(6):12–13

Davies C 1995 Gender and the professional predicament in nursing. Open University Press, Buckingham

Department of Health 1997 The new NHS. Modern, dependable. The Stationery Office, London

Department of Health 1998a The Health of the Nation – a policy assessed. The Stationery Office, London

Department of Health 1998b Health Services Circular 1998/021: Better health and better health care – implementing 'The new NHS' and 'Our healthier nation'. The Stationery Office, London

Department of Health 1998c Our healthier nation. The Stationery Office, London

Department of Health 2000 The NHS Plan. The Stationery Office, London

Department of Health 2002a Liberating the Talents. The Stationery Office, London

Department of Health 2002b Shifting the Balance of Power. The Stationery Office, London

Department of Health and Social Security 1980 Careers in clinical nursing: report of a chief nursing officer's working party. Department of Health and Social Security, London

Hart C 1996 The great divide. International History of Nursing Journal 1(3):5–17

Merrison Report 1979 Royal Commission on the National Health Service. HMSO, London

Ministry of Health 1959 The welfare of children in hospital – a report of the committee (chairman: Sir H Platt). HMSO, London

O'Keefe E, Ottewill R & Wall A 1992 Community health: issues in management. Business Education Publishers, Sunderland

Rafferty A 1995 Unpublished work. In: Kitson A 1997 John Hopkins address: Does nursing have a future? Image – The Journal of Nursing Scholarship 29(2):111–115

Rafferty A 1996 The politics of nursing knowledge. Routledge, London

Royal College of Nursing 1977 Evidence to the Royal Commission on the NHS. Royal College of Nursing, London

Salmon Report 1966 Report of the committee on senior nursing structure. HMSO, London

Salvage J 1985 The politics of nursing. William Heinemann, London

Scott C 1998 Specialist practice: advancing the profession? Journal of Advanced Nursing 28(3):554–562

Whiting M 2003 Improving Numbers. Guest editorial. Paediatric Nursing 15(1):3

Witz A 1992 Professions and patriarchy. Routledge, London

World Health Organization (WHO) 1978 Health for all by the year 2000. World Health Organization, Copenhagen

Chapter 2

1888–2004: A historical overview of community children's nursing

Mark Whiting

KEY ISSUES

- Community children's nursing has a complex history dating back to the middle of the nineteenth century.
- Much of the history of the provision of formal community children's nursing can be closely linked to the emergence and development of both district nursing and health visiting.
- The rapid growth of community children's nursing in the 1980s and 1990s seems to have occurred more as a result of the pioneering spirit of individual practitioners than as a consequence of identifiable social policy reform.

INTRODUCTION

This chapter is concerned with the historical development of community children's nursing in the UK. Particular attention will be focused upon the emergence, during the closing years of the nineteenth century, of a community nursing service for children based within the Hospital for Sick Children, Great Ormond Street (GOS), London. This period is of particular note because it was around the same time that the forebears of the current district nursing and health visiting services were becoming established (Stocks 1960, Owen 1982). Consideration will then be given to the early years of the NHS, focusing on published accounts of service developments in Rotherham, Birmingham, Paddington, Southampton, Edinburgh, Gateshead, Oxford and Brent. An overview of service provision in 1988 will provide a summary of service development up to that date.

The care of the sick child has moved steadily in recent years from being almost exclusively the responsibility of the hospital (Oppé 1971) towards the community (NHS Executive 1996a). This has been reflected in very significant reductions in the length of time for which children are admitted to hospital, from an average of around 2 weeks at the time of the Platt Report (Ministry of Health 1959) to a little over 2 days by the early 1990s (Audit Commission 1993). Inpatient hospital care has been envisioned in the future as being required for only the most acutely or seriously ill members of society and it has been suggested that, in consequence, community healthcare will provide for a much broader range of needs (DoH 1997a). This is a far cry from the situation that existed in the middle of the nineteenth century.

EARLY DAYS

The first children's hospital to be established in the UK was the Hospital for Sick Children, GOS, London in 1852 (Kosky & Lunnon 1991, Lomax 1996). However, over 100 years earlier, Thomas Coram had established the Foundling Hospital, also in London. Coram, a retired sea captain, had been appalled at the numbers of dead and dying babies to be found on the streets of London and set about interesting the Government, the Anglican Church and members of the ruling classes in providing financial support for a 'hospital' that was to provide the necessary care for these babies or 'foundlings', many of whom were the illegitimate children of the poor. Coram's attempts to interest the authorities in providing funds for his proposals were largely unsuccessful and initial funding for the hospital came predominantly from charitable rather than state sources.

The hospital was soon overwhelmed by the demand for admission of 'foundlings' (Lomax 1996). Franklin (1964) reported that, in spite of wealthy patronage there were insufficient funds to meet the demands of the large numbers of babies who were often abandoned at the hospital entrance. The hospital's governors eventually appealed to the House of Commons for financial support. The Government donated £10 000 to the hospital on the condition that for an initial period of 6 months no infant should be refused admission. In the event, unregulated admissions continued for nearly 4 years, often with dire consequences. Of 14 934 babies admitted to the hospital between 1756 and 1760 only 4545 survived (Franklin 1964). Lomax (1996 p 4) suggests that state intervention was, in part, responsible for the discrediting of the hospital, leading to accusations that, by agreeing to accept all children arriving at its doors, it encouraged 'irresponsibility and immorality'.

The Foundling Hospital was concerned primarily with providing protection and education for children rather than with the provision of medical or nursing care. However, in 1852, when Charles West opened the first Hospital for Sick Children in GOS, there was a clear recognition of the need specifically to provide both medical and nursing expertise. The establishment of the hospital at GOS preceded what can only be described as a tidal wave of activity in the establishment of children's hospitals in the UK. By the turn of the century, there were over 30 children's hospitals and upwards of 50 children's convalescent homes. In addition, many general hospitals had formally dedicated one or more wards exclusively for the care of children (Lomax 1996).

One of the original aims of the GOS Hospital for Children was 'to train girls for a few months to enable them to be effective as children's nurses in private families' (Lomax 1996 p 8). However, whilst this may have been the intention of Sir Charles West, it was not until the mid 1870s that formal proposals to develop a private domiciliary nursing service were made to the hospital's management committee.

> *'Some consideration took place on the reference in Dr West's paper to the training of nurses proposed by the Lady Superintendent in visiting hospital out-patients at their own homes, under the regulations suggested by Dr West and coincided in by the Lady Superintendent. The majority of the Medical Officers were in favour of the plan being made trial of for 6 months, but the lay members of the committee were unanimously opposed to the extension of the work of the hospital beyond the walls.'*

(Hospital for Sick Children 1874)

Despite this initial reticence, by 1880 a scheme to supply trained private nurses was in preparation, and by 1888 a private domiciliary nursing service was operating from the hospital (Hunt & Whiting 1999). In order to treat sick children at home, it was clear that professional supervision was required. Lomax (1996) suggests that many of the early children's hospitals provided a domiciliary visiting service (staffed by the hospital physicians) when they first opened; however, many were forced to abandon this both because of the 'expenses involved and because of opposition from both hospital and general physicians' (p 12). It is unclear how many of the hospitals actually employed nurses to visit children in their own homes, although of the 11 children's hospitals in London by the turn of the century only the Victoria Hospital in Westminster and GOS are recorded as so doing (Lomax 1996). In addition, whilst a small number of the provincial children's hospitals had initially provided some home nursing services free of charge, most of these services rapidly became available on a fee-paying basis only, effectively a private outreach nursing service.

For some families, district nurses were available even when the families could not afford to pay for their services. Indeed, it is clear that one of the original intentions of William Rathbone, who had been responsible for the introduction of district nursing in the 1850s, was to provide a nursing service in the community for those (adults and children) who were unable to pay for hospital care. However, Lomax (1996 p 12) suggests rather disparagingly that this was 'to some extent at the expense of divorcing institutional practice from domiciliary care'. A further issue that militated against the development of the outreach nursing service concerned the expenses involved in the training of the nurses, which were incurred within the overall costs of running hospitals. This money was derived largely from donations to the hospitals and as such it was intended to fund the provision of care for the poor. It was certainly not intended to provide for the training of 'private nurses' available only to those who could pay for their services.

From the outset, the private nursing service based at GOS Hospital was staffed by nurses who had been 'trained' in the nursing of children (Wood 1888). Wood (1888 p 507) was very single minded in her insistence that 'sick children require special nursing, and sick children's nurses require special training'.

A register of the nurses providing a private nursing service in patients' homes was commenced in 1888, and included the names of nine nurses, perhaps the earliest recorded team of Community Children's Nurses (CCNs) (Hunt & Whiting 1999). The team of nurses provided for children with a wide range of needs, including those arising from acute infectious disease, chronic nutritional failure and orthopaedic and general surgical problems. Care was ordinarily provided on a 'live-in' basis, and whilst this was often quite short term (for perhaps three to seven days), some children received continuing care from one or more nurses over periods of several months.

The private nursing service was a great success, generating significant sums of money for the hospital and undergoing considerable expansion during the early years of the twentieth century. By 1938, 30 nurses were employed, each of whom had been required to be trained by GOS Hospital in the care of sick children (Hospital for Sick Children 1936) and each of whom provided full-time nursing care to one single child at a time (with a waiting list of children as soon as one of the nurses became 'free'). However, in 1948, the implementation of the NHS Act 1946 brought the GOS Hospital for Children into the 'welfare state' and thus required the dissolution of the private nursing service. On 14 March 1949, the last remaining member of the nursing staff, who had been caring for a child requiring long-term care, returned to the hospital from duty in the community.

COMMUNITY CHILDREN'S NURSING IN THE EARLY YEARS OF THE NHS

The period from the middle of the nineteenth century up to the inception of the NHS in 1948 was a time of significant expansion and development of both district nursing and health visiting services. In addition to bringing the 'voluntary' and 'municipal' hospitals together under the umbrella of the NHS, the 1946 Act also made arrangements for the statutory provision by health authorities of both district nursing and health visiting services.

A detailed history of the development of health visiting, dating back to the establishment of the Manchester and Salford Sanitary Reform Association in 1852 can be found in the work of Owen (1982). Whilst much of the work of health visitors has always been concerned with the health of children, the provision of 'hands on' nursing care to sick children had never been a significant feature of their work (Clark 1981, While 1985).

The history of district nursing, which has been traced back to the appointment, in 1859, of a single nurse in Liverpool by William Rathbone, has been reviewed in detail by Stocks (1960). The original intentions of the district nursing services were focused in meeting the needs of the 'sick poor', and it is clear that in the latter years of the nineteenth century the care of sick children in their own homes formed a significant part of the nurses' caseload (Rathbone 1890). Baly et al (1987 p 189) suggest that, up to the 1920s, 'much of the district nurse's work was involved in caring for children with infectious diseases'.

The requirements of the NHS Act 1946 for the newly created health authorities to 'secure the attendance of nurses on persons who require nursing in their own homes' (para III section 25) and to 'make provision in their area for the visiting of persons in their homes by visitors to be called health visitors' (part III section 24[1]) represented, in large areas of the UK, little more than the formal realignment of pre-existing services into the new structures of the NHS. However, no specific arrangements were made within the Act for the nursing of children in the community. The extent to which either district nursing or health visiting services were providing care to sick children in the community at the time of the Act is unclear, although it is likely that the number of sick children for whom such services might be provided was very small indeed. Subsequent studies of district nursing (Dunnell & Dobbs 1982) and health visiting (Clark 1981) suggest that this situation remains.

THE CHILDREN'S NURSING UNIT IN ROTHERHAM

The first recorded appointment within the NHS of a nurse involved exclusively in the care of sick children was in Rotherham in 1949 (Gillet 1954). This service was introduced to address concerns relating to a high rate of infant mortality in the preceding winter that was considered to have arisen 'largely due to cross-infection in hospital' (p 684). The service was initially staffed in 1949 by a single Queen's Nursing Sister who had undertaken a 'postgraduate course covering children's diseases' (p 684) and this was supplemented with a second appointment later in the year. Referrals to the service were made by the local general practitioners (GPs) and a major element of the work of the nurses was concerned with the care of children with acute infections. In 1952, one-third of the referrals to and visits undertaken by the nurses were of this nature (Table 2.1).

Gillet confidently asserted that the service contributed significantly to an improvement in the infant mortality rate in the Rotherham district, although no specific evidence to support this claim was provided. He did, however, identify four additional advantages of the services as (Gillet 1954 p 685):

- *'the child remaining at home in familiar surroundings is less likely to fret;*
- *the danger of cross infection is lessened;*
- *the mother is encouraged to help in the nursing of the child and the health teaching to parents and relatives done in these cases is considerable;*
- *the call on hospital beds for sick children has been reduced.'*

A similar list of potential advantages was identified for the domiciliary Nursing Service for Infants and Children in Birmingham and the St Mary's Paediatric Home Care Project in Paddington, London, both of which were established in 1954. No further published reports of the Rotherham service beyond the mid 1950s have been traced, although reference to the service is made in the Report of the Committee on the Welfare of Children in Hospital (Ministry of Health 1959).

Table 2.1 Referrals to and visits undertaken by Rotherham Community Children's Nursing Unit in 1952

Diagnosis	No. of cases	No. of visits
Pneumonia	67	537
Bronchitis	119	990
Gastroenteritis	6	62
Measles	23	197
Measles and pneumonia	9	76
Measles and bronchitis	1	1
Scarlet fever	1	1
Chickenpox	1	7
Pemphigus	3	11
Ophthalmia neonatorum	1	12
Whooping cough	5	56
Whooping cough and pneumonia	1	3
Poliomyelitis	1	3
Total of infectious cases	238	1956
Total of non-infectious cases	475	3881

Source: Gillet (1954).

THE CHILDREN'S HOME NURSING SERVICE IN BIRMINGHAM

Partly in response to the success of the Children's Nursing Unit in Rotherham, and as a result of a collaborative venture between the Birmingham Health Committee, the House Committee of the Children's Hospital, the Local Medical Committee and the Local Executive Council, a children's home nursing service was established in Birmingham in October 1954. Initially, the service was focused upon 'an area containing a population of about 100 000, around the Children's Hospital and two district nursing centres' (Smellie 1956 p 256). A 'state registered nurse with district training' (Morris 1966) from each of the district nursing centres was appointed specifically to care for children in the community and, before taking up their posts, each nurse spent a week of orientation in the Children's Hospital to familiarise themselves with both current inpatient care and to meet members of the ward and outpatient nursing teams. The nursing staff worked in close collaboration with the local GPs (initially 27 GPs were involved) (Howell 1974) and in the first year of their work visited 454 children in their own homes, undertaking a total of 3295 visits. The major focus of the nurse's work was in the management of acute infectious disease. The work was focused largely on the general practice population, but also included a number of children for whom early hospital discharge had been facilitated. Evening visits by the nurses were identified as being the 'most important in allaying the worries and anxieties of the mothers, so that there have been very few emergency calls during the night' (Smellie 1956 p 256).

By 1962 the service expanded to four nurses, and in order to provide a comprehensive service a senior member of the team was seconded to undertake night duty. The team undertook a total of 10 936 visits in 1962. Close collaboration with the general practice population was seen as key to the success of the service, with 39 GPs using the service regularly and 15 occasionally (Howell 1974). In addition, strong links were established with both the health visiting services and with the Birmingham Children's Hospital (Morris 1966). This collaboration is further highlighted in the pattern of referrals to the service reported by Robottom (1969), who noted that, of 1047 referrals made to the service from May 1967 to April 1968, 777 were from GPs, 241 were from hospitals and 29 from health visitors. At the time of Robottom's report, the nurses working in the service were formally identified as 'paediatric nurses', and Robottom herself was certainly a Registered Sick Children's Nurse (RSCN). However, in 1974, only three of the five members of the team were RSCNs (Howell 1974).

In 1969, Robottom had noted that only two nurses were working in the service. She recommended that 'for a more effective Children's Home Nursing Unit the first need is an increased paediatric nursing staff. The child population of the city is approximately 257 000: 10 paediatric nurses in addition to the existing two would enable this service in its present form to cover the whole city on a basis of one nurse per 20 000 children.' (Robottom 1969 p 312).

By 1974, four of the five nurses working in the service were 'attached' to one of the four hospitals containing paediatric beds within the Birmingham area (Howell 1974). At this stage there had been a significant shift in the work of the nursing team away from the care of children with acute problems and towards those with more long-standing nursing needs. This was accompanied by a reduction from 92% referrals by GPs in 1960, to only 43% in 1973.

THE PADDINGTON HOME CARE SCHEME

A 'home care scheme' was introduced in Paddington in April 1954, and was staffed initially by a trained 'paediatrician and three nurses with paediatric training' (Lightwood 1956 p 13). Although the nurses worked closely with the district nursing services, it would appear that none of the original members of the scheme had actually trained as district nurses themselves. The scheme was initiated because a review undertaken within the paediatric department at St Mary's Hospital had found that 'nearly a quarter of children in hospital during the review period were admitted for conditions which could have been managed at home if the doctors had possessed the facilities and experience required, and that there were other children whose stay in hospital could have been shortened' (Lightwood et al 1957 p 313).

The establishment of the Home Care Scheme was supported by the Local Medical Committee, the County of London, the Paddington and St Marylebone District Nursing Association, the County Council, the local medical officers of health and the constituent hospitals of the St Mary's Hospital group. It was established with three clear aims (Lightwood 1956):

1. Improving cooperation between hospital staff and family doctors.
2. Avoidance of admission to hospital for sick children.
3. Cutting the cost of inpatient treatment by providing a cheaper alternative whilst maintaining high standards.

The work of the team was very similar to that reported in Rotherham and in the early years of the Birmingham scheme, with a major concentration on the management of symptoms and the care of children with acute febrile illness. Lightwood et al (1957) even described the management in the home (including lumbar puncture) of a 12-week-old infant with meningococcal meningitis.

From the outset and throughout the 50 years of its existence to date, the staff of the scheme has included both RSCNs and registrar or consultant grade paediatricians. It has been argued that the availability of medical staff within the scheme made it very different to those in Birmingham and Rotherham (McClure 1960). However, it is perhaps of rather more than academic interest that, in spite of considerable publicity of the scheme over the years, including multiple publications in reputable medical journals, the model of joint medical and nursing provision developed in Paddington has never been replicated elsewhere in the UK.

The major work of the home care scheme was based, at the outset, upon referrals made by the local GPs and, more often than not, this was followed up by a joint visit between the GP, paediatric registrar and nursing sister. Bergman et al (1965 p 317) suggested: 'Home care is an extramural ward of the hospital' although whether the GPs involved with the scheme shared this view is unclear.

In the first 10 years of the service, 1882 of a total of 2923 referrals were made by GPs. Of these referrals, 2497 children were nursed at home following assessment by the home care registrar, with only 165 children being admitted to hospital (Bergman et al 1965). Table 2.2 shows the diagnostic groups of the children referred to the scheme during the first 10 years, with the five most common medical diagnoses being acute respiratory and infectious problems and accounting for almost two-thirds of all referrals. By the mid 1970s, however, as with the Birmingham service, there had been a definite change in the nature of the workload of the home care team towards children with more chronic problems (Jenkins 1975), a pattern that persists to the present day (Whiting 1994).

'THE WELFARE OF CHILDREN IN HOSPITAL'

The above-titled report from the Ministry of Health (1959) provided the first official endorsement of the development of community nursing services for sick children. The report recognised the emerging acceptance within the nursing and medical professions of the potential psychological harm

Table 2.2 Diagnostic groups of children referred to the Paddington Home Care Scheme 1954–1964

Diagnosis	No. of cases
Upper respiratory	594
Lower respiratory	548
Contagious disease	324
Gastroenteritis	233
Otitis media	206
Feeding problems	194
Pulmonary collapse	93
Urinary infection	89
Fever of unknown origin	59
Tuberculosis	52
Postoperative care	44
Congenital heart disease	37
Rheumatic fever	29
Central nervous system disorders	27
Poliomyelitis	13
Skin disease	10
Behaviour disorders	10
Miscellaneous	637

Source: Bergman et al (1965).

that might arise in children as a result of hospitalisation and recommended that 'children should not be admitted to hospital if it can possibly be avoided' (Ministry of Health 1959 para 17). The report further observed 'too few local authorities as yet provide special nursing services for home care of children and the extension of such schemes should be encouraged' (Ministry of Health 1959 para 18).

Whilst it is fair to say that many of the report's recommendations pertaining to the care of children in hospital have been implemented successfully, the proposals for expanding community nursing provision for children fell on very deaf ears indeed. There are no published reports of the establishment of new community children's nursing services until 1969.

AN INITIATIVE IN PAEDIATRIC DAY-CASE SURGERY IN SOUTHAMPTON IN 1969

A paediatric home nursing service was introduced in November 1969 in Southampton (Atwell et al 1973). The service was developed to support the newly established Centre for Paediatric Surgery for the Wessex Region in the Southampton Children's Hospital. In developing the service there was a clear statement of intent to avoid unnecessary overnight stays in hospital for children as well as a pragmatic approach to the need to optimise the use of beds and cots in the paediatric unit.

The development of the service was supported jointly by the consultant paediatric surgeon, the senior nursing officer in the community and the local medical officer of health. Initially, two nurses, who held qualifications in both district nursing and sick children's nursing, were appointed to provide follow-up in the community of children who had undergone day surgery. Gow & Atwell (1980) reported that the hospital was providing ten children's day lists per week (seven general surgical, one dental, one orthopaedic and one medical); however, the service rapidly developed its scope of operation to incorporate follow-up of children requiring inpatient care for medical and surgical problems as well as referrals from GPs, health visitors and social workers (Gow 1976).

A PROGRAMME OF INTEGRATED HOSPITAL AND HOME NURSING CARE FOR CHILDREN IN EDINBURGH

Three distinct, but complementary, children's home nursing initiatives were introduced in Edinburgh between 1969 and 1972 (Hunter 1974, 1977). The first initiative, in 1969, involved the appointment of a children's nursing sister within the outpatient department who was responsible for the provision of an outreach service from the Royal Hospital for Sick Children, in order to support the parents of children with 'long-term disability' (including diabetes mellitus or coeliac disease) or congenital abnormality (including cleft lip) (Hunter 1974).

The second service development in Edinburgh involved the secondment to the hospital of a district nursing sister who was already trained as a sick children's nurse. The focus of the nurse's work was in caring for children who had been referred to the hospital either for inpatient care or for outpatient assessment of predominantly acute problems. Hunter (1974) observed that in the month before the nurse's appointment only four children had received care from the district nursing service, but during the first year of the attachment of the district nursing sister to the hospital 2400 visits were paid to children, increasing to 5700 visits in 1972 when a second sister was appointed. A major focus of the nurses' work was in supporting the management of medication regimens including the administration of drugs by injection. In addition, the management of burn and scald injuries was a significant area of work.

The third element of the Edinburgh scheme initially involved a research project, but rapidly led to the appointment of a nurse working flexibly between the hospital ward, outpatient department and the community and focused on the care of children with cystic fibrosis. By 1974 each of these services had developed considerably, and were also supplemented by two further appointments of district nursing sisters covering the north side of Edinburgh and the county of East Lothian (Hunter 1974). In 1986 Campbell wrote: 'We are all very committed to our home care nursing programme and I for one know that in home care I have the best job in the NHS' (Campbell 1986 p 307).

A SCHEME TO PROVIDE HOME NURSING CARE FOR SICK CHILDREN IN THEIR OWN HOMES IN GATESHEAD

A children's home nursing scheme was established in Gateshead in 1974, following the appointment of two district nurses who were 'retrained' in the hospital care of children (Hally et al 1977, Jackson 1978), although the nurses working with the scheme retained, as the major focus of their work, an 'adult' patient caseload. It is not altogether clear from these published accounts whether or not the nurses were actually registered as sick children's nurses, although the authors suggest that, in the absence of such qualifications or 'equivalent experience', 'a longer and more formal period of retraining is desirable' (Hally et al 1977 p 764). The Gateshead scheme was very much focused upon children at the interface between hospital and community care, with close involvement of GPs and hospital-based paediatricians. Referrals to the scheme were only accepted on the basis that the children would otherwise have been admitted to hospital or would have required a longer stay in hospital. Consequently the children referred to the scheme were almost exclusively suffering from acute 'paediatric' problems. No further published reference to the scheme beyond 1978 has been found.

A DIABETIC CLINIC FOR CHILDREN IN OXFORD

In 1973, a children's diabetes clinic was established at the John Radcliffe Hospital in Oxford. The following year a community nursing sister, qualified as both a health visitor and a registered sick children's nurse, was appointed to the team from the community nursing budget in order to facilitate the care of children with newly diagnosed diabetes mellitus and to provide ongoing care for children with established diabetes. The nurse was based within the hospital and provided an outreach service exclusively to children with diabetes (Smith et al 1984). This service represented a new development within community children's nursing, that of community outreach nursing, within a clearly delineated area of disease-specific practice.

BRENT'S INTEGRATED PAEDIATRIC NURSING SERVICE

In 1974, the NHS underwent its most radical reorganisation since its inception. One clear objective of the reorganisation was that, within the newly configured district health authorities, services that had been traditionally described as either 'hospital' or 'community' should be fully integrated. Smith (1977) provides a detailed account of how representatives of three nursing divisions within Brent District Health Authority ('hospital', 'midwifery' and 'community') had each argued that a proposed integrated children's unit should be located within their own division. After much deliberation a decision was finally made to locate the unit within the community nursing division. It was further agreed that this unit would include inpatient and outpatient paediatric facilities, the special care baby unit, school nursing and health visiting.

In 1976, two 'home nurses' and two liaison health visitors were appointed within the newly integrated services (McLetchie 1977). By 1981 the service had expanded to include three sister-grade registered sick children's nurses and in this year the role of the team was extended to provide a follow-up service for children attending the accident and emergency department (Glucksman et al 1986). In 1982–1983, 556 children who were referred following attendance in the accident and emergency department were visited by the community children's nursing team. The nurses made a total of 1271 visits (average of two visits per child: 351 children (63%) received only one follow-up visit, and the maximum number of visits per child was five). Approximately 40% of the children were referred for follow-up of a minor medical problem, 30% were for removal of sutures and the remaining 30% for soft tissue injuries including burns and scalds (Glucksman et al 1986).

'FIT FOR THE FUTURE'

In 1973 the Secretary of State for Social Services brought together, under the chairmanship of Professor Donald Court, a Committee whose terms of reference were: 'To review the provision made for health services for children up to and through school life; to study the use made of these services by children and their parents and to make recommendations' (DoH and Social Security 1976 p 397).

The Committee produced its final report in 1976. Amongst its many recommendations, those that are of perhaps greatest interest include the proposal to develop a 'distinct group of nurses called child health visitors, who would combine preventive and curative nursing responsibility for children' (Chapter 7, recommendation 5), and the suggestion that the child health visitor 'should be assisted in her work in surgeries, health centres and home nursing by a child health nurse who would have paediatric training' (Chapter 7, recommendation 7). In making these recommendations the Court Committee was clearly cognisant of earlier developments in the provision of nursing services to sick children in the community. They observed 'nursing support for sick children in the community is currently an underdeveloped area and in terms of its commitment to practical aid and education for parents of sick children, what we are proposing is in many ways a new nursing service' (para 12.16 p 182).

As with many of the recommendations arising from the Court Committee the responses to these particular proposals were very limited indeed. A policy review group established under the auspices of the National Children's Bureau (NCB) to review progress in implementing 'Court', observed: 'There has been no lack of committees, reports and studies on these subjects. We have been most unimpressed by the action that has arisen as a result of these studies and deliberations' (NCB 1987 p 10).

THE 1980s

Despite the strong endorsements and recommendation of the Court Report, no new community children's nursing services were established for several years. A study of community children's nursing services undertaken by Starbuck in 1981 noted the 'recent establishment' of a home care service for children in Rochdale involving a district nurse and health visitor but there are no published records of this service. Two subsequent studies received a negative response from the health services in Rochdale when seeking to confirm details of the service (Catchpole 1986, Whiting 1988). Whiting in 1985 (p 5) considered the journey towards provision of a nationwide community children's nursing service; the ways in which existing services had been established, the local and national needs that have prompted their development and methods by which it may be possible to channel resources into nationwide provision (Box 2.1).

Box 2.1 Summary of Whiting (1985) 'Building a nationwide community paediatric nursing service'

- The nursing care of children is best provided by a children's nurse wherever the child is to be cared for.
- 'Resistance to the development of community children's nursing schemes comes from many sources. Fears of those who would stand in the way of progress are without foundation.
- Those health visitors who see the sick children's nurse working in the community as unnecessary must accept that the needs of children who are acutely ill or are suffering more chronic disease are best met by qualified children's nurses. Any areas of overlap between the two groups are minimal and far more acceptable than to leave glaring gaps in the services provided.
- District nurses who feel aggrieved at the loss of the younger age group from their case loads should certainly agree that sick children need … children's nurses and must accept that neither the SRN/RGN qualification or the district nurse training equips the individual nurse to meet the unique needs of the sick child.'
- Reluctance to develop community children's nursing services on financial grounds is misplaced. CCNs are appearing all over the country as more and more districts realise that nursing children in their own homes is less expensive than nursing them in hospital.
- Recognition of this economic reality provides an ideal standpoint from which to launch the concept of community paediatric nursing … but the justification for nursing sick children in their own homes is not based merely upon the fact that it 'saves money'.
- The disruption that hospitalisation can cause for the sick child and family is largely preventable.
- CCNs were under increasing pressure to justify their existence and encouraged to 'expand services and prepare for the day when a country-wide community children's nursing service is no longer an idealistic pipedream but is an essential practical reality'.

In 1986, Catchpole undertook a survey of community children's nursing service provision in England and suggested that there had been a significant expansion in service provision during the early 1980s. The survey identified ten new services established between 1983 and 1986 (Table 2.3).

Table 2.3 Paediatric community nursing services established from 1983 to 1986

Location	Year established
Swindon	1983
Sutton	1984
Surrey	1984
Nottingham	1984
Manchester (North)	1984
Hartlepool	1984
Blackburn	1985
Northampton	1985
Stockport	1985
Portsmouth	To commence 1986

Source: Catchpole (1986).

Catchpole suggested that one significant feature of the new services was that five out of ten of them were based in hospitals, although most of the long-established services were community based. She also observed that a number of the services that were configured within the community nursing services actually had a base in the hospital paediatric department: 'They all have one common aspect however, which differentiates the service from that of the adult district nursing service and that is they offer an extension of hospital work into the patient's home' (Catchpole 1986 p 23).

In 1988, a national census of community children's nursing provision (Whiting 1988) suggested that the growth in service development described by Catchpole had been sustained. Whiting (1988) identified a total of 24 services in England in January 1988 (Boxes 2.2 and 2.3).

Box 2.2 Community children's nursing teams in England in 1988 (Whiting 1988)

- Aylesbury
- Brighton
- Doncaster
- Isle of Wight
- Northampton
- North Staffordshire
- Paddington
- Southampton

- Basingstoke
- Carshalton
- Ealing
- Kettering
- North Birmingham
- Nottingham
- Salisbury
- South Birmingham

- Brent
- Central Birmingham
- Enfield
- Milton Keynes
- North Manchester
- Oxford
- Scunthorpe
- Stockport

> **Box 2.3** Summary of data (Whiting 1988)
>
> - Eighteen teams based in hospital children's wards/departments
> - Five teams based in community settings
> - Forty-five staff employed as CCNs
> - Referrals to teams predominantly from children's wards
> - Most teams received referrals from range of hospital/community-based agencies
> - All 23 teams provided care both to children with chronic diseases and with acute 'medical' problems
> - Eighteen teams provided care to children with physical handicap/learning disabilities
> - Nineteen teams followed up non day-case surgery
> - Eleven teams provided day surgery follow-up
> - Eleven 'teams' had only one nurse
> - Five teams had two nurses
> - Five teams staffed by three nurses
> - Largest team had seven nurses
> - Larger teams more likely to be involved in post-surgery follow-up
> - The 11 teams that featured a single nurse provided daytime only care, District Nurses often provided cover at other times
> - Larger teams able to provide more extensive cover, small number of teams with three or more staff able to provide a visiting service at weekends
> - Two services provided '24-hour care'

In addition, 33 districts gave details of plans to establish community children's nursing services; four of these services were actually in the final planning stages and were 'up and running' by April 1988 (Tables 2.4–2.6). The research confirmed that the services in Rotherham, Rochdale and Gateshead, referred to above, were no longer operating.

Whilst it is evident that, in 1988, there was tremendous diversity in the practice of the community children's nursing services, there was also a core of clinical activity which clearly delineated the care of children in the community from other areas of nursing practice. The formal recognition of this emerging area of practice by the establishment, in 1988, of a Paediatric Community Nurses Forum within the Royal College of Nursing (RCN) illustrates how far things had progressed from the situation in 1983 when there were only seven services in the whole of England.

1988–2004

As is widely documented, there has been a dramatic expansion in both the number of teams and the average size of those teams (Fig. 2.1).

The establishment of the Community Children's Nursing Forum was a watershed event, bringing together, for the first time, CCNs from across the UK. At this time, CCNs were most usually referred to as Community Paediatric Nurses – CPNs. The title 'Community Children's Nurses' was subsequently adopted partly in order to avoid any possible confusion with

Table 2.4 Major referral sources to 23 community children's nursing teams

Referral source	No. of teams
General hospital children's ward	22 (96%)
Health visitor	21 (91%)
General practitioner	19 (83%)
Special care baby unit (SCBU)	18 (78%)
General hospital outpatients department	17 (74%)
Children's hospital children's ward	13 (57%)
School nurse	13 (57%)
Social worker	11 (48%)
General hospital casualty department	10 (43%)
Children's hospital outpatients department	9 (39%)
Children's hospital casualty	6 (26%)
Source: Whiting (1988).	

Table 2.5 Illustration of the frequency with which each of the 23 community children's nursing services reported their involvement in the care of children with a range of medical conditions

Condition	No. of teams ($n = 23$)
Respiratory conditions (e.g. asthma)	20 (87%)
Children with stomas (e.g. tracheostomy, gastrostomy, ileostomy)	18 (78%)
Cancer or leukaemia	17 (74%)
Congenital orthopaedic problems	17 (74%)
Eczema and other skin disorders	15 (65%)
Enuresis or encopresis	15 (65%)
Congenital cardiac problems	15 (65%)
Acute medical problems (e.g. non-specific infections, gastroenteritis)	14 (61%)
Diabetes mellitus	14 (61%)
Renal problems (e.g. nephrotic syndrome)	10 (43%)
Blood dyscrasias (e.g. haemophilia, thalassaemia, sickle cell disease)	9 (39%)
Source: Whiting (1988).	

Table 2.6 Activities forming a part of the community children's nursing team's caseload

Activity	No. of teams ($n = 23$)
Teaching aspects of practical care to parents and children (e.g. giving injections, nasogastric feeding)	23 (100)
Support to families of children dying at home	22 (96)
Teaching of other professional colleagues	22 (96)
Education of children and parents with specific medical problems (e.g. diabetes, asthma)	22 (96)
Postoperative wound care	19 (83)
General health education	19 (83)
Administration or supervision of medication (not intravenous)	19 (83)
Dressings or wound care following trauma (e.g. scalds, lacerations)	18 (78)
Administration of intravenous drugs	12 (52)

Values in parentheses are percentages. Source: Whiting (1988).

Fig. 2.1 Number of CCN teams: United Kingdom (1954–2004). (Based on both historical data (up to 1988) and the RCN Directory of Community Children's Nursing services from 1988 to 2004.)

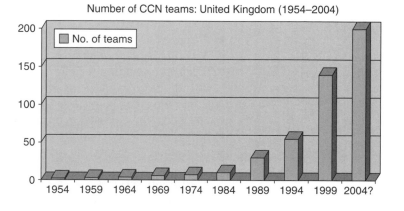

Number of CCN teams: United Kingdom (1954–2004)

Community Psychiatric Nurses, also CPNs (Langlands 1990). The initial aims of the forum were based on a recognition of the need for CCNs to develop effective communication networks with each other in order to facilitate the sharing of both clinical expertise, for example 'Guidelines on intravenous therapy for children in the community' now in its third edition (RCN 2001), and also the experiences of the practical 'nuts and bolts' of establishing new services. Over the years, this second objective has been achieved in large part through the publication of both a succession of directories of Community Children's Nursing Services (16th edn) (RCN 2004), providing contact details of community children's nursing teams and summary details of the teams' work. The forum has also produced a series of documents that have offered advice and direction for those wishing to develop local services (Tatman et al 1994, RCN 1996, 2000, 2002).

During this period the need to expand community children's nursing provision was supported by a number of Government publications including 'The welfare of children and young people in hospital' (DoH 1991), 'Children first' (Audit Commission 1993), 'The children's charter' (NHS Executive 1996b) and 'Child health in the community' (NHS Executive 1996a). In addition, a number of evaluative studies of provision provided strong endorsement of services, particularly from the perspective of the parents (Holden et al 1991, Bosanquet et al 1994, Jennings 1994, Smith et al 1996, Peter & Torr 1996). Several commentators have mapped the development of services during this period (Tatman & Woodroffe 1993, Kelly et al 1994, Whiting 1995, Carter 2000, Eaton 2000, 2001, Whiting et al 2001, Parker et al 2002, Cramp et al 2003). One recurring theme in the literature is the variation in the way that services are provided. No two services are exactly the same. This is despite the fact that the establishment of a number of teams has been preceded by many months of painstaking research, with prospective service managers visiting existing teams across the UK, in order to identify the 'right model' for local services development. Eaton's research in 2001 identified six models. The range of models now includes:

- Hospital-based 'generalist' outreach services
- Hospital-based services comprising a number of 'specialist' nurses
- Community-based teams who are not specifically aligned with a single Primary Care Trust
- Primary Care Trust-based teams
- Ambulatory care or assessment unit and hospital-at-home services
- Services (including respite) for children with life-limiting illnesses including community-, hospital- and hospice-based services
- Continuing care teams (see Chapter 22)
- Specialist nurses based in tertiary referral centres
- Services based in Child Development/Sure Start Teams
- Community neonatal services.

In addition, services are configured in different ways depending upon the extent to which they support children who fall into each of the following seven categories (Health Committee 1997a):

- Children with long-standing (chronic) physical ill health/long-term nursing needs
- Supporting children with disabilities
- Children with life-limiting illness/terminal care
- Neonatal and post-neonatal care/children with complex disabilities presenting at birth
- Acute illness/nursing needs
- Children needing emergency treatment (surgery/trauma/orthopaedic care) to assist early discharge
- Children undergoing 'planned' surgery.

Some services are provided on weekdays during office hours, others operate a 24-hour/7-day-a-week service and all points in between. This diversity in services provision has some merits. It could be argued that the major drivers in service development are the demands of local service users and that differences between services are determined by variations in local demands. However, such inconsistency in the organisation, nature, extent and clinical focus of service provision cannot be explained entirely by differences between the needs of local populations. The House of Commons Health Select Committee (HSC) (Health Committee 1997a) concluded that it was 'highly undesirable that there should be such local disparities in the provision of community children's nursing services and we are not convinced that there is a logical explanation for this' (p xlix).

Both the House of Commons HSC (Health Committee 1997a) and a recent systematic review of community children's nursing provision (Parker et al 2002) identified the absence of systematic evaluation of the differences between services and concluded 'We very much regret that no research has ever been conducted on the most cost effective way of providing the nursing service that children and their carers in the community need' (Health Committee 1997a p xlix). 'We have been able to find no completed robust evaluation of generic paediatric home care services in the UK' (Parker et al 2002 p 81).

A possible explanation for the variation in services provision lies in the dynamic nature of the NHS at the time of most rapid growth in community children's nursing provision, the last 15 years. The period at the end of the 1980s and through the early 1990s, saw a number of key changes which are relevant in the context of the provision of services.

The publication of Casey's initial articulation of the partnership model in 1988 (Casey 1988, Casey & Mobbs 1988) and its later refinement (Casey 1993, 1995) struck a chord with British children's nurses, mirroring many of the philosophical underpinnings of the family-centred care model developing in the United States (Ahman 1994a, 1994b). It linked closely with the imperatives of The Children Act (1989) in respect of professionals and parents working together to promote the health and well-being of children and, in so doing, recognised and valued child and family perspectives on care. Parents have been very supportive of community children's nursing and the adoption of the partnership philosophy by children's nurses has been a crucial factor in the shifting of care between hospital and the community.

With the introduction of Project 2000 (UK Central Council 1986) pre-registration nursing education took a dramatic shift in focus towards the community. This was followed in 1994 by the rationalisation of the community nursing courses which existed prior to this time and the introduction of the Specialist Practitioner programmes in Community Children's Nursing (UK Central Council 1994) (see Chapter 8).

The introduction of the Griffiths' reforms and the concepts of 'purchasing' and 'provision' in the NHS created a market economy which encouraged those responsible for services delivery to find creative ways of delivering cost-efficient services (DoH 1988, 1989a, 1989b). This led to the establishment of both stand-alone hospital and stand-alone community

Trusts and the introduction of GP fundholding. During the early 1990s there was very rapid growth in community children's nursing provision, with services developing within both hospital and community Trusts in approximately equal numbers. The introduction of GP fundholding, including the creation of 'total fundholding practices' had no clearly discernible effect upon the growth in service availability during this period (see Figure 2.1).

In 1992 the DoH (England) made available a total of two million pounds to be used for the development of a series of pilot projects for children with life-limiting illness. In total 52 projects were funded of which 15 involved researching or development of community nursing services for children (NHS Executive 1998a). At the end of the pilot projects, the funding of a number of the services was continued by the host Trust in which the services had been based. This represented the start of a significant pattern of investment in the development of community nursing services for children with life-limiting diseases. It was followed in 1998, by the creation of eight Diana Community Children's Nursing teams in England (one in each of the new Regions) and the funding of programmes of CCN education in Wales, Scotland and Northern Ireland (NHS Executive 1998b). The funding of the eight teams of CCNs in England was renewed in 2002 and in January 2003 the New Opportunities Fund (NOF) provided 48 million pounds of investment for the development of community services for children with life-limiting ill-nesses, including £15.3 million for palliative care in hospices and £26.6 million for home-based respite services (NOF 2003). The aggregated effect of this significant investment in the care of children with life-limiting ill-nesses remains to be seen, however there can be little doubt that this has fundamentally influenced the work of CCNs and will do so for several years to come.

The Clothier Report (Clothier et al 1994) focused the attention of those responsible for commissioning the education of children's nurses. The report, combined with the recommendations of the DoH report on the 'Welfare of children and young people in hospital' (1991) and the subse-quent Audit Commission investigation which culminated in the prod-uction of 'Children First' (1993), has given rise to a dramatic increase in the numbers of children's nurse education places. Glasper & Charles-Edwards (2002) identified that between 1986 and 2001, the numbers of nurses in training for the children's nursing part of the register increased from 747 (6.2% of the General Nursing total) to 1668 (19.6% of the Adult Nursing total). Undoubtedly this has led to a significant increase in the numbers of children's nurses working across a range of practice settings, including in the community. Although there are no up-to-date figures in relation to the total number of CCNs currently employed, the House of Commons HSC reported that, by May 1996, 495 CCNs were employed in England (a 1000% increase since 1988).

The House of Commons HSC was established in 1996. Its overall terms of reference were: 'To consider the specific health needs of children and adolescents and the extent to which those needs are adequately met by the National Health Service' (Health Committee 1997b p v). In order to help shape the focus of its work, the Committee sought the views of professional and voluntary organisations as to possible subjects which might form the central themes of its deliberations. The RCN identified the provision of community children's nursing services as one of a number of key issues. The RCN was invited to provide written evidence to the Committee specifically in relation to community children's nursing provision and was then invited to nominate CCN representatives to provide oral evidence to the Committee and to answer questions arising from its enquiries. This formed part of the evidence heard by the Committee in respect of child health services provision in the community and much of this evidence appeared verbatim in the subsequent report and recommendations of the committee (Health Committee 1997a). It noted: 'At present less than 50% of the country is covered by a comprehensive CCN service, and fewer than 10% of children have access to a 24 hour service' (Health Committee 1997a p xviii) and continued:

> 'We regard it as highly undesirable that there should be such local disparities in the provision of CCN services and are not convinced that there is any logical explanation for this ... It is a cause of serious concern that only fifty per cent of health authorities purchase Community Children's Nursing Services ... for many years there has been a nursing service available to all adults in their own homes. We consider that, as a matter of principle, sick children need and deserve no less.'

(Health Committee 1997a p xix)

The Committee made five specific recommendations concerning the services that ought to be available (Health Committee 1997b p xv):

> '(a) All children requiring nursing intervention should have access to a community children's nursing service staffed by qualified children's nurses, supplemented by those in training, in whatever setting in the community they are being nursed.
> (b) This service should be available 24 hours a day, seven days a week.
> (c) Every GP should have access to a named CCN.
> (d) Information about the services should be easily available to all relevant healthcare professionals and voluntary organisations.
> (e) Coordination between agencies and professionals should be regarded as a necessary part of providing a good service.'

Ordinarily when a Select Committee issues a report, the Government is required to provide a formal response to the House of Commons within 3 weeks. However the publication of the HSC reports coincided with the dissolution of the Conservative Government in February 1997. The incoming Labour Government did not provide a response to the reports until October of that year. In its response it stated that 'The Government is committed to developing a new NHS Charter which concentrates on the quality and success of treatment. The high level Advisory Group, which will assist the government in this task will be made aware of these recommendations' (DoH 1997b p 20). A succession of broad social policy initiatives has set the scene for the National Services Framework (NSF) for Children.

'The New NHS. Modern, dependable' (DoH 1997a) outlined the Government's plans for the NHS over a 10-year term. In 'A first class service' (DoH 1998) the quality framework of 'clinical governance' was introduced alongside the proposals to create a series of NSFs. 'The NHS Plan' (DoH 2000) heralded the largest single investment the NHS had ever seen. In 2001, the publication of 'Shifting the balance of power' (DoH 2001a) signalled a sea-change in NHS funding, with the stated intention that by April 2004, 75% of funds would be directed through the new Primary Care Trusts who would take on full responsibility for commissioning healthcare on behalf of their local populations. It was against this background that the Children's Taskforce was launched in 2001 (DoH 2001b) with clear responsibility to produce the children's NSF by 2003/4. The first stage of that framework was launched in April 2003 (DoH 2003) and the full NSF is yet to be published. CCNs have been involved in a number of the External Working Groups supporting the NSF, including work focused upon 'the ill child' and 'disabled children' in order to ensure that the 'high level Advisory Group' is very clearly aware of the issues which the HSC so succinctly identified in relation to the provision of community children's nursing services. Only time will tell how successful their efforts have been.

CONCLUSION

Community children's nursing has come a long way since the late 1880s. Many models of community children's nursing have developed and many titles have been used to describe those practitioners. Registered children's nurses, working in community settings and providing care for children require the particular skills and knowledge of those nurses if they are to achieve optimal health. There is, however, a central core to that practice, the work of the CCN, which defines and delineates that practice and makes it unique. Although there is much that is still to be achieved, and the concerns expressed by the Health Committee (1997a) make it clear that this is the case, CCNs have come a long way on their journey to provide a nationwide community children's nursing service (Whiting 1985).

REFERENCES

Ahmann A 1994a Family centred care: the time has come. Pediatric Nursing 20(1):52–53

Ahmann A 1994b Family centred care: shifting orientation. Pediatric Nursing 20(1):113–117

Atwell J, Burn J M B, Dewar A K & Freeman N V 1973 Paediatric day case surgery. Lancet ii:895–897

Audit Commission 1993 Children First: A Study of Hospital Services. HMSO, London

Baly M E, Robottom B & Clark J M 1987 District Nursing, 2nd edn. Heinemann, London

Bergman A B, Shrand H & Oppe T E 1965 A pediatric home care program in London – ten years' experience. Pediatrics 36:314–321

Bosanquet N, Connoly M, Hart D & Dzapasi L 1994 Paediatric Nursing Service – North Middlesex Hospital: Integrating the A&E Department Service for Children with the Paediatric Home Care Nursing Service. Health Policy Unit, Department of General Practice, Lisson Grove Health Centre, London

Campbell M 1986 Community nurse – a typical day. British Journal for Nurses in Child Health 1(10):307

Carter B 2000 Ways of working: CCNs and chronic illness. Journal of Child Health Care 4(2):66–72

Casey A 1988 A partnership with child and family. Senior Nurse 84:8–9

Casey A 1993 Development and use of the partnership model of nursing care. In: Glasper E A & Tucker A (eds) Advances in Child Health Nursing. Scutari Press, London

Casey A 1995 Partnership nursing: influences on involvement of informal carers. Journal of Advanced Nursing 22:1058–1062

Casey A & Mobbs S 1988 Partnership in practice. Nursing Times 84(44):67–68

Catchpole A 1986 Community Paediatric Nursing Services in England: 1985. Unpublished results, Oxford Polytechnic

Clark J 1981 What do Health Visitors do? A Review of the Research 1960–1980. Royal College of Nursing, London

Clothier C, MacDonald C A & Shaw D A 1994 The Allitt Inquiry. HMSO, London

Cramp C, Hughes N & Dale G 2003b Children's home nursing: results of a national survey. Paediatric Nursing 15(8):3–43

Department of Health 1988 Community Care: Agenda for Action. The Griffith's Report. HMSO, London

Department of Health 1989a Working for Patients. HMSO, London

Department of Health 1989b Caring for People: Community Care in the Next Decade and Beyond. HMSO, London

Department of Health 1991 The Welfare of Children and Young People in Hospital. HMSO, London

Department of Health 1997a The new NHS. Modern, dependable. The Stationery Office, London

Department of Health 1997b Government response to the reports of the Health Committee on Health Services for Children and Young People, session 1996–97: 'The Specific Health Needs of Children and Young People' 307-1; 'Health Services for Children and Young People in the Community, Home and School' 314-1; 'Hospital Services for Children and Young People' 128-1; 'Child and Adolescent Mental Health Services' 26-1. The Stationery Office, London

Department of Health 1998 A first class service: quality in the new NHS. The Stationery Office, London.

Department of Health 2000 The NHS plan: a plan for investment; a plan for reform. The Stationery Office, London.

Department of Health 2001a Shifting the balance of power within the NHS – securing delivery. The Stationery Office, London

Department of Health 2001b Children's Taskforce: an introduction. The Stationery Office, London

Department of Health 2003 Getting the right start: National Service Framework for children: standards for hospital services. The Stationery Office, London

Department of Health and Social Security 1976 Fit for the future. The report of the Committee on Child Health Services, vol 1. HMSO, London

Dunnell K & Dobbs J 1982 Nurses Working in the Community. HMSO, London

Eaton N 2000 Children's community nursing services: models of care delivery. A review of the UK literature. Journal of Advanced Nursing 32(1):49–56

Eaton N 2001 Models of community children's nursing. Paediatric Nursing 13(1):32–36

Franklin A W 1964 Children's hospitals. In: Poynter F N L (ed.) The Evolution of Hospitals in Britain. Pitman, London, p 103

Gillet J A 1954 Children's nursing unit. British Medical Journal 684:1954

Glasper E A & Charles-Edwards I 2002 The child first and always: the registered children's nurse over 150 years. Part two. Paediatric Nursing 14(5):38–43

Glucksman E, Tachakra S S, Piggott S & Lea H 1986 Home care team in accident and emergency. Archives of Disease in Childhood 61:294–296

Gow M A 1976 Domiciliary paediatric care in Southampton. Queen's Nursing Journal October:192, 205

Gow M A & Atwell J 1980 The role of the children's nurse in the community. Journal of Pediatric Surgery 15(1):26–30

Hally M A, Holohan A, Jackson R H, Reedy B L E C & Walker J H 1977 Paediatric home nursing scheme in Gateshead. British Medical Journal 1(6063):762–764

Health Committee 1997a House of Commons Select Committee. Health services for children and young people in the community: home and school. Third report. The Stationery Office, London

Health Committee 1997b The specific health needs of children and young people. Second Report. The Stationery Office. London

Holden C E, Puntis J W L, Charlton C P L & Booth I W 1991 Nasogastric feeding at home: acceptability and safety. Archives of Disease in Childhood 66:148–151

Hospital for Sick Children 1874 Medical Committee minutes, volume 6: Special meeting of the joint committee – March 18. Archives of the Great Ormond Street Hospital NHS Trust, London

Hospital for Sick Children 1936 General rules for the private nursing staff. Archives of the Great Ormond Street Hospital NHS Trust, London

Howell M 1974 Domiciliary care of sick children in Birmingham – its history and development. Presented to the Annual Conference of the National Association for the Welfare of Children in Hospital (NAWCH), NAWCH, London

Hunt J & Whiting M 1999 A re-examination of the history of children's community nursing. Paediatric Nursing 11(4):33–36

Hunter M H S 1974 A Programme of Integrated Hospital and Home Nursing Care for Children. Presented to the Annual Conference of the National Association for the Welfare of Children in Hospital (NAWCH). NAWCH, London

Hunter M H S 1977 Paediatric hospital at home care: 1. Integrated programmes. Nursing Times Occasional Papers 10 March: 33–36

Jackson R H 1978 Home care for children. Journal of Maternal and Child Health March: 96, 98, 100

Jenkins S M 1975 Home care scheme in Paddington. Nursing Mirror 27 February:68–70

Jennings P 1994 Learning through experience: an evaluation of hospital at home. Journal of Advanced Nursing 19:905–911

Kelly P J, Taylor C & Tatman M A 1994 Hospital outreach or community nursing. Child Health 2(4):160–163

Kosky J & Lunnon R J 1991 Great Ormond Street and the Story of Medicine. Granta Editions, London

Langlands T 1990 Meeting future needs. Paediatric Nursing 2(3):8–9

Lightwood R 1956 The home care of sick children. The Practitioner 177:10–14

Lightwood R, Brimblecombe F S W, Reinhold J D L, Burnard E D & Davis J A 1957 A London trial of home care for sick children. Lancet 9: 313–317

Lomax E M R 1996 Small and Special: The Development of Hospitals for Children in Victorian Britain. Wellcome Institute for the History of Medicine, London

McClure C R 1960 The St Mary's Hospital home-care for sick children scheme. Public Health 74(8):313–316

McLetchie C 1977 Specialist in home care: paediatric home nurse. Internal report. Brent Health District, London

Ministry of Health 1959 The welfare of children in hospital – report of the committee (chairman Sir H Platt) HMSO, London

Morris I 1966 Nursing children at home. Nursing Times:1653–1656

National Children's Bureau 1987 Investing in the future: child health ten years after the Court Report – a report of the Policy and Practice Review Group. National Children's Bureau, London

National Health Service Executive 1996a Child health in the community. A guide to good practice. The Stationery Office, London

National Health Services Executive 1996b The patient's charter: services for children and young people. The Stationery Office, London

National Health Services Executive 1998a Evaluation of the pilot project programme for children with life threatening illnesses. The Stationery Office, London

National Health Services Executive 1998b Diana Children's Community Nursing Teams Health Service Circular 1998/1999

New Opportunities Fund 2003 Lottery rolls-out £70 million relief for hospices and carers. Single biggest investment in children's palliative care. Online. Available: www.nof.org.uk 14 September 2004

Oppé T 1971 Home care for sick children. British Journal of Hospital Medicine 5(1):39–40, 43–44

Owen G M 1982 Health visiting. In: Allen P & Jolley M (eds) Nursing, Midwifery and Health Visiting since 1900. Faber and Faber, London, p 92

Parker G, Bhakta P, Lovett C A, Paisley S, Olsen R, Turner D & Young B 2002 A systematic review of the costs and effectiveness of different models of paediatric home care. Health Technology Assessment 6:35

Peter S & Torr G 1996 Paediatric hospital at home: the first year 8(5):22–23

Rathbone W 1890 Sketch of the History and Progress of District Nursing from 1859 to the Present Date. Macmillan, London

Robottom B 1969 The contribution of the children's nurse to the home care of children. British Journal of Medical Education 3(4):311–312

Royal College of Nursing (RCN) Paediatric Community Nurses Forum 1996 Buying paediatric community nursing: an RCN guide for purchasers and commissioners of health care. RCN, London

Royal College of Nursing (RCN) Community Children's Nursing Forum 2000 Community Children's Nursing: promoting effective teamwork for children and their families. RCN, London

Royal College of Nursing (RCN) 2001 Administering intravenous therapy to children in the community, 3rd edn. RCN, London

Royal College of Nursing (RCN) Community Children's Nursing Forum 2002 Community Children's Nursing. Information for primary care organisations, strategic health authorities and all professionals working with children in community settings. RCN, London

Royal College of Nursing (RCN) 2004 Directory of Community Children's Nursing Services 16th edn. RCN, London

Smellie J M 1956 Domiciliary nursing service for infants and children. British Medical Journal i:256

Smith J 1977 Brent's integrated paediatric nursing unit. Nursing Mirror 4 August: 22–24

Smith J, Hughes A & Wiles R 1996 Loddon NHS Community Trust: paediatric community nursing team – service evaluation. College of Health, London

Smith M A, Strang S & Baum J D 1984 Organisation of a diabetic clinic for children. Practical Diabetes 1(1):8–12

Starbuck C 1981 Nursing care of children in the community. BSc nursing dissertation, University of Manchester

Stocks M 1960 A hundred years of district nursing. Allen and Unwin, London

Tatman M & Woodroffe C 1993 Paediatric home care in the UK. Archives of Disease in Childhood 69:670–680

Tatman M, Kelly P, Dryden S, Sappa M, Sidey A, Whiting M & Burr S 1994 Wise decisions: developing paediatric home care teams. Royal College of Nursing, London

The Children Act 1989 HMSO, London

UK Central Council for Nursing, Midwifery and Health Visiting (UKCC) 1986 Project 2000: A new preparation for practice. UKCC, London

UK Central Council for Nursing, Midwifery and Health Visiting (UKCC) 1994 The future of professional practice – the Council's standards for education and practice following registration. UKCC, London

While A E 1985 Health visiting and health experience of infants in three areas. PhD thesis, University of London

Whiting M 1985 Building a nationwide community paediatric nursing service. Nursing Standard October 17:5

Whiting M 1988 Community paediatric nursing in England in 1988. MSc thesis, University of London

Whiting M 1994 40 years on and still a viable product. At Home: The Newsletter for Homecare Therapy Initiatives Caremark, Leyburn, Yorkshire

Whiting M 1995 Nursing children in the community. In: Campbell S & Glasper A (eds) Whaley and Wong's Children's Nursing. CV Mosby, London

Whiting M, Greene A & Walker A 2001 Community Children's Nursing – Delivering on the 'Quality Agenda'? In: Sines D, Appleby F and Raymond E (eds) Community Health Care Nursing. Blackwell Science, Oxford

Wood C J 1888 The training of nurses for sick children. Nursing Record 6 December: 507–510

Chapter 3

A 'new' National Health Service

Sean Mountford and David Widdas

with a contribution from:

Sharon Linter

KEY ISSUES

- Principal factors influencing service provision for children and young people.
- Structure of the new National Health Service.
- Children's National Service Framework.
- Child protection.
- Integration of children's services.
- Influencing commissioning priorities.

INTRODUCTION

The way the NHS is organised is undergoing change at an unprecedented level and it is unlikely it will ever again be a truly 'static' organisational system. There is now an expectation of partnerships with other organisations, such as social services and education, and a developing 'concordat' or partnership agreement with the independent sector.

The art in understanding the structure of the NHS is therefore not to worry about either the detail or the actual names of anyone within the structure but to try instead to understand the broad concepts as to what the various 'parts' are meant to do and where the power lies. The reason why an idea as to how the overall structure of the NHS works at a clinical level is needed is to understand where to go to create change in order to improve the delivery of clinical service.

Resources within the overall NHS in terms of money, staff and equipment are finite and decisions about what is more or less important in terms of where these limited funds should go are made by setting priorities at all levels. Priority setting is now undertaken by commissioners based within Primary Care Trusts (PCTs) and in some cases by specialist agencies for areas that are highly specialised such as transplant surgery.

In an attempt to move out of yearly agreements that inhibited long-term planning there is now a 3-year planning cycle developed through 'Local Delivery Plans' (LDPs) agreed by the PCTs and provider organisations such as the acute hospitals or the private sector. For the first time these LDPs offer opportunities for a longer-term planning cycle. However the impact of this is limited by the constant yearly financial cycle that inhibits an entrepreneurial approach by the pressure to always break even each year.

Deliverers of clinical services must know how to influence these priorities as they will have a profound effect on the services that are delivered both in terms of resources (staff, equipment, environment, etc.) and on the actual type of clinical service, i.e. preventive or treatment interventions used on a day-to-day basis (these are also influenced by professional bodies such as the Royal College of Nursing, Royal College of Paediatrics and Child Health). The Government are committed through policy to involve clinicians in planning decisions. This is embodied within the formation of the Professional Executive Committees (PECs) within PCTs who are charged with shaping services within local areas. Nurses and other professional groups have a legitimate right to be part of the PEC.

PRINCIPAL FACTORS INFLUENCING SERVICE PROVISION FOR CHILDREN AND YOUNG PEOPLE

The four themes central to the new NHS

The four themes, although they appear 'political' speak, are broadly important but do not have to be understood in detail (DoH 1997).

Box 3.1 Themes of the new NHS

- Developing partnerships and cooperation for appropriate healthcare (integrated/patient centred/clinically and cost effective).
- Abolition of the internal market and the contracts/transactions associated with it, in favour of less costly/more equitable system (based on longer-term service agreements within a framework of a jointly agreed health improvement programme).
- Building on the best of the many initiatives in primary care spawned during the 1990s to create a health service with primary care at its centre.
- Tackling inequalities in the light of the public health agenda and the Government paper 'Our healthier nation' (DoH 1998a).

Changes in the health of children and young people and society's needs

These changes include:

- The five outcomes identified by children and young people: (1) being healthy (enjoying good physical and mental health and living a healthy life style); (2) staying safe (being protected from harm and neglect and growing up able to look after themselves); (3) enjoying and achieving (getting the most out of life and developing broad skills for adulthood); (4) making a positive contribution (to the community and to society and not engaging in antisocial or offending behaviour); and (5) economic wellbeing (overcoming socio-economic disadvantages to achieve their full potential in life) (Department for Education and Skills 2003).

- A 'health' system which provides the 80% of children who will need virtually no medical 'illness' services with excellent primary and preventive care.
- Ensuring that the 15% of children's straightforward illnesses are treated using effective and evidence-based interventions (e.g. children with asthma).
- Ensuring that the 3% of children who have illnesses that are complex and difficult to treat (e.g. cystic fibrosis, cerebral palsy, complex congenital heart disease) have this treatment using appropriate technology combined with the highest standards of humane care.
- Opening up the ethical debate on the 2% of children with very complex illnesses or disability as to whether they should be allowed to suffer the consequences of doctor interventions (e.g. complex genetic disorders, severe cerebral palsy).
- Dealing with the much greater parental expectations, especially from those who have greater direct access to medical information using the World Wide Web, but accepting that there will also be a greater gap between the 'haves and have nots' of this information.
- The need to ensure a far greater parental (and child, where possible) input in discussions on management of sick and disabled children.

Actual structure of the new NHS

Starting at the top of the NHS, and probably of least direct importance to most clinicians in their day-to-day work, is the Department of Health (DoH) (the political arm of the service) and the NHS Executive (the business arm). At the very top is the Secretary of State for Health and ministers who are responsible for certain related subjects, such as public health, women's health, resources and waiting lists. Children's services are one part of the NHS Executive. The NHS Executive is responsible for a number of different departments (directorates) only one of which is 'Health Services'. The Health Services Directorate is again broken down into a number of different departments, only one of which is 'Health Services for Young People and Women'. Young people, in this case, includes children.

The NHS Executive has been streamlined. In England the majority of NHS Executive business is now managed through Strategic Health Authorities (SHAs) that overview performance and development. In Wales, Scotland and Northern Ireland variations of different health service structures operate. Of much more importance to clinicians is the structure of PCTs and how they relate to service development at a local level (see Box 5.2). Again, there will be variations in the structures and concepts laid out below for Wales, Scotland and Northern Ireland. PCTs have two main roles as commissioners of all local health services and providers of some specific services including community children's nursing.

Key principles to commissioning in the new NHS

- Promoting partnership – between the SHA, PCT, NHS Trusts and General Practitioners (GPs), via the PCTs, using an 'open and transparent approach' to sharing financial position and prospects.

- Developing service and financial frameworks – in consultation with GPs, other key professionals and local interests. PCTs collate all commissioning intentions through the production of a framework document for their area, (involving the public by including local people, service users and carers) using wide informal consultation on developing services and the financial framework.
- Developing service agreements – having developed frameworks, service agreements include:
  - what services are provided in terms of scope and activity
  - setting quality standards
  - defining the funding
  - monitoring arrangements.
- Developing longer-term agreements – by the use of multi-agency and interdisciplinary partnerships.

Partnerships and teams in commissioning

The discussion document 'Partnership in Action' (DoH 1998b) proposed legislation to improve strategic planning between health services and social services in order to improve joint commissioning and service provision. The DoH proposed to do this by having pooled budgets between health and social services deployed under a lead commissioner for certain areas of common health and social services provision. The low take up of these schemes has led to the formation of the concept of Children's Trusts.

However, in the area of overall health commissioning and priority setting, there are still a great many complex and unanswered questions that include:

- Who defines needs (e.g. Public Health, management of the SHA, PCTs, Government, the public)?
- Who defines appropriate and effective interventions (e.g. Public Health, clinicians, DoH)?
- Who defines priorities (e.g. Government, Public Health, executive of the local SHA, PCT clinicians, the public)?
- Who ensures change takes place (e.g. management of the local SHA, PCT)?
- Who monitors changes and quality (e.g. management of the local SHA, Public Health, PCTs)?

Local Delivery Plans

LDPs provide a strategic approach to developing the health of a population at PCT level and are adopted from previous contracting processes. The plans cover all age groups and are developed by the Directors of Public Health within PCTs. They are central to the commissioning process. The implementation of the National Service Framework (NSF) is key to content of delivery plans. The NSF will be a major driver for commissioning children's services for the next 10 years and remains an integral component of LDPs.

CHILDREN'S NATIONAL SERVICE FRAMEWORK

NSFs were established to improve services through the setting of national standards. They use evidence-based knowledge and are aimed at improving quality and tackle existing variations in care. NSFs have already been published for mental health, coronary heart disease, older people's services and diabetes. The children's NSF responds to some of the key challenges that have faced children's health and social care services, for example:

- Learning from Bristol (2001): the report of the public inquiry into children's heart surgery at the Bristol Royal Infirmary.
- The Victoria Climbie inquiry: the report into her abuse and death (Laming 2003).

The next NSFs to be published will cover children's services, renal services and long-term conditions as defined within the NHS plan (DoH 2000).

The children's NSF has three main aims:

- improving services
- tackling equalities
- enhancing partnerships.

It is designed to put children and young people at the centre of their care, building services around their needs as described in the document 'Emerging Findings' (DoH 2003a). This document defines the work of the children's NSF planning teams to date and is a recognition of the key importance of children in our society. Emerging Findings identifies the key themes of the NSF as:

- illness prevention and health promotion
- early identification and intervention of disease and disability
- empowerment, self management and family support
- child-centred care
- women-centred care
- transition and growing up
- safeguarding children from harm
- equitable access to services for all children and pregnant women.

Unlike other NSFs the children's NSF is producing broad standards as opposed to targets. These standards aim to provide greater flexibility to plan locally to meet local priorities and to foster innovative solutions to problems. The children's NSF benefits from an unprecedented level of service and user involvement and is made up of working groups:

- The Acute Module Phase 1 – Hospital Services
- The Acute Module Phase 2 – The Ill Child, children with long-term conditions and children with acute and/or minor illness in all settings
- maternity
- mental health and psychological well-being of children and young people
- children in special circumstances
- disabled children and long-term chronic conditions
- the ill child
- healthy children and young people
- medicines.

The findings of each working group, together with a wide range of consultation exercises run by the National Children's Bureau, are to be published as chapters within the final NSF document.

In addition to individual working groups within the NSF there are additional groups, common and accessible to all of the working groups, that underpin the overall work of the NSF. These additional groups are:

- Research and Development – to underpin standards and set priorities for future research.
- Clinical Governance – to embrace clinical governance and the recommendations/requirements of the National Institute of Clinical Effectiveness.
- Workforce – the Children Care Group Workforce Team aims to take a national view on health and social care workforce pressures and priorities. This group also addresses skills competencies workforce.
- Information management and technology – developing information and technology including an integrated care record service.

CHILD PROTECTION

Victoria Climbie came to Great Britain for a better life. During the 11 months she lived in England she suffered terrible abuse resulting in her death. The Climbie Inquiry produced 108 recommendations for health, social services, local authorities and the police based on multiple weaknesses identified within their operating systems (Laming 2003). The inquiry summarised the weaknesses as:

- a lack of professional standards of practice
- a gross failure of all systems involved
- widespread organisational malaise
- inappropriate focus of management
- lack of accountability.

This emotive inquiry supports practitioners in evaluating local child protection practice and in challenging areas of concern and summarises the following recommendations:

- clear lines of accountability with no doubt or ambiguity as to who is responsible from the top to the bottom of each system involved
- success of management based on outcomes for people not bureaucratic activity
- effective support involving multi-agency working with each agency fully carrying out their distinctive responsibilities
- the appropriate implementation of existing law
- information passed in a clear way to other agencies with a two-way dialogue about uncertainties and free exchange of information within the NHS
- a national children's database that effectively follows children through all systems and agencies and between all regions
- referral criteria should only be used after an assessment of suitability of referral, degree of risk and urgency of response has been made
- temporary staff supported and supervised by personnel with in-depth local knowledge
- supervision as a key principle to good practice
- practical, manageable, reasonably sized procedures available to all front-line staff.

INTEGRATED CHILDREN'S SERVICES

The Victoria Climbie Inquiry provided clear evidence of a lack of joint working within children's services. The Government believes a way of dealing with the accountability issues raised by Laming is in greater integration between involved services (Department for Education and Skills 2003). However the report cautioned against blurring between organisational roles (Laming 2003).

The Government will legislate to create a Director of Children's Services within each local authority. This role will lead to a single director with responsibility for education, social services and delegated functions from other areas, for example health, housing and leisure. The Government also wishes to see, within local authorities, a lead council member for children. This is the first step in a vision of greater integration of children's services within their preferred option of Children's Trusts.

Children's Trusts are designed to help tackle a range of identified problems including difficulties with:

- sharing information between services to identify children with multiple risks
- ensuring that children do not receive multiple, sometimes duplicate, assessments from different agencies involved
- focusing spending to provide intensive support in a more coherent way, rather than a large number of agencies spending small amounts of money on the same child
- harnessing the resources of the voluntary, community and private sectors
- broadening the focus so that service coverage extends beyond core priorities
- coordinating plans, partnerships and strategies across agencies
- developing a strategic needs analysis of the overall needs of children within an area
- workforce planning especially when new services create new demands on different parts of their workforce
- identifying a single person with overall accountability for improving services for which the Trust is responsible
- organising their services around the needs of children rather than for the convenience of providers (DoH 2003b).

A Children's Trust enables organisations to join together in a local partnership to commission and deliver services to children, in particular to children with a combination of health, education and social care needs (DoH 2003b). This widens the focus of service delivery to include health, social services and education. The Government has so far avoided being prescriptive on the structure of Children's Trusts. It is currently allowing pilot sites to develop around identified key features (Box 3.2).

The required minimum level for integration of health provision between services will be the 'children's delivery plan' agreed by the local Director of Children's Services. The preferred developmental model is the delegation of commissioning and the transfer of budgets to Children's Trusts (Department for Education and Skills 2003, 2004). Unless community children's nursing services are contracted from the PCT this could

> **Box 3.2** Key features of Children's Trusts
>
> ■ Short- and long-term objectives for being healthy, staying safe, enjoy-ing and achieving, making a positive contribution, economic wellbeing (Department for Education and Skills 2003)
> ■ A Director of Children's Services
> ■ Single planning and commissioning function with pooled budgets
> ■ Co-located services
> ■ Multidisciplinary teams
> ■ Key worker system
> ■ Common assessment framework and information system
> ■ Joint training modules
> ■ Shared child protection policy
> ■ Shared arrangements for interfacing with other services (DoH 2003b)

result in Community Children's Nurses (CCNs) being employed by their local authority alongside their colleagues from social services and education.

Children's Trusts will be accountable to the Director of Children's Services. Currently the legal framework and flexibilities within The Health Act 1999 are being used to set up pilot Children's Trusts (DoH 2003b). There are legislative plans to ensure partnership working but the implementation of Children's Trusts remains voluntary (Department for Education and Skills 2003, 2004). However each area is required to estab-lish local 'safeguarding children's boards' across health, social services and education replacing existing Area Child Protection Committees and it is expected that these will be chaired by the Director for Children's Services.

Current health, education and social service inspections will be replaced by an integrated children's inspectorate with particular emphasis on how well services work together (Department for Education and Skills 2003, 2004). The NSF is a pan-children's services approach and will require joined up commissioning, planning and funding in order to succeed.

INFLUENCING COMMISSIONING PRIORITIES

General factors

Most of what has been commissioned in the past will continue to be com-missioned in the same way in the future. This is because the overall num-ber of individual activities being commissioned in the field of paediatrics and child health runs into hundreds, if not thousands, and the time involved in reviewing the evidence that even one or two of these activ-ities should be increased, decreased, ceased or changed is enormous.

Furthermore, there is the realisation that some decisions about service delivery need to be made nationally. Decisions about screening pro-grammes (e.g. for hearing defects in children) should be made nationally because: (a) of quality issues, (b) of funding issues, (c) of equity of access issues and (d) the science is complicated. The way to influence these national decisions is for CCNs to try to get elected on to the relevant committee, for example the National Screening Committee.

Specific ways to influence

Primary Care Trusts – need to be informed and influenced by clinicians working in the field so that they:

- understand and support parents in their role as the primary health carers of children
- support primary prevention initiatives relative to childhood illnesses (e.g. immunisations, 'back to sleep' campaigns)
- understand and act on the social context of child health in cooperation with local council services
- use contemporary information relative to effective interventions in the field of child health
- understand the prevalence of childhood disability and the community management needed to care for these children
- have a basic understanding of the 'rights of the child' and child protection issues.

Local Delivery Plans – must include features relative to the health of children and young people. This can be achieved by clinicians:

- working with the PCT's Director of Public Health to ensure that the needs of children and young people are addressed in the LDPs
- learning from the NHS Modernisation Agency ways of demonstrating service development needs based on the real needs of children and their families, evidence and data.

Nationally
- Writing about concerns and priorities to the relative Royal Colleges with copies to other relevant organisations.*
- Writing to local members of parliament with copies to other relevant organisations.*
- Working with relevant voluntary organisations such as the Association for Children with Life-threatening or Terminal Conditions and their Families to produce best practice guidance and obtain media coverage.*
- Posting views on the NSF for children's website.

CONCLUSION

Although the NHS is a huge and complex organisation its final 'activities' are provided by clinicians at field level, such as CCNs who are preventing ill health and treating illness in the population so as to create a final 'product' which is a healthier nation. In developing health services and setting priorities it is therefore essential that (1) the voice of the child and family is heard, (2) the voice of the whole of society (which pays for

---

*Under a previous Government, Trusts put 'gagging clauses' into many NHS workers' contracts. Check Trust whistle-blowing policy and with your union before 'going public'.

the activity and product via taxes) is heard and (3) the voice of the 'worker' who carries out the activity that produces the product is also heard.

To this third end, CCNs need to understand where they can be most effective in influencing the priorities given to services for children and young people and their families and the relative health outcomes resulting from these services.

REFERENCES

Department for Education and Skills 2003 Every Child Matters. The Stationery Office, London

Department for Education and Skills (DfES) 2004 Every Child Matters: next steps. DfES Publications, Nottingham

Department of Health 1997 The new NHS. Modern, dependable. The Stationery Office, London

Department of Health 1998a Our healthier nation. The Stationery Office, London

Department of Health 1998b Partnership in action. A discussion document. The Stationery Office, London

Department of Health 2000 The NHS Plan: A Plan for Investment – A Plan for Reform. The Stationery Office, London

Department of Health 2003a Getting The Right Start: The National Service Framework for Children, Young People and Maternity Services – Emerging Findings. The Stationery Office, London

Department of Health 2003b Children's Trusts. The Stationery Office, London

Laming 2003 The Victoria Climbie Enquiry. The Stationery Office, London

Learning from Bristol 2001 The report of the public inquiry into children's heart surgery at the Bristol Royal Infirmary 1984–1995. The Stationery Office, London

The Health Act 1999 The Stationery Office, London

The editors would like to acknowledge the contribution made by Aidan Macfarlane in the previous edition of this book, which has been used as a foundation for this chapter.

Chapter 4

Role of the community children's nurse in influencing healthcare policies

Sue Burr with Julie Hughes

KEY ISSUES

To maximise the potential to influence healthcare policies community children's nurses need to:

- Ensure that the needs of children and their families are always the focus of their activities
- Embrace the methodology for seeking the user perspective and recognise the value of consumer views in planning and delivering community children's nursing services
- Acknowledge an individual responsibility to participate in the formulation and implementation of healthcare policy at local, national and international level
- Identify opportunities and be knowledgeable about the processes available
- Develop a broad vision of children's health and the societal and governmental factors that impinge on health and healthcare provision
- Actively seek to work with others across professional and organisational boundaries
- Have confidence in their knowledge and skills, be informed, actively disseminate good practice, reveal inequalities, be assertive and persistent.

INTRODUCTION

Healthcare policy should incorporate the specific needs of different groups within the population, ensuring that the most vulnerable groups receive particular consideration. Children and young people are one of the most vulnerable groups but, in an NHS focused on the physical health needs of adults, the specific needs of children, particularly those with continuing complex health needs, are frequently ignored.

Community children's nurses (CCNs) must ensure that the needs of the children are central to all their activities and take an active role in reminding others of that fact. Management and organisational structures and processes should support the meeting of needs and they should recognise the voice of the service user to ascertain those needs.

Healthcare policy is formulated by Government at both national and local levels. In this complex society a myriad of factors influences the Government's policy making, but first and foremost all nurses need to acknowledge that they have a professional responsibility to influence healthcare policy.

WHY NURSES SHOULD INFLUENCE NATIONAL HEALTHCARE POLICY

Nurses are the healthcare professionals who have both the most intimate and continuous contact with people, whether in the promotion of health, during sickness, rehabilitation or bereavement. They are the largest group of healthcare professionals nationally and internationally. Logically, nurses' influence on healthcare policy should be crucial to its development, but too often nurses neither seek nor have influence.

Nursing organisations have recognised the importance of the nurse's role in policy making. The International Council of Nurses (ICN) (1985) issued a policy statement that included the following:

> '*ICN strongly believes that international organisations and national governments should recognise the expertise of professional nurses and utilise it in policy making and the planning of health services. ICN also believes that active participation of professional nurses in policy making at all levels of health is essential*.'

In the mid 1980s Dame Sheila Quinn and Trevor Clay, both Vice Presidents of the ICN and respectively President and General Secretary of the Royal College of Nursing (RCN), continually urged nurses to 'get political' and to utilise their power within the political system.

In the UK all nurses are required by the Nursing and Midwifery Council (NMC) Code of Professional Conduct (NMC 2002) to protect the public and to provide a good quality of care to patients. To do so, nurses must be involved in both the shaping and implementation of policy. The Code also requires nurses to be advocates for their patients. This is particularly pertinent for nurses caring for the most vulnerable groups in society, of which children are one. The RCN's Charter (RCN 1916) includes 'promoting the advancement of the science and art of nursing for the benefit of patients'. To do that RCN members have to influence national and local healthcare policy.

Whilst nursing organisations have clearly stated the importance of nurses being involved in shaping healthcare policy, individual nurses have been slow to respond. This gives cause for concern because the reluctance of nurses has resulted in others taking the initiative and nursing issues being marginalized. Interestingly, nurses are increasingly recognising their role in empowering patients/clients but remain reluctant to use the same processes to empower nursing.

NURSES' RELUCTANCE TO PARTICIPATE IN POLICY MAKING

Many factors influence healthcare policy. These include the values of society, its culture, the socio-economic situation, the political ideology, and the power of professional and consumer groups. The Government's actions will be further influenced by practical considerations such as the size of its majority and the date of the next general election. Several of these factors particularly affect the nursing profession, for example the traditional role of women in a profession where the majority of members are female. The hierarchical culture of nursing has perpetuated the myth that healthcare policy is the responsibility of senior managers, with little acknowledgement by nurses in clinical practice of their responsibility.

The power of the male-dominated medical profession and, until recently, nurses' limited educational opportunities, have contributed to their reluctance to influence policy, although by the sheer size of numbers nurses should be able to exert considerable power. Clay (1987) recognised that they have been slow to acknowledge that power, too often expending energy disagreeing amongst themselves.

The radical changes in nursing education should assist all nurses to recognise their responsibility to influence policy and to identify and utilise the increasing opportunities available. The RCN Association of Nursing Students' resolution to RCN Congress in 1997 'that this meeting of RCN Congress supports the introduction of political education as an integral part of pre-registration courses' was passed with a good majority and marks a watershed.

The political perspective for nurses is slowly being integrated throughout nursing curricula and initiatives such as the Leading and Empowering Organisations programme and the RCN clinical and political programmes are key examples (Antrobus 1998, 2003, Antrobus & Kitson 1999, Cunningham & Kitson 2000, Woolnough & Faugier 2002). Whilst evaluation from these programmes is awaited it is anticipated that they should make a real difference in nurses' confidence to influence healthcare policy. It is important to convince all nurses of their responsibility to influence policy whatever the post held or healthcare setting in which they practice. Nurses at the client/patient interface have as much to contribute as senior managers who, too often, are remote from clinical practice.

CHILDREN, CHILDREN'S NURSES AND HEALTHCARE POLICY

Children's lack of political power, alongside the traditional view that caring for children is suitable employment for women not able to undertake more responsible work, is reflected in the low status and value attributed to children's nursing. The Health Committee (1997 para 15 p viii) states: 'It would be fair to conclude that until recent years, insufficient attention was paid to the need to train nurses to deal with the specific health needs of children.' and 'Likewise, insufficient effort appears to have been made to capitalise on the skills of qualified children's nurses' (para 16 p viii).

The DoH's response (1997) states: 'We acknowledge that past shortages of qualified children's nurses have limited the opportunities for the health service to benefit from their skills. As the number of children's nurses increases their skills can be utilised in many more areas of healthcare for children and young people'.

It is important to remember that studies from the Briggs Report (Briggs 1972) to the present time (Glasper & Charles-Edwards 2002) show no shortage of applicants wishing to undertake pre-registration programmes in children's nursing. Similar interest is apparent for post registration programmes in many specialised aspects of children's nursing including community children's nursing. The restricted opportunities, funding and failure to acknowledge the value of nurses educated to meet the specific needs of children have been very slow to be recognised by those who hold power within the nursing profession. Decisions regarding the educational needs of nurses vary across the four countries of the UK though the principles are similar. In England decisions are taken at Workforce Development Confederation (WDC) level (within Strategic Health Authorities) in discussion with education officers from within the Trusts and Primary Care Trusts (PCTs). It is essential that nurses appreciate the role of the WDC (or with Scotland, Wales and Northern Ireland of the appropriate body commissioning education), also that they are aware of who the appropriate children's nursing education representatives are to enable them to express the needs of children's nurses. This requires children's nurses to be particularly active in recognising and contributing to workforce planning as well as policy formulation and implementation to ensure that the specific needs of children are appropriately considered.

Recognising the educational needs of nurses wishing to work with children is essential considering that children and young people comprise almost a quarter of the population. Despite this the Chair of the Select Committee on Health noted in introducing the debate on the Committee's Report on 25 March 1998 (House of Commons 1998) following its Inquiry into Services for Children and Young People 'it is rare for the House of Commons to debate any issue concerning children'. The presence of about ten Members of Parliament (MPs) for the debate was a marked contrast to both the 'standing room only' for a debate on fox hunting a few weeks earlier and the full House debate through the night of 24 March on whether public schools could retain the right to beat pupils.

Over a decade ago, the Government recognised that women and women's issues needed an advocate within government if equality with men's issues was to be achieved. Children who have no vote are in an even less fortunate position. Children's issues, even those relating to health, are scattered throughout many ministries, often at the bottom end of each department's agenda. Whilst governments proclaim the importance of children's health for the nation's future, it is traditionally the most junior Minister of Health who is given responsibility for children.

To address the difficulties of fragmentation and lack of advocates, the Health Committee (1997) recommended the setting up of a subcommittee of cabinet for children, similar to that for women. The governmental response at that time (DoH 1997) was: 'We have no plans to set up a Cabinet Sub-Committee on Children and Young People'. This was in contrast to Scotland and Wales where, following the 1997 general election, a minister with specific responsibility for children was appointed. To date it would seem that the Commissioner for Children in Wales appears to be making a real difference and the appointment of a Minister for Children in England is welcomed. The Children's Bill (to be published late 2004) contains a requirement for an independent champion for children in the form of a Children's Commissioner. However, the English Commissioner appears less independent than the Welsh counterpart. It is an unfortunate fact that many long-recommended changes in services for children have been ignored until a tragedy occurs.

Emotion and rhetoric are commonly applied to issues concerning children, with the media keen to utilise a 'good' child story or picture. Politicians are commonly seen kissing babies at election rallies but it is rare for any political manifesto to actually refer to children. Despite politicians seeking these positive emotive opportunities it has taken significant tragedies to motivate the Government to react to the need for improved and integrated services for children (see Chapters 3, 5 and 22). CCNs must remain vigilant as, despite the Government's commitment to address the needs of children's services, the situation remains that many of the health professionals, including nurses, providing care for children have not undertaken any specific education programme in the needs of sick children.

In recognising the need for vigilance it is valuable to review the current political structure for children's services in England and recognise the positive opportunities that this offers. The NHS plan published in 2000 sets out a radical programme of reform for the NHS and Social Services (DoH 2000). The children's Taskforce is one of the ten taskforces established to turn that plan into a reality and the Taskforce is chaired by the National Clinical Director for Children (DoH 2002a). Taskforce members include front-line staff and those involved in planning and developing children's services across health and social care. The Taskforce aims to deliver real improvements for children's services and a major programme of work that oversees this is the National Service Framework (NSF). The NSF is developing new national standards to ensure better access and smoother progression in the provision of services for children (see Chapter 3). Whilst this is encouraging it is important to note that in the response to the Kennedy Report the Secretary of State promised mandatory standards within the NSF (DoH 2002b). However, that promise was then withdrawn.

There is a mechanism for auditing quality that nurses must familiarise themselves with if their voice is to be heard. In April 2002 ministers in England announced that quality measurement would be upheld by two parallel working bodies. The Commission for Social Care Inspectorate and the Commission for Health Audit and Inspections hold the remit to improve the quality of health and social care. One strategy for achieving this would be to measure compliance with NSF standards (DoH 2003a). The other three countries in the UK are observing the developments in England as they devise their own auditing and quality-measuring strategies. The anticipated Children's Bill includes plans for an integrated inspections framework across health, education and social services.

Other elements of the work of the Taskforce include continuing work on the 'quality protects' initiative. 'Quality protects' is a key part of the Government's wider strategy for tackling social exclusion and working with disadvantaged and vulnerable children. It is important to note that the DoH have produced an action plan to increase the involvement and participation of children and young people in developing children's services (DoH 2002c). The National Clinical Director for children actively encourages professionals, carers and children to contribute their voice and this openness must be reciprocated. A further significant development for children's services is that all Trusts must now have a named individual taking responsibility for children's services. However this individual is not required to have a children's services background and in practice therefore will often have a limited knowledge of the needs of children and their families.

It has been recognised that services need to be child-focused and coordinated across social services, health, education, housing and other agencies at a local level. A 'children at risk' review took place in 2002 and recommended piloting a new children's Trust model for integrated services (DoH 2003b). These models aim to create a service model that recognises and facilitates the complex multi-agency work needed to provide services for children. CCNs must be influential in this process. Despite encouraging developments children's nurses must not become complacent but persist in influencing policies, and driving the Government agenda, that genuinely benefit children and their families (see Chapter 3).

Following the Allitt enquiry (DoH 1994) the Government reinstated an earlier guidance which stated that there should be at least two qualified children's nurses on duty 24 hours a day in all hospital children's departments and wards. Unfortunately such directives are not mandatory and many of the health professionals, including nurses, providing care for children have not undertaken any specific education programmes in the needs of children. Furthermore, no such directive applies to the care of sick children in the community, despite being a recommendation following the review of children's services by the House of Commons Health Committee (1997). As a consequence there has been a lack of understanding and commitment by commissioning and purchasing authorities to meet the needs of sick children and their families in the community in some areas.

SPECIFIC DIFFICULTIES FOR COMMUNITY CHILDREN'S NURSES

Community children's nursing services have met additional obstacles in their attempts to influence policy. The historical context has been outlined in the opening chapters of this book. Health visitors and school nurses have had strong advocates for their services within professional organisations whereas CCNs have not (see Chapter 10).

Parents and children's healthcare staff have been keen to adapt the pattern of care to meet children's psychological and changing clinical needs and to develop community children's nursing services. Staff in community services for children, traditionally focused on maintaining health, have resisted these developments. Indeed, this was reflected in the research commissioned by the English National Board (Procter et al 1998). The study included interviews with managers of services, parents, nurses and other medical professionals. Whilst there was recognition of the skills of the

CCN there was no clarity on where they might fit into a Primary Care setting.

As the Health Committee (1997 para 160 p xlviii) in its third report, 'Health services for children and young people in the community: home and school' was able to conclude:

> 'Children's health services at present are too often based on traditional custom and practice or indeed on professional self-interest. Children's health services must be needs led, not based on historical patterns or the self-interest of provider groups.'

CCNs have lacked a power base within professional organisations as they have not enjoyed any significant strategic service planning, particularly within the existing and varying structure of community services. Consequently appropriate educational preparation, or the lack of it, has been a major difficulty. The community children's nursing strand of the community specialist practitioner programme has not been wholly endorsed and supported by workforce planners who are unable to recognise the role (see Chapters 8 and 9).

In summary, CCNs have encountered difficulties in influencing healthcare policy for children because:

- Children are not politically powerful.
- Children's nurses in general, but specifically CCNs, have lacked a power base, corporate identity and strategic direction within the nursing profession (see Chapter 10).
- Nurses working in the community and health visitors, for reasons unrelated to improving services for sick children, have historically not welcomed the development of community children's nursing services.
- Despite repeated Government recommendations that community children's nursing services should be universally established, no strategy has been formulated, no specific model advocated, little research undertaken, limited finances allocated, only limited governmental initiatives undertaken and no directives regarding the implementation of guidance issued.
- Community children's nursing teams are often small in number with management of the service being the responsibility of those with no practical experience in the field.
- As community children's nursing services have evolved there has been no definitive structural guidance for the profession and teams have developed on an ad-hoc basis (Eaton 1998).
- Specific education for CCNs has only been available since 1996. Furthermore, this only became available as a result of persistent lobbying of the English National Board for Nursing and Midwifery and the United Kingdom Central Council (UKCC) by the emerging body of CCNs supported by the Community Children's Nursing Forum within the RCN.

It is therefore hardly surprising that some 40 years since the Government recommended the rapid expansion of community children's nursing services (Ministry of Health 1959) there is still in excess of 20% of UK regions without a service (RCN 2004). As the Health Committee

(House of Commons 1997a para 49 p xix) concluded: 'For many years there has been such a service for adults, sick children need and deserve no less'.

CHANGING TIMES

John F Kennedy reminded us that 'change is the law of life. And those who look only to the past or present are certain to miss the future'. Change is often painful and for CCNs seems exceedingly slow. However, change is central to the present Government's activities. The Labour Government, elected in 1997, has introduced a mass of legislation affecting healthcare, and if only they recognise and utilise them, nurses have many opportunities to influence these changes. The Government's white paper for England 'The new NHS. Modern, dependable' (NHS Executive 1998a), and similar documents in the other three countries of the UK, provides a clear impetus for nurses in clinical practice to influence new patterns of organising, providing and evaluating care. A central vision is the direct link between increasing the participation of NHS staff in decision making in relation to the implementation of policy. The Children's Taskforce and the external working groups of the NSF are working examples of this vision. The Government's commitment to collaboration across all services, and the desire to crush the existing bunker mentality ever present among health and social care professionals that creates tensions and threatens innovation, are key objectives for the NSF working groups (Williams & Sibbald 1999). However this change from hierarchy to shared governance is radical and nurses will need assistance to become informed and active participants.

The term 'shared governance' means different things to different people. Professional organisations have provided guidance for their members (RCN 1998). It aims to increase the formal participation of nurses in the decision-making process. The evaluation of shared governance within healthcare, particularly in the UK, is limited at present.

Whilst the Government is currently proclaiming increased power to localities, a tight central control is maintained. The power of the medical profession remains clear but the tide is turning with the introduction of nurse prescribing in 1999 and subsequent developments with the extended nurse-prescribing programme for Nurse Practitioners and Consultant Nurses in 2002 (DoH 1999a). The reference in the white paper 'Making a Difference' to a career pathway for nurses wishing to stay in the clinical field is being recognised through the introduction of Nurse Consultant posts (DoH 1999b). Examples include three such posts within community children's nursing. Evaluation of these posts may indicate their scope for political influence within the community children's nursing profession.

The regulation of healthcare professions has never been debated so publicly. The public inquiry into the deaths of infants following cardiac surgery at Bristol Royal Infirmary (Learning from Bristol 2001) will potentially mark a watershed for the accountability of healthcare professionals and general managers. The establishment of a National Institute of Clinical Excellence in England, the work of the Clinical Resource and Audit Group and development of clinical guidelines through the Scottish

Intercollegiate Guidelines Network in Scotland, will enable national standards to be formulated and audited. Nurses, particularly CCNs, must be ready for these changes and identify and embrace the opportunities that will arise.

HOW CAN COMMUNITY CHILDREN'S NURSES INFLUENCE HEALTHCARE POLICY?

Having acknowledged a professional responsibility to influence change, the opportunities to do so must be identified and utilised. Whilst different governments will introduce a range of changes, which will vary in the four countries within the UK, the mechanisms and opportunities for CCNs will continue to be available.

Developing a broad vision

Finding time to develop a vision can be very rewarding and represents a real basis for developing a strategy to take community children's nursing forward. CCNs should remember that vision, leadership and influencing skills are not the prerogative of those who hold senior positions. Every individual CCN has a responsibility for such a role.

Reflective practice is 'politically correct' terminology and obviously important to professional development, but developing a vision requires some lateral thinking from a range of perspectives. Many community children's nursing services have developed from a handful of very committed nurses who have worked extremely hard, in isolated circumstances, to develop services with little opportunity to reflect on wider health issues. This can result in a somewhat narrow understanding of children's changing health needs and the services needed to meet them. CCNs, indeed all nurses, must develop a broad vision if they are to provide holistic, good-quality and cost-effective standards for their patients/clients. Associated skills such as profiling the community and assessing need in conjunction with available resources are addressed in Chapter 18.

Community children's nursing, whilst expressing concern at the fragmentation of care received by children and families, has not always been proactive in working with others. The Government has made its position clear on the need for multidisciplinary and multi-agency working (NHS Executive 1998b). CCNs need to be familiar with relevant publications and incorporate them into their vision of community children's nursing services and adapt their practice accordingly.

Box 4.1 Developing a vision

- Have you ever made time to consider your vision for community children's nursing?
- What aspects of your role excite you?
- Where are the gaps in service? What frustrates you? How could the difficulties be resolved?
- Have you/your team members critically analysed the difficulties/ formulated an action plan for resolving them?
- Is poor communication at the root of many of the frustrations?

Know the facts

To influence policy it is crucial to be familiar with the facts relevant to the specific aspect of the policy you wish to influence. These should be produced in a clear, concise document that details the advantages and disadvantages of your proposal over the present situation. Cost-effectiveness, efficiency, equitable provision, consumer preference and accessibility must be considered carefully. CCNs are often in the situation of attempting to influence those who have little insight into the specific needs of children and their families and of the role of the CCN.

It is helpful if the main arguments are documented in a summary with particular attention paid to the business plan (see Chapter 18). Knowing the facts must not be confined to a narrow professional perspective. CCNs must acquaint themselves with wider issues such as organisational change and identify who holds the power both directly and indirectly:

- Does your proposal fit the political or local health agenda?
- Has your manager been asked or asked you to comment on a consultation document?
- Is change, maybe a reconfiguration of services, being considered?
- Is increased consumer choice evident?
- Does an influential person (e.g. chair of the Trust or local MP, or a group such as Patient Advice and Liaison Service (one of several organisations committed to public involvement), or the Trust's lead for children's services) have a particular interest?

If your business proposal is controversial careful preparation before presenting to management will pay dividends. Presentation of papers and posters at professional conferences and articles in professional journals to disseminate examples of good practice and information will reinforce your arguments. This exercise can assist in refining your proposals. Seek appropriate opportunities to present your case. If not successful the first time, don't give up. Reflect on the event, seek assistance in analysing what happened and why you were not successful, then prepare for another attempt. The 'drip, drip' effect applied in a variety of ways can, in the long term, be very effective.

Use the facts

Acquiring the facts is essential but of little use if not used to improve services for children. There are many formal and informal mechanisms and opportunities available to CCNs, some very familiar, others such as the parliamentary processes less so.

The parliamentary process

Whilst the local MP's surgery should be familiar to all nurses, mechanisms such as Early Day motions or the facility to have questions asked in the House may not be. RCN parliamentary officers are keen to assist members in familiarising themselves with the opportunities available.

The 'All Parliamentary Select Committee on Health' is an important mechanism, which nurses have been slow to use. Select committees, set up in 1979 to shadow the work of each Government department, undertake inquiries into specific issues, utilising written evidence submitted by interested individuals and groups. The committee then invites a small number of individuals and groups to give oral evidence before the whole committee.

The Health Select Committee's first inquiry into Services for Children and Young People was undertaken in 1996, and published reports in 1997 (House of Commons 1997a, 1997b). The RCN's Community Children's Nursing Forum utilised the opportunity by submitting written evidence and being invited to give oral evidence. The Third Report 'Health services for children and young people: home and school' (Health Committee 1997) is a rich source of information for all CCNs as well as providing an excellent example of how practising CCNs can influence national healthcare policy. The NSF has provided further opportunities.

Responding to topical issues

Topical issues may not present in a clear way and CCNs, who do not have a strong power base, need to be particularly vigilant and imaginative to identify and utilise opportunities. For example, the Government's invitation to submit proposals to commemorate the life of Diana, Princess of Wales, was not an obvious opportunity for CCNs to raise the profile of the children and their families who would benefit from a community children's nursing service. CCNs used the House of Commons Select Committee on Health's shock at the paucity of community children's nursing services and the NHS Executive Report 'Evaluation of the pilot project programme for children with life threatening illnesses' (NHS Executive 1998c) to support the RCN's formal proposal that community children's nursing services would be a fitting tribute to Diana, Princess of Wales. This 'topical issue' enabled the RCN to inform and influence both the decision makers and the general public of the importance of providing community children's nursing services.

Responding to consultation documents and inquiries

Responding to consultation documents is a proven way of influencing policy, whether at local or national level. The RCN Community Children's Nursing Forum was shocked that the UKCC consultation document on the future education and practice of community nursing (UKCC 1993) made no reference whatsoever to services for children who required nursing care in the community. The large working group responsible for its preparation did not include a registered children's nurse. The Forum's strong response to the consultation paper, and the publicity achieved, resulted in the definitive document acknowledging community children's nursing as one of eight distinct specialities of community nursing and open only to registered children's nurses (UKCC 1994).

Some opportunities to influence policy are not so clear. For example, the Royal Commission on 'long-term care' (Sutherland 1999) has been interpreted by many as concerning only the elderly. Unfortunately, although the Commission planned to include a range of client groups, it had time to report only on services for the elderly. However, the opportunity to submit written evidence regarding children was utilised and thus raised the specific difficulties for children. Clinical advances have resulted in an increasing number of children with complex clinical needs reaching adolescence and adulthood. Agreed criteria for continuing care for children are rare and there is considerable evidence that many families receive little assistance, particularly in areas without a community children's nursing service (see Chapter 22). The RCN Community Children's Nursing

Forum therefore set up a joint working party with the RCN Children with Disabilities Group to focus on specific issues of concern, and submitted evidence to the Royal Commission. In addition to collaborating with fellow professionals it is important that CCNs recognise the benefits of working closely with all parties involved in children's services and initiating and accepting invitations to participate with these groups at local and national levels.

Collaborative working   Whilst Florence Nightingale achieved considerable influence on healthcare policy as an individual, we live in a very different world. Working collaboratively in the interests of a common aim, to achieve more equal, effective and efficient services for children and their families, is the way forward. That aim must be discussed overtly and understood before joint working is attempted. Collaborative working has been common rhetoric for some years and in 1998 working in partnership became politically correct (NHS Executive 1998b). The reality is that, since the establishment of the NHS until the present time, there has been little evidence of working across professional boundaries. Change may not be easy, but is essential if services are to be improved. This will be recognised in the education of health and social care professionals with the greater and shared emphasis on the need for inter-professional education. The vision is to 'ensure professions learn from and about each other to improve collaboration and quality of care' (Centre for Advancement of Inter-professional Education 1997 bulletin no.13).

Support for community children's nursing from paediatricians, paediatric surgeons, paediatric sections of the organisations representing the professions allied to medicine, and particularly from consumer groups has exerted increasing influence on healthcare policy and will continue to do so. Much of the evidence submitted to the House of Commons Select Committee relating to CCNs and the difficulties encountered by families when a community children's nursing service was not available was provided by consumer organisations. This formal and unsolicited support from so many organisations surprised the RCN's Community Children's Nursing Forum and led to it working with organisations such as Action for Sick Children, Contact a Family and Barnardo's.

It is clear that community children's nursing services need to identify where their allies are, both nationally and locally. Local organisations are particularly important because they vary considerably between localities and usually have excellent local networks, which may be very supportive to families and community children's nursing services.

The Diana Community Children's Nursing Teams focus on working together, whether that be within health services or between health, social services, education and the voluntary sector (NHS Executive 1998d). This philosophy is clearly reflected in the Resource Pack entitled 'Sharing the Care' (English National Board & DoH 1999). Having defined funding, these teams are able to cut across the traditional boundaries that prevent continuity and cost-effective, efficient care, which cause so much frustration not only to the children and their families but also to staff and volunteers. This provides a model for the future and, once again, CCNs will have been at the forefront of breaking down unhelpful traditional boundaries and changing practice in order to enhance the care of sick children and their families.

CONCLUSION

Children's lack of political power coupled with the small number of CCNs and their lack of power have added to the difficulties in influencing policies. Nurses are slowly acknowledging their responsibility to influence healthcare policy, becoming familiar with the mechanisms available and more confident and competent in their actions concerning healthcare policy. CCNs have achieved much, particularly considering their small number and the many obstacles experienced. There remains much to achieve, but change is evident.

The Government's choice of community children's nursing teams, led by registered children's nurses with a community qualification, is a fitting tribute to the life of Diana, Princess of Wales and marked a watershed in the development of community children's nursing. It also provides CCNs with opportunities to influence healthcare policy.

CCNs must look beyond the immediate frustrations of day-to-day clinical practice and resolve, both as individuals and as members of a small group of nurses, to become actively involved in shaping healthcare policy at local, national and international level, to ensure that tomorrow's children and their families will have the benefit of a universally accessible community children's nursing service wherever they live. As Clay (1987) reminded us: 'participation in the political life of the country is the alternative for individual nurses to the silent frustration of the past or industrial action'.

REFERENCES

Antrobus S 1998 Political leadership in nursing. Nursing Management 5(4):26–28

Antrobus S 2003 What is political leadership? Nursing Standard 17:43

Antrobus S & Kitson A 1999 Nursing leadership: influencing and shaping health policy and nursing practice. Journal of Advanced Nursing. 29(3):746–753

Briggs A 1972 Report on the Committee on Nurse Education. HMSO, London

Centre for Advancement of Interprofessional Education (CAIPE) 1997 Principles of inter-professional education: A definition. CAIPE bulletin no. 13. CAIPE, London

Clay T 1987 Nurses, power and politics. Heinemann, London

Cunningham G & Kitson A 2000 An evaluation of the RCN's clinical leadership development programme – Part 1. Nursing Standard 15(12):34–37

Department of Health 1994 The Clothier Report. HMSO, London

Department of Health 1997 Government response to the Reports of the Health Committee on Health Services for Children and Young People, Session 1996–97: 'The specific health needs of children and young people' (307-I); 'Health services for children & young people in the community, home and school' (314-I); 'Hospital services for children & young people' (128-I); 'Child and adolescent mental health services' (128-I). The Stationery Office, London

Department of Health 1999a Review of prescribing, supply and administration of medicines. Final report. The Stationery Office, London

Department of Health 1999b Making a Difference. The Stationery Office, London

Department of Heath 2000 The NHS Plan: A Plan for Investment – Plan for Reform. The Stationery Office, London

Department of Health 2002a Children's Taskforce: An introduction to the 3rd edition. Online. Available: www.dh.gov.uk 14 September 2004

Department of Health 2002b Learning from Bristol; The DoH response to the report of the public inquiry into children's heart surgery at the Bristol Royal Infirmary Online. Available: www.dh.gov.uk/bristolinquiryresponse.htm March 2004

Department of Health 2002c Listening, hearing and responding. DoH action plan: Core principles for the involvement of children and young people. Online. Available: www.dh.gov.uk/scg/actionplaninvolveyoung2002.htm March 2004

Department of Health 2003a Emerging findings: Getting the right start: The NSF for children, young people and maternity services. The Stationery Office, London

Department of Health 2003b Children's Trust Guide. Online. Available: www.dh.gov.uk/childrenstrust/index.htm March 2004

Eaton N 1998 Community children's nursing; An evaluative framework. Journal of Child Health Care 2(4):170–173

English National Board for Nursing Midwifery and Health Visiting (ENB) & Department of Health 1999 Sharing the Care. Resource pack for Diana, community children's nursing teams. ENB, London

Glasper EA & Charles-Edwards I 2002 The child first and always: the registered children's nurse over 150 years. Part two. Paediatric Nursing 14(5):38–43

Health Committee 1997 Third report. Health services for children and young people in the community: home and school. House of Commons session 1996–97, minutes of evidence and appendices. The Stationery Office, London

House of Commons 1997a Health Select Committee. Session 1996–1997. Second report. The specific health needs of children. The Stationery Office, London

House of Commons 1997b Health Select Committee. Session 1996–1997. Children's health. Minutes of evidence vol II, and appendices vol III. The Stationery Office, London

House of Commons 1998 Debate on children's health, 25 March 1998, Hansard. The Stationery Office, London

International Council of Nurses (ICN) 1985 Policy statement. Nurses' involvement in health care policy. ICN, Geneva

Learning from Bristol 2001 The report of the public inquiry into children's heart surgery at the Bristol Royal Infirmary 1984–1995. The Stationery Office, London

Ministry of Health 1959 The welfare of children in hospital. HMSO, London

National Health Service Executive 1998a The new NHS. Modern, dependable. Department of Health, London

National Health Service Executive 1998b Partnership in action (new opportunities for joint working between health and social services). Department of Health, London

National Health Service Executive 1998c Evaluation of the pilot project programme for children with life threatening illnesses. Department of Health, London

National Health Service Executive 1998d Diana children's community nursing teams. Department of Health, London

Nursing and Midwifery Council (NMC) 2002 Code of Professional Conduct. NMC, London

Procter S, Biott C, Campbell S, Edward S, Redpath N & Moran M 1998 Preparation for the developing role of community children's nurse. English National Board for Nursing, Midwifery and Health Visiting, London

Royal College of Nursing (RCN) 1916 Royal College of Nursing Charter. RCN, London

Royal College of Nursing (RCN) 1998 Guidance for nurses on clinical governance. RCN, London

Royal College of Nursing (RCN) 2004. 16th edn. Directory of Community Children's Nursing Services. RCN, London

Sutherland S 1999 With respect to old age: long term care, rights & responsibilities. The Stationery Office, London

UK Central Council for Nursing, Midwifery and Health Visiting (UKCC) 1993 Consultation on the Council's proposed standards for post-registration education. UKCC, London

UK Central Council for Nursing, Midwifery and Health Visiting (UKCC) 1994 Future education and practice of community nursing. UKCC, London

Williams A & Sibbald B 1999 Changing roles and identities in primary health care: exploring a culture of uncertainty. Journal of Advanced Nursing 29(3):737–745

Woolnough H & Faugier J 2002 An evaluative study assessing the impact of Leading Empowered Organisations Programme. Nursing Times Research 7(6):412–427

Chapter 5

Improved integration within public and community health

Lynn Young, Anna Sidey and David Widdas

KEY ISSUES

- The developing health agenda for integrated services.
- Integrated nursing teams.
- The development and function of Primary Care Trusts.
- Opportunities for Community Children's Nurses.
- Health Action Zones, Healthy Living Centres and Sure Start.

INTRODUCTION

Since 1998 nurses have experienced a whirlwind of reorganisation, the rapid development of new structures, numerous projects, pilots and initiatives and a move towards working within a very different culture. The explosion of ideas, aspirations and re-juggling of traditional hierarchies have collectively caused turbulence to be the norm. Change is now expected and has become constant and commonplace. Government continues in its determination to transform the public sector through major modernisation programmes in the hope that all parts of it, for example health, transport and education work together and become 'fit for purpose' in the twenty-first century.

THE DEVELOPING HEALTH AGENDA FOR INTEGRATED SERVICES

The health agenda is clear. Bold and expensive efforts are being made in order to reduce health inequalities, improve healthcare services and the public health and diminish social exclusion. Nurses, particularly those who work in the community, are at the forefront of this formidable public health movement, much of which is focused on improving the health of children (DoH 1999a). The belief that healthy children have a good chance of growing into healthy adults leads to the assertion that healthy adults are more likely to contribute to the nation's economy as they tend to earn regular incomes, pay tax and rear self-sufficient healthy families. It therefore makes economic, as well as moral sense, to focus attention and valuable resources on children.

Nurses have their own professional responsibilities in terms of influencing policy development and challenging practice. These are essential if nurses are to adapt in a positive way to the changing environment, make their full contribution to the improvement of children's health and effectively manage the evolving workforce.

Government strategy is aimed at promoting the regeneration of self-reliant and cohesive communities. The Government's radical and new policies, the English health reforms described in the white paper 'The new NHS. Modern, dependable (DoH 1997a) and the equivalent papers for Scotland, Wales and Northern Ireland (DoH 1997b, 1997c, 1999a) are of particular interest to the nursing profession. A tidal wave of Government initiatives, aimed at developing improved integrated services, has flooded the NHS and the community at large. These include 'Making a Difference: strengthening the nursing, midwifery and health visiting contribution to health and healthcare' and 'Saving Lives: our healthier nation' (DoH 1999b, 1999c). The themes underpinning 'Making a Difference' are:

- nurses, midwives and health visitors at the heart of the NHS modernisation agenda
- the challenges facing the nursing and midwifery professions
- a strategic direction for nurses, midwives and health visitors
- strengthening and modernising the contribution of nurses toward improved public health and health services.

Current health and social reform is forcing greater integration between health, social services, education and the independent sector. The sheer size of the nursing workforce and the fact that it functions in all settings means that nurses are well placed to take the lead in improving the integration of services. It is also significant that for some years many nurses have worked hard to improve integration with their colleagues and other professional groups and disciplines. The catalyst to strive for improved integration is the growing awareness that there has, in the past, been an inability of care agencies and informal carers to work closely together. This has resulted in the focusing of attention on the needs of the service and its employees rather than those of the patients and their families. It is a salutary lesson to those who provide services that when a child dies or is harmed as a result of abuse, the subsequent public inquiry often reveals that far from being neglected by professionals a large number of different disciplines had been involved (Laming 2003). Following the tragic death of Victoria Climbie and the subsequent Laming Inquiry, the Department of Health (DoH) published guidance 'What to Do if You're Worried a Child is Being Abused' (DoH 2003). This was disseminated to every registered nurse with the aim of encouraging anyone who suspects child abuse to take the appropriate action at the earliest possible opportunity.

Members of the public when they need a range of different services may find themselves in what they perceive as the middle of confusion and chaos, different rules, exasperating funding systems, conflicting philosophies, unidentifiable budgets and a group of people, who, whilst maybe doing their best as individuals, fail to connect with one another. Progress on integrating services can be depressingly slow, but in a number of areas positive change is being achieved, for example the 'Sure Start' initiative (Department for Education and Employment 2001).

The Cumberlege Report described examples of inspirational community nursing services but also offered constructive recommendations on how practice and primary healthcare services could be improved (DoH and Social Security 1986). The Report called for the development of strong primary healthcare teams that would profile the needs of their populations and agree upon action plans aimed at improving health and health services. While the word 'integration' is not used in the report, over a decade later it is interesting to note that many of the recommendations, relevant to improving integration, are being implemented.

Present Government policies are a catalyst for further integration. Developing improved integrated services is high on the present health and social care agenda. Government is striving to build a system of integrated care, based on partnership, by removing false barriers and helping different organisations to work together in order to improve care for the public (DoH 1998a). The English discussion document 'Partnership in Action' (DoH 1998a) made proposals to improve the integration of health and social care services and therefore their performance. The Government white paper 'Modernising social services' (DoH 1998b) continued the drive to integrate services including education. 'Every Child Matters' moves this agenda forward again. It proposes closer integration between health, social services and education, improving joint working with health and raising the potential of social services, education and health into becoming one Children's Trust (Department for Education and Skills 2003, 2004).

It can be both difficult and challenging to achieve improved integration between carers and professionals and the organisations in which they work, but there is now reason to be optimistic. Current policies and initiatives, together with the commitment of those involved, have potential for improving the lives of the most vulnerable members of our communities. Community nurses have been listened to. Their particular efforts to integrate the different nursing disciplines and improve integration between the Primary Care Trust (PCT), general practice, health and social care and the acute and primary healthcare sectors, are impressive. Working in the community can be complicated and frustrating, especially when there is a failure to coordinate services. Nurses know that, once at home, people do not fit neatly into boxes for the convenience of services.

Integration is defined as the 'the harmonious combination of the different elements' (Oxford University Press 2002). The elements of the community are complex. The responsibility lies with service providers to distance themselves from social and professional tribalism and to concentrate more on what needs to be done and how problems can best be solved.

Long before the present Government's plans for the NHS, community nurses in a number of areas had been seeking ways to improve primary healthcare through the development of strong and robust integrated nursing teams. Following the restructuring of the NHS and social care services, nurses working in integrated teams are in a strong position to take the lead in implementing improved services within their locality. They are well placed to show others, such as General Practitioners (GPs) and social service personnel, the way forward in line with the Government's aspirations described in 'The new NHS' (DoH 1997a), the discussion document 'Partnership in Action' (DoH 1998a) and 'Every Child Matters' (Department for Education and Skills 2003, 2004).

INTEGRATED NURSING TEAMS

'Integrated nursing brings together the different skills, knowledge and expertise of a team of nurses so that priority needs can be met and a comprehensive service provided within a community' (Young & Poulton 1997). A number of nurses who have helped to develop integrated teams report that success can depend very much on the commitment shown by GPs and management. When this happens, extraordinary change can be achieved. One powerful key to change is the ability of nurses to shift their attention from caseload-specific activities and traditional titles to the health needs of the local population and ways in which the team can best promote health gain. The following principles can help guide nurses through the process of improving integration:

- The team's desire to improve the quality of care and treatment drives motivation.
- Stronger integration brings benefits to nurses in terms of improved job satisfaction and raised morale.

The Birtley Community Nursing Team in Newcastle comprises those who, among a large number of nurses, have successfully developed integrated teams and documented their experiences of providing services to the local population. One of their projects was to improve the child health clinic by tackling issues such as waiting times, the appointment system, the facilities and parental involvement and satisfaction. The child health clinic is now run by a GP, Health Visitor (HV), Nursery Nurse and two Practice Nurses, although the GP and HV times have now been reduced. The evaluation of this project has demonstrated that the desired outcomes appear to have been achieved by the team. They also developed a 'clinical supervision project' for child protection following dissatisfaction expressed by nurses with the existing system (Birtley Community Nursing Services 1998).

The NHS Executive document 'Evaluation of the pilot project programme for children with life threatening illnesses' offered much information on a 5-year series of pilot projects into the study of services for children with life-threatening illnesses. The Conservative Government started the programme in 1992 and an evaluation took place in 1997 (NHS Executive 1998). The main conclusions drawn following the evaluation are shown in Box 5.1.

> **Box 5.1** Care of children with life-threatening illnesses (NHS Executive 1998)
>
> - Each district should have a senior health service appointment to coordinate services for children with life threatening illnesses.
> - The role of key worker should be made explicit and be enhanced. The key worker should be the first point of contact and be responsible for coordinating services for the family (see Chapter 23).
> - Families need community children's nursing services and these nurses need to be team members in order for them to be supported and for workload and stress to be shared.
> - Respite care services and community children's nursing services should be well integrated and under one management structure (see Chapters 22 and 23).
> - Social care services should also be integrated with community children's nursing services.

THE DEVELOPMENT AND FUNCTION OF PRIMARY CARE TRUSTS

The UK is committed to a public health programme that diminishes health inequalities and social exclusion. There is a consensus that improved inter-agency and professional integration will make a valuable contribution to achieving the programme's aims. While considerable efforts are being made to achieve improved integration, the UK has developed four national health services. Political devolution has resulted in each country having its own white paper on health. 'The new NHS' (DoH 1997a) is the English paper, Scotland has 'Designed to care' (DoH 1997b), Wales has 'Putting patients first' (DoH 1997c) and Northern Ireland's paper is 'Fit for the future' (DoH 1999a). While the principles and intentions described in the four white papers are similar, they differ in language, organisational development and the position of nurses in the new commissioning structures.

PCTs are the new vehicle for health commissioning and are the bedrock of 'The new NHS'. They are as much about new behaviour as new structures. Different skills and expertise from those used within GP fundholding and the internal market are needed in order to achieve improved healthcare services. Developing a fully integrated health and social care service is first and foremost in the minds of PCT members regardless of their discipline. They work closely with local councils, social services and voluntary organisations to improve the health of children.

> **Box 5.2** Aims of Primary Care Trusts
>
> - Improved health/reduced health inequalities.
> - Improved primary healthcare/general practice.
> - Improved integration between health/social care services.
> - Improved services for the most vulnerable groups in the community.
> - Formulating local development plans.
> - Implementing clinical governance.
> - Commissioning a range of secondary care services.
> - Delivering primary care services.

OPPORTUNITIES FOR COMMUNITY CHILDREN'S NURSING

Community children's nurses (CCNs), with their knowledge and experience, have the opportunity to influence local health policy and help to design integrated services for children. They are able to do this through the work of the PCT professional executive committee, the PCT board, clinical governance groups and teams charged with implementing the National Service Framework (NSF) for children. CCNs are in a strong position to be involved in the strategic planning function of the PCT and the development of services. They can do this by:

- collecting, correlating and disseminating information which identifies the health needs of local children
- providing evidence of services currently available to children and identifying gaps in service provision
- comparing this information with national targets, anticipated healthcare needs of children and service quality/performance data
- proposing priorities for new children's services
- planning how to work with local people and their children and service providers in order to improve health and healthcare
- using this information to influence the local delivery plan.

Community nurses are now alongside their GP colleagues in the driving seat of the NHS. Their experience of developing integrated teams are an asset to the PCT boards and act as a catalyst for achieving improved integration across all sectors. Nurses once again demonstrate that the success of the health and social care systems depends, to a large extent, on them taking the lead in policy, management and organisational developments as well as direct patient care. Nurses have the ability to bring both clinical knowledge and the human experience to the PCT board. This will result in more effective service development and improved integration in line with Government aspirations.

HEALTH ACTION ZONES

'Health Action Zones are partnerships between the NHS, local authorities, community groups and the voluntary and business sectors to develop and implement a health strategy to deliver within their area measurable improvements in public health and in the outcomes and quality of treatment and care' (DoH 1998a).

Health Action Zones (HAZs) are concerned with developing an integrated approach to tackling certain problems that are adversely affecting a section of the population. The overall aim is for the health of the worst off in our communities to improve at a faster rate than that of the general population. Artificial barriers, which impede integration and therefore standards of care, are broken down. Action is taken to prevent ill health, improve health and reduce health inequalities. England has 26 HAZs.

CCNs working within an HAZ should be involved in all child health initiatives and work alongside other disciplines, such as HVs, Midwives, School Nurses and colleagues in education and social services. An example is the Beacon Community Regeneration Pilot in Penwerris, Cornwall which achieved remarkable success. Penwerris inspired other initiatives and achieved specific outcomes. They included:

- post-natal depression reduced by 70%
- child protection registrations reduced by 58%
- fear of crime reduced by 87%
- central heating and insulation to 900 homes
- violent crime reduced by 52%
- burglaries reduced by 34%
- vehicle crime reduced by 22%
- unemployment reduced by 69% (Barnes et al 2001).

HEALTHY LIVING CENTRES

During 1998 the Government announced that National Lottery money could be spent on health, along with other good causes. A total of £300 million was ring-fenced to fund a number of community projects throughout the UK that focused on helping people to improve their own health and wellbeing. As a result the Healthy Living Centre (HLC) initiatives developed. These are concerned with improving the quality of life for individuals by increasing independence and their ability to live with dignity.

HLCs benefit from the involvement of the community and the cooperation of all stakeholders, private and public, in order to have a positive impact on the health of individuals. Businesses, schools, local authorities, PCTs, general practices and the voluntary sector build on their existing relationships and, in partnership, develop an integrated approach to tackling health inequalities.

Of particular interest to CCNs is the Rock Trust HLC in Edinburgh that received a grant of £500 000 to help improve the health of young people. A partnership of seven agencies called 'Underground', committed to the health and welfare of young people, reaches out to them so they can make better use of available services. A self-contained flat has been transformed into a large space which provides a café, crèche, library facilities and a whole range of other services from a team of different disciplines including dietician, librarian, midwife, sexual health nurse, dentist, podiatrist and optician. There are opportunities to learn Samba drumming and benefit from a selection of complementary therapies, such as reiki, shiatsu and acupuncture.

CCNs working within an HAZ are likely to have an HLC as their work base rather than the traditional hospital or health centre. There are opportunities for CCNs to participate actively in the drive to further develop integrated services for children and their involvement will make a major contribution to achieving better health for all children.

SURE START

Sure Start is an example of how Nurses, Midwives and HVs working with social care and education have helped to transform the lives of disadvantaged parents and their children. Sure Start has developed since 1999 following the findings of the Treasury-led Comprehensive Spending Review on Services for Children Under Eight. The main aim of

Sure Start is to improve the life chances of young children in disadvantaged areas. It does this by providing new services where they are most needed but also by ensuring that, within each Sure Start locality, services that do exist are better coordinated.

The key objectives of Sure Start are to coordinate, streamline, add value, be flexible, responsive and involve parents as active participants instead of passive recipients. The Sure Start centres facilitate partnerships across the health economy (Department for Education and Employment 2001).

CONCLUSION

This chapter is an introduction to the wider picture of health and attempts to inspire and provoke CCNs to question their attitudes and approaches to working practices, the nursing profession and how well they integrate with other disciplines. The initiatives and developments referred to are examples of services where the strength of integration and partnership working is the key to bringing better health and higher quality of life to those people who suffer most from social deprivation. National priorities have been set, which include the modernisation of primary healthcare and improving services for children. CCNs are pivotal to the delivery of Government community health initiatives concerned with services for children. Ministers are determined to force different agencies to cooperate, in particular health, education and social care services. However, the principles of integration must underpin all care, whether the child is part of a Sure Start programme within an HAZ or receiving acute and highly technical care in the local intensive care unit.

REFERENCES

Barnes M, Sullivan H & Matka E 2001 Building capacity for collaboration: The national evaluation of Health Action Zones. University of Birmingham

Birtley Community Nursing Services 1998 Birtley community nursing services to people in and around Birtley. Portfolio of evidence. Birtley Community Nursing Services, Birtley

Department for Education and Employment (DfEE) 2001 Sure Start. A guide for 4th wave programmes. DfEE Publications, Nottingham

Department for Education and Skills 2003 Every Child Matters. The Stationery Office, London

Department for Education and Skills (DfES) 2004 Every Child Matters: next steps. DfES Publications, Nottingham

Department of Health 1997a The new NHS. Modern, dependable. The Stationery Office, London

Department of Health 1997b Designed to care. The Stationery Office, London

Department of Health 1997c Putting patients first. The Stationery Office, London

Department of Health 1998a Partnership in action. A discussion document. The Stationery Office, London

Department of Health 1998b Modernising social services. The Stationery Office, London

Department of Health 1999a Fit for the future. The Stationery Office, London

Department of Health 1999b Making a Difference: strengthening the nursing, midwifery and health visiting contribution to health and health care. The Stationery Office, London

Department of Health 1999c Saving Lives: Our Healthier Nation. The Stationery Office, London

Department of Health 2003 What to do if you are worried a child is being abused. The Stationery Office, London

Department of Health and Social Security 1986 Neighbourhood nursing – a focus for care. The Cumberlege Report. HMSO, London

Laming 2003 The Victoria Climbie Inquiry. The Stationery Office, London

National Health Service Executive 1998 Evaluation of the pilot project programme for children with life threatening illnesses. The Stationery Office, London

Oxford University Press (OUP) 2002 The Shorter Oxford English Dictionary. OUP, Oxford

Young L & Poulton B 1997 Integrated nursing teams can influence locality commissioning. Primary Health Care 7(10):8–10

Chapter 6

Working in partnership with the voluntary sector

Peter Kent

KEY ISSUES
- What is the voluntary sector?
- How the voluntary sector is funded and managed.
- Services available and how to assess their value.
- How to contact the voluntary sector.
- How to work alongside or in partnership with voluntary organisations.
- The future of the voluntary sector.

INTRODUCTION

Community children's nurses (CCNs), along with many other health professionals, will work with voluntary organisations from time to time. This may involve little more than obtaining information on behalf of a family but may equally extend to a close, formal working relationship where decisions are made collaboratively and responsibility is shared. To get the best from this relationship a sound understanding of the voluntary sector and how it is organised, managed and funded is required. This chapter provides an overview, rather than a comprehensive historical description of the voluntary sector in the UK and aims to give the reader sufficient understanding to enable good working relationships to be developed that will be of benefit to children and their families. The current relationship with the state, particularly the health service, will be considered, including the implications for joint working in the mixed economy of care. The chapter concludes with a brief consideration of what the future may hold for voluntary and statutory sector partnerships.

THE VOLUNTARY SECTOR

The voluntary sector is a term invented in the late 1970s (Harris & Rochester 2001) and although the sector is difficult to define it is, nevertheless, possible to provide a snapshot of the sector today that will enable effective working relationships to be developed. A voluntary organisation is essentially one that does not owe its existence to some statutory means. No law or Act of Parliament says it must exist; it exists because someone wants it to and has some objective they believe can be achieved by getting together with others and taking collective action. Charities, for example, are voluntary organisations, but not all voluntary organisations are charities. Not-for-profit organisations are often voluntary organisations as too are non-governmental organisations. However, not all will be charities, some will not be voluntary bodies at all and may be private organisations. The size and history of voluntary organisations is equally diverse. Some are national bodies with thousands of members, others comprise a small group of local people with a shared interest or need (Kendall & Knapp 1996). The Treasury in a cross-cutting review, The Role of the Voluntary & Community Sector in Service Delivery (HM Treasury 2002), estimated that 70% of voluntary organisations operate at local level and that there are approximately half a million voluntary and community groups in the UK. The National Council for Voluntary Organisations (NCVO) estimates that 140 000 general charities in the UK had a total income of £15.6 billion in 2000/01 (NCVO 2002).

STRUCTURE AND FUNDING OF VOLUNTARY ORGANISATIONS

Management of voluntary organisations varies. Small local organisations may be run entirely by a committee of volunteers and employ no paid staff. Large national bodies will have sophisticated management structures that reflect their status as multi-million-pound enterprises. Some organisations rely solely on volunteer staff. This has little to do with the size of the organisation. Small organisations are just as likely to have few volunteers as a large national body and some of the largest charities have vast numbers of volunteers, for example the St John's Ambulance Brigade or the Red Cross. The number deployed can have as much to do with the nature of the service provided, or the pool of people available as potential volunteers, as with the internal structure of the organisation.

Raising the funds to sustain a voluntary organisation can consume a good deal of time and effort. Much of the income will be from voluntary donations, donations made by the general public and others, from membership subscriptions or as a result of organised events. Organisations that have existed for some time will usually have investment income and income from legacies. The smaller, and newer, the organisation the more likely it will be to rely on voluntary income. The number of people involved in fundraising will depend on a number of factors, not least the size of the organisation. Staff in smaller organisations can find themselves spending considerable time fundraising, including having to raise their own salaries.

A major source of income is, of course, the state. In 2000/01 NCVO estimated that almost 30% of UK voluntary sector income came from Government and that in England alone state funding amounted to £3.7 billion with the NHS contributing 16.1% towards that total, local authorities 30.7% and central Government 53.2% (NCVO 2002). Traditionally funding for the voluntary sector came in the form of grants, either one-off payments or funding spread over a number of years. For organisations working in the field of health and social care, an important source of funding has been the DoH's Section 64 programme. This is a general 'power to fund' under section 64 of the Health Services and Public Health Act 1968 (DoH 1968) that enables the Secretary of State for Health to make grants to voluntary organisations in England and Wales whose activities support the DoH's policy objectives relating to health and personal social services. Not all organisations are eligible for such grants and there have always been more applicants than recipients. Section 64 project grants are awarded primarily for projects that have national significance and funding is provided for a maximum of 4 years. Core grants are made only to national organisations that can demonstrate their work fits in strategically with the DoH's objectives and funding is at a fixed cash level for 3 years. Nevertheless, many major national organisations do continue to receive renewals of core grants, which suggests in the final analysis that the decisions can have political considerations (Davis-Smith et al 1995, Palmer & Hoe 1997).

COMMISSIONING AND CONTRACTING

The most significant development in the relationship between the statutory and voluntary sectors in the past 20 years has been the move to contracting and purchasing of services based on a relationship differing very little from similar relationships in the private sector. The concept of purchasing or commissioning health and personal care services (the mixed economy of welfare) was initiated by the Thatcher Conservative Government, which wanted to introduce a contract culture to the welfare state and divided the health service into purchasers and providers (DoH 1989). The overall aim was to reduce the scale of governmental activity in the welfare state and change its role from direct provision of services to that of planning, monitoring and regulating services provided by other sectors.

The Labour Government elected in 1997 introduced a new structure based on Primary Care Groups (PCGs), rather than General Practitioner (GP) fundholders, and in local government replaced compulsory competitive tendering with the concept of best value, but has otherwise continued the general political direction of travel (DoH 1997). Namely, that the welfare state should no longer be the provider of first resort and there should be no automatic assumption that the NHS or Local Authorities (LAs) should provide the majority of healthcare and personal social services. A key shift, however, has been the manner in which resources are distributed. Health Authorities and their successors, the PCGs, have been replaced by Primary Care Trusts (PCTs) in England and by analogous primary care organisations in Scotland, Wales and Northern Ireland. PCTs are accountable to Strategic Health Authorities and are charged with developing an alternative means of improving the quality of care patients receive, described as 'partnership working'. Partnership working requires a wide range of care providers to be brought together including the private sector, social services and voluntary sector and PCTs are expected, through partnership working, to tackle health inequalities, the inverse care law, social exclusion and other health needs (Starey 2003).

LAs will provide fewer services directly and will be seen increasingly as commissioners on behalf of their communities. The Government believes the result will be a more competitive environment governed by measurable standards of value for money and quality of service enshrined in the commissioning criteria. The subsequent contracts and service agreements will also be subject to scrutiny, review and renewal. This should serve both to maintain competition and as a brake on health and social care spending, which the Government seeks to limit without explicit rationing of resources or services.

There have been two contradictory impacts on the voluntary sector. Firstly, the voluntary sector's role in welfare provision has expanded and instead of complementing, supplementing or providing an alternative to the state, voluntary organisations are increasingly taking responsibility for 'mainstream' services. Secondly, although the sector's status is enhanced, many organisations feel they are 'junior partners' in the relationship and that they compete as providers and contractors to sell services to government purchasers (Harris & Rochester 2001). However, despite the increasing emphasis on performance levels and quality of service in the contractual relationship, there are no national quality standards for the voluntary sector, and quality assurance can vary significantly (Levaggi 1996, George 1997).

WHAT VOLUNTARY ORGANISATIONS DO

In the health sector, voluntary organisations run hospices, ambulances, paramedic services, counselling services, childcare and services for the elderly, provide advice, support and information and employ nurses, physiotherapists, social workers and doctors. Generally speaking the services have sought to complement those of the health service. Grant-making trusts and other charities can make grants to individuals in need of equipment, financial hardship or respite care. Most take pride in their professionalism. An organisation that depends on volunteers can deliver a professional service just as well as an organisation employing predominantly salaried staff. The important distinction is the organisational culture and attention to procedures governing selection, training, supervision, confidentiality, monitoring and evaluation. Organisations may exist to provide a single service that meets a particular need, usually among a very specific group of people, while others may provide a wide range of services for broad categories. A number of organisations exist to meet the particular needs of specific minority ethnic, religious or cultural communities. Such organisations may have developed as a response to a need that is unique to that community or because services in the past have not been sufficiently responsive to minority community needs or because a service can be better provided by an organisation that has evolved from within a particular community. There are organisations that exist in one location only and others that are national bodies with local branches or groups enjoying varying degrees of autonomy. Before deciding whether to use an organisation's service it is important to assess its ability to deliver that service in a manner and context that meets appropriate standards of professional practice. This can be carried out in much the same way as assessing the suitability of services within the NHS before making a referral. The most important criterion is to establish that the people running the service or organisation do so in a manner that is broadly consistent with your own, your employer's and your professional body's views of good practice (Harvey & Philpott 1996). A good example is the independent national guidance for palliative care services (Association for Children with Life-threatening or Terminal Conditions and their Families & Royal College of Paediatrics and Child Health 2003).

CONTACTING THE VOLUNTARY SECTOR

Most areas will have a Local Council for Voluntary Service (LCVS), or similarly titled body, that both represents and supports local voluntary organisations. The NCVO will know the name and contact details of the LCVS in any particular area. The NCVO will also have information about national organisations that have local branches or regional offices and it publishes a directory of voluntary organisations (Voluntary Agencies Directory 2003). Organisations sharing a particular interest or operating in a particular service area often collaborate, forming umbrella groups. Larger umbrella groups also employ their own staff who can be an invaluable source of information and support. However, voluntary organisations, especially small community groups, will not always be aware of what is available from the health service or the relationship between health, social services and education, and CCNs can play a key role in coordinating services, encouraging dialogue and partnership working.

WORKING WITH THE VOLUNTARY SECTOR

Entering a partnership with a voluntary organisation is in principle much the same as conducting any other relationship. It requires confidence in the partner's ability, trust in their integrity and commitment and agreement to work together in a manner that is based on an explicit understanding of the rights and responsibilities of the partners. The economic, cultural and political environments in which the organisation exists need to be understood. The limitations that exist owing to finance or small numbers of trained staff must be recognised. Clearly, some forms of partnership working will be informal and may involve little more than superficial contact from time to time with, for example, an information service or helpline. Other partnerships will require the agreement reached to be confirmed in writing. This can help not only with the management of the relationship but also provides others with a clear picture of what was agreed and with whom responsibility for particular aspects of the partnership lies. CCNs can perform a valuable role linking the voluntary sector at local level with the health service.

The Commission for Patient and Public Involvement in Health (CPPIH), established in January 2003, has, among its five main functions, responsibility for recruitment and appointment of patients' forums. The role of the forums is to ensure local people have a direct say in the monitoring and development of services in their local NHS trusts, including the PCT. The CPPIH transition advisory board has recognised that many people find committees and formal structures off-putting and has recommended the forums develop new ways of working with individuals and community groups. With their combination of hands-on-experience, and experience and understanding of both children's needs and health service structures, CCNs may be ideally placed to assist voluntary organisations to participate in planning and developing services.

Many organisations will be very familiar with contracts or service agreements between purchasers and providers and both operate in and understand the mixed economy of care. They will deliver services according to clearly prescribed criteria and in a manner laid down by the commissioning authority. Their ability to move beyond the boundaries of their contract or agreement may, however, be limited. Their obligations to the purchaser need to be understood in case they compromise the partnership, and the nature of the service can change, or even terminate, if the purchaser negotiates new terms when the contract is reviewed. An informal partnership will be based largely on personal relationships, and requests for support or a service will be negotiated equally informally on a day-to-day or case-by-case basis. Where a contractual basis for the partnership exists, negotiations will be much more formal and may involve intermediaries, such as commissioning managers (Palmer & Hoe 1997).

The Government is reorganising children's services by combining health, education and social services into Children's Trusts (DoH 2003a). The Trusts will have pooled budgets and management structures and the Government aims to achieve fully integrated services for child protection, family support, services for looked after children, family placement and leaving care by the end of 2005. There is no set model for Trusts and the guidance issued to pilot trusts referred to some or all services for 0–19-year-olds provided by local education authorities, social services and health. Trusts, therefore, can cover as many, or as few, services as is considered appropriate locally. The Government has also created the position of a Minister for Children in the Department for Education and Skills. This will bring together services formerly spread across several Government departments. The Minister's responsibilities will include Sure Start, early years, childcare, Connexions, the Children and Young People's Unit, the Teenage Pregnancy Unit and the Family Policy Unit. The Minister will take over responsibility for children's services from the DoH but not for children's health services. The Government is also developing a National Service Framework (NSF) for children, young people and maternity services (DoH 2003b) (see Chapter 3). The voluntary sector's role in the external working groups has been advisory.

CASE STUDIES

Leicester parents of disabled children established a Parent and Carers Council in 1999 with the support of Contact a Family, a national umbrella organisation that encourages parent support groups at local, regional and national levels. The aim is to foster a greater understanding and sharing of experiences through first-hand knowledge of being carers of children with special needs. Volunteer parents give practical advice, assist with form filling or letter writing, provide support and act as advocates for families. The Council raises the needs of the family members with appropriate service providers, gathers information from parents and carers to highlight problems and distributes leaflets to organisations in the local area. The Leicester Council has 500 members and a further 400 on the mailing list. Another in Calderdale has 60 members and a further 40 on the mailing list. Both Councils received grants from the health service, social services and the education authority that enabled them to establish themselves. Calderdale has received funding from the Children's Fund to pay for a project worker and an administrator whilst Leicester has submitted a proposal to the Home Office for a coordinator.

Local health professionals, including the CCN, have found the council a key reference point and have been able to draw on the members' expertise to influence local decision-making and provide parents of newly diagnosed children with appropriate support.

FUTURE OF THE VOLUNTARY SECTOR

The Government has published two major reports in the early years of the new century that may have profound implications for the voluntary sector. The first, Private Action Public Benefit (The Strategy Unit Report 2002) reviewed the legal and regulatory framework within which charities and the not-for-profit sector conduct their activities. The report made a number of proposals for reform of charity law and status that would, the report argues, improve the range of legal forms enabling organisations to be more effective and entrepreneurial, develop greater accountability and transparency and ensure independent, fair and proportionate regulation. A charity would be redefined as an organisation that provides a public benefit that has one or more charitable purposes. A list of 12 charitable purposes is proposed that will clarify and modernise the definition of what is charitable. A new legal form for social enterprise would be introduced known as the Community Interest Company and a new form of incorporated body specifically for charities introduced, the Charitable Incorporated Organisation.

The second report was the Role of the Voluntary and Community Sector in Service Delivery: A Cross Cutting Review (HM Treasury 2002) which set a timetable for changes to be made in the relationship between voluntary sector service providers and statutory sector purchasers. It also announced the establishment of a new investment fund called 'future builders' that will provide a one-off 3-year investment of £125 million to assist voluntary and community organisations in their public service work. The implication for some is that, despite assurances from the Government that the sector will not have to sacrifice its independence or be forced into delivering public services, it may be left with little choice. However, given that the majority of charities currently carry out their work with little or no money from the state it would be premature to conclude that the contractual relationship will come to dominate the sector to the exclusion of all others. Nevertheless, organisations that are significant providers of services in the field of health and social care are increasingly likely to have major contractual relationships with commissioning authorities. They will also be in a competitive environment where they compete not just with other voluntary organisations but the public and private sectors too. It is argued too that without incentives to award contracts to medium-sized voluntary organisations with strong links to local communities there is a risk commissioners will prefer to contract with national charities with whom they have established relationships. The history and diversity of the voluntary sector, however, suggests that most organisations will adapt and many will prosper. As with most socio-economic changes, the organisations in the middle may experience the most severe squeeze. They may find themselves unable to compete effectively for contracts with major national organisations that can offer economies of scale and equally unable to fund their activities solely from donations and traditional fund-raising methods. Given that funding, for example from LAs, can be cut with little notice, organisations that depend heavily on a single contract are likely to be especially vulnerable.

CONCLUSION

The voluntary sector can justifiably be referred to as the third sector of the economy. It employs an estimated 500 000 people (full-time equivalents) and the 140 000 general charities in the UK had a total estimated income of £15.6 billion in 2000/01. Voluntary organisations are also significant providers of health and social care services. Indeed, it would be difficult to envisage the NHS without the thousands of voluntary organisations working alongside the statutory sector. To obtain the most appropriate care for children and their families, CCNs need to learn about the organisations working in their field and how their services are made available. They can be powerful agents for change, working collaboratively and playing a key role in developing new partnerships and services. Collaborative working can be a purely informal arrangement between nurse and colleague in a voluntary organisation, or may be based on the contractual arrangement between commissioning authority and voluntary organisation. In many cases there will be a mixture of arrangements, reflecting the mixed economy of care. If CCNs are to ensure that children receive the best possible service they need to understand this relationship, have an appreciation of the political and financial context within which it is set and some understanding of the changes that could take place as a consequence of government initiatives.

Good practice will be founded on understanding, trust and confidence in each other's ability to work together in the interests of the people that matter most: the children and those who care for them. The voluntary sector is already a major partner in the delivery of health and social care services. However, the relationship between the sector and the health service has changed significantly in the past decade and many voluntary organisations are now contracted to provide services and must negotiate with health and local authorities in much the same way as the private sector. Opportunities for partnership at local, regional and national level exist and are encouraged by central Government. Nevertheless, such opportunities require careful preparation and, like all relationships, take time to develop. Once established, however, partnerships can make a lasting contribution to the quality of life enjoyed by children.

REFERENCES

Association for Children with Life-threatening or Terminal Conditions and their Families (ACT) & The Royal College of Paediatrics and Child Health 2003 A Guide to the Development of Children's Palliative Care Services, ACT, Bristol

Davis-Smith J, Rochester C & Hedley R (eds) 1995 An Introduction to the Voluntary Sector. Routledge, London

Department of Health 1968 Health Services and Public Health Act. HMSO, London

Department of Health 1989 Working for patients. HMSO, London

Department of Health 1997 The new NHS. Modern, dependable. The Stationery Office, London

Department of Health 2003a Children's Trusts. Online. Available: www.dh.gov/help/publications.htm 13 January 2004

Department of Health 2003b Getting the right start: National Service Framework for Children. Emerging Findings. The Stationery Office, London

George M 1997 On the spot. Community Care 1202:23

Harris M & Rochester C 2001 Voluntary Organisations and Social Policy in Britain. Palgrave, Basingstoke

Harvey C & Philpott T (eds) 1996 Sweet Charity: The Role and Workings of Voluntary Organisations. Routledge, London

HM Treasury 2002 The Role of the Voluntary and Community Sector in Service Delivery: The Stationery Office, London

Kendall J & Knapp M 1996 The Voluntary Sector in the United Kingdom. Manchester University Press, Manchester

Levaggi R 1996 NHS contracts; an agency approach. Health Economics 5(4):342–352

National Council for Voluntary Organizations (NCVO) 2002 The UK Voluntary Almanac. NCVO, London

Palmer P & Hoe E (eds) 1997 Voluntary Matters: Management and Good Practice in the Voluntary Sector. Directory of Social Change, London

Starey N 2003 The Challenge for Primary Care. Radcliffe Press, Oxford

The Strategy Unit 2002 Private Action, Public Benefit: A Review of Charities and the Wider Not-For-Profit Sector. The Cabinet Office, London

Voluntary Agencies Directory 2003 National Council for Voluntary Organizations, London

Chapter 7

Working in partnership with education

Phillippa Russell

KEY ISSUES

- Current Government policy and new opportunities for partnership between community children's nursing and education services.
- The importance of early identification of special educational needs and the connections between social disadvantage and educational difficulties.
- Working with children, their families and schools: what community children's nursing services can contribute to the education of children with special healthcare needs or disabilities.
- Recognising the diversity of special healthcare needs which schools and families now endeavour to meet in the community (including the increase in children who are 'technologically dependent' with multiple complex healthcare needs).

INTRODUCTION

The House of Commons Health Committee's (1997) report on the specific health needs of children and young people set a new agenda for partnership between the NHS and education services. The Committee strongly endorsed the role of community children's nurses (CCNs) and envisaged a more diverse role within the education system than that of the current school nursing services (sections 13–15). The same committee also noted the changing pattern of disability and chronic medical conditions in children, with increasing numbers of children with complex needs requiring health-specific nursing advice or care in school settings.

The past few years have seen an unprecedented interest by central Government in improving standards in education. The key theme of 'excellence for all' acknowledges that schools and education authorities alone cannot make a difference to the life chances of children and young people. 'Emerging Findings' from the National Service Framework (NSF)

(DoH 2003) clearly identify partnership between different agencies as crucial to the improvement of children's life chances and essential in maximising social and educational inclusion for children with disabilities or special healthcare needs. Such cooperation can function at different levels but will, importantly, offer new opportunities to community nursing services to work in partnership with families and schools. A particular challenge will be the growing number of children with disabilities and associated healthcare needs attending mainstream settings. The need for advice and practical assistance around healthcare needs is a frequent barrier to disabled children's access to child care and after-school activities and a major concern for parents (Department for Education and Skills 2002a, 2002b). The Government's green paper 'Every Child Matters' (Department for Education and Skills 2003) also underlines the need to ensure better 'joined-up services' and multi-agency working to improve the life chances (and safety and wellbeing) of vulnerable children.

HEALTH INEQUALITY AND EDUCATIONAL AND SOCIAL DISADVANTAGE

The same years have seen growing concern about health inequality and social and educational disadvantage. H Graham (1999), in her keynote address to the Community Practitioners and Health Visitors Conference, noted that 'Inequalities in health occupy a central place in the history of health visiting and school nursing, with the professions established at the end of the nineteenth century as part of a wider public health strategy. At the end of the twentieth century health inequalities are again top of the public health agenda.'

Education is important for the future wellbeing of children and families and 'Our healthier nation' (DoH 1998) cites schools as a key health setting. Whilst health-related education is obviously a key factor, general educational attainment is also fundamental as it opens the door to making healthy choices and raising expectations. As Graham (1999) observed, there is a 'long shadow of disadvantage', which means that children born into poorer circumstances experience more material, psychological and educational risks. The National Child Development Study clearly demonstrates the cumulative consequences of disadvantage in terms of educational achievement as well as future socio-economic and health status in adult life (Davie et al 1999). The Government has established a Social Exclusion Unit to endeavour to address the root causes of social, educational and health inequality. However, solutions will be complex and will require partnerships at local level between a wide range of community services.

There is growing interest in early identification and intervention in terms of preventing subsequent educational failure. The Government's 'Sure Start Programme', launched in 1999 and now providing Sure Start programmes in 500 areas, targets resources at the most disadvantaged communities and provides evidence of the powerful and influential role for health visitors and community nurses working in partnership with education and social services. As the Acheson Report (1998) observes 'Education is a traditional route out of poverty for those living in disadvantage ... education can play an important role in reducing health inequalities by ensuring that children are equipped with the knowledge they need to achieve a healthy life'. Acheson (1998) envisages community health services and schools working in partnership to address healthy living and thereby improve educational achievement. Importantly, the report mirrors the key messages in the Sure Start Programme about involving parents (in particular mothers) in contributing to their children's wellbeing (Department for Education and Employment 2001). 'Wellbeing' is very relevant to educational achievement. The contribution of health visitors to young children's learning through home visiting programmes is validated by Robinson (1999) in a review of the research literature on the effectiveness of domiciliary health visiting. Russell (1999) reviewed the research literature on the connection between disability and disadvantage and the effectiveness of early intervention and home visiting programmes for parents. She drew similar conclusions about the positive role of community nurses such as Portage home visitors and parent educators and advisers in helping parents to be active partners in the care and education of children with disabilities or special educational needs. 'Together from the Start' (DoH & Department for Education and Skills 2003) highlights the importance of multi-agency working and introduces the 'Family Service Plan' to minimise bureaucracy and ensure clarity about the respective and mutually supportive roles of professionals in supporting individual children with disability and their families.

PARTNERSHIPS BETWEEN COMMUNITY NURSING SERVICES AND EDUCATION: WHAT KINDS OF ROLES?

The Special Educational Needs Code of Practice (Department for Education and Employment 1999) set the scene for a partnership approach to assessing special educational needs. Community nursing services can have an important role to play, not only in clearly identifying any special health needs that will directly affect a child's education, but in working to support parents in helping their own children and in listening to and supporting the children themselves. The involvement of children in assessment and decision making can be very challenging but it can also be positive. Russell (1998) in a review of policy and practice in involving disabled children in decision making notes the role of community nurses as 'health advocates' for disabled or sick children and the value of making children active partners in their care and education programmes.

The contribution of community children's nursing services to raising parents' expectations and contributing to their children's educational progress and overall development is illustrated by Townsley et al (2003). They note the potential of health visitors and other community nurses as parent advisers, providers of practical advice and assistance and key players in promoting high-quality integrated services for children with complex special needs.

The following two case studies illustrate the impact of a disability or special healthcare need upon children's education and personal growth and development. They also demonstrate the potential for community children's nursing services to contribute to assessment and problem solving in educational settings.

> **Case Study 7.1**
>
> Emily aged 13, has moderate learning disabilities, diabetes and epilepsy. She attends a mainstream school with additional support. Her mother has long-term mental health problems and difficulty with Emily's diet and insulin management. Emily has had two petit mal seizures because of failure to take her medication appropriately. Her small size and irritable behaviour, if her blood sugar levels rise, have made her a constant target for minor bullying and attendance at school is irregular. There is concern about her relationship with a fellow male pupil because of her immaturity and need for affection.

> **Case Study 7.2**
>
> Nabwl is 7. He has a rare degenerative condition and a gastrostomy and his mobility is decreasing. He is a lively child and anxious to continue to attend school with his friends. He has recently started to have episodes of incontinence that cause him acute embarrassment. His respite carers feel they can no longer offer him short-term breaks because of a lack of clarity about their legal liability for his care. They are also concerned about carrying out procedures they feel might lead them to being accused of child abuse because of an absence of local guidance on invasive care.

Emily and Nabwl have very individual special educational and healthcare needs. They also illustrate the challenges and the opportunities for community nursing services to support vulnerable children in education.

PRACTICAL HELP WITH MANAGING CHILDREN WITH MEDICAL CONDITIONS IN EDUCATIONAL SETTINGS

Emily's poor attention and her behaviour at school have improved significantly because:

- A CCN (Diabetes) has worked with her to give her greater responsibility and confidence in managing her diabetes.
- Liaison with the practice nurse at the family's health centre also ensured that Emily's mother was more vigilant about her daughter's diet and encouraged her to self-inject.
- The practice nurse has also introduced Emily's mother to a local support group for parents of children with special needs and put her in touch with the British Epilepsy Association. Both organisations have given her helpful written information, videos and practical advice. Emily's mother has admitted to feeling that epilepsy is stigmatising and hoping that the seizures were 'just febrile convulsions'. She now feels more confident through seeing other parents coping positively.
- Emily was fond of sweets and sometimes stole sweets and biscuits from her class. This behaviour resulted in much of the teasing, which in turn caused her to drop out of school. The school nurse was able to include diabetes in a 'health awareness' programme at the school and to encourage Emily's class to understand her frustration at the deprivation of sweets and to give her some support.

Emily's behaviour has improved. Liaison between the school and community children's nursing services has made the school's current Personal Health and Social Education programme more accessible to a child with a learning disability. Emily's relationship with her former 'boyfriend' is now as a 'friend' only and she is enjoying more social activities with her peer group at school. Most importantly, the CCN has worked with the school to enable greater confidence and ensure that Emily's diabetes, as well as her epilepsy, is acknowledged within her individual education plan and within her Statement of Special Educational Needs (SENs). Emily now has an individual Health Plan and feels more confident (and responsible) for her own health and her treatment. She has decided to join a British Diabetic Association young people's group to meet others who are also living with a medical condition and who, like her, sometimes have problems with diet and medication. The school has now introduced an anti-bullying policy and this includes explicit reference to children with disabilities or other special needs. It has also recognised the importance of acknowledging its new duties not to discriminate against disabled pupils (SENs and Disability Act 2001) and to develop an 'accessibility plan' to improve access and inclusion over time across the school. The SENs and Disability Act 2001 introduces a new Part 4 on disability duties in education. The definition of disability covers a range of medical conditions as well as specific disabilities.

Nabwl's disability and his need for a high level of personal and nursing care present particular challenges. Initially there was ambivalence in his special school about providing the level of technical support that he required because of issues of legal liability. Nabwl's mother was frequently requested to come into school to supervise his feeding and personal care. The pressures upon her were so heavy that she developed depression. A CCN resolved the difficulties by:

- working with the specialist community children's nursing team who supervised his care to agree a protocol for his personal care
- agreeing a 'whole-school policy' regarding invasive care procedures and specifying his needs within his Statement of SENs. The school and the community children's nursing service drew upon guidelines from recent research and development (Servian et al 1998, Lenehan & Carlin 2003) in developing agreements for all concerned
- providing training and support for his learning support assistant and in drafting her job description. The assistant has nursing experience and can in turn advise and support on the day-to-day management issues of other children with special care needs.

As a consequence:

- The Primary Care Trust has agreed that, because of Nabwl's special needs, the school will have regular support from a CCN who will work closely with teachers, parents and others to ensure that there is a carefully integrated programme.
- Because Nabwl's education and home care can be planned together, the difficulties with the 'short break' carers have been resolved and he

now spends two nights a week with his link family. He enjoys sharing their family life and his mother's health has improved because she has additional time to share with her other children. The integrated management approach also ensures that the right equipment is available at home, school and the respite carers.

Children with complex disabilities and their families are becoming more common in community services. The NSF Emerging Findings (DoH 2003) report that there is a marked increase in the numbers of children with complex multiple disabilities. The numbers of ventilator-dependent children have increased by 77% since 1997 (Barnardo's 2003). Most of these children live in a family home. Beresford (1998) notes that 70% of parents with a disabled child report problems with their housing and note the negative impact this has on their quality of life.

Commentators outline the challenges these children and their families present to services, whilst emphasising that good-quality community nursing support can enable them to participate actively in educational and other activities (Servian et al 1998, Townsley & Robinson 1999). The Social Services Inspectorate (1998) notes the impact on all services of the increasing number of children with complex disabilities and medical needs. This publication commends the role of nurses in training and supporting a range of carers in schools and community services and cites a training programme as a useful example.

CONCLUSION: THE NHS AND EDUCATION – MESSAGES FOR THE FUTURE

The debate about inequality and educational achievement highlights the growing importance of community nursing services working with parents and children in schools. Findings from the NSF Emerging Findings on Disabled Children (DoH 2003) acknowledge the importance of these services and their special role in supporting children with disabilities or health problems. The evidence about the value of early intervention creates a range of opportunities for health visitors and other community nurses in developing their skills in supporting and educating parents, and in ensuring that the growing number of children with complex disabilities and special needs are properly supported by community services. The special contribution of CCNs relates to their ability to:

- work directly with children and families in their local communities (which is of particular importance for 'hard to reach' families who seldom attend hospital or other appointments)
- develop good working relationships with other local professionals in health, education and social services, which facilitates partnership approaches when children and families have multiple needs
- offer a non-stigmatising and acceptable service
- provide practical advice and offer solutions to day-to-day problems (many schools in particular say that they often need advice on very practical difficulties relating to the care or management of a child, for which they would prefer a 'named person' in the locality).

'Together from the Start' (DoH & Department for Education and Skills 2003) highlights the importance of families having multi-agency 'Family Service Plans' and the creation of 'Key Workers' to coordinate services for children with more complex needs (see Chapters 22 and 23). CCNs, who frequently have long-term relationships with families, may also provide this role or at least support other professionals providing care coordination and support on an on-going basis for parents. A parent commented:

> 'When you have a disabled child, you collect a 'Noah's ark' of professionals. Your whole life is taken over. My life was saved by community nurses. They visited me at home. They enjoyed a good laugh (well, we would have cried if we hadn't laughed!). And they really helped John's teachers to understand why he was sometimes so difficult, how they could meet his care needs. It was such practical sensible help. It made us feel we had a future. You need a good friend if you have a disabled child.'

The green paper 'Every Child Matters' (Department for Education and Skills 2003) sees integrated teams of health and education professionals, social workers and others as essential to safeguarding vulnerable children and improving the life chances of all children and young people. The green paper envisages radical reforms in children's services that will 'sweep away legal, technical and cultural barriers to information sharing so that for the first time, there can be effective communication and partnership between everyone with a responsibility for children'. These proposed changes offer new opportunities (and challenges) for community nursing services. They offer real hope of better multi-agency working and 'joined-up services' to help children and families.

REFERENCES

Acheson D 1998 Independent inquiry into inequalities in health. The Stationery Office, London

Barnardo's 2003 Breathing Space. Community support for children on long term ventilation. Barnardo's, Essex

Beresford B 1998 Housing unfit for children: housing, disabled children and their families. The Policy Press and Joseph Rowntree Foundation, York

Davie R, Butler N & Goldstein H 1999 From birth to seven: a report of the National Child Development Study in association with the National Children's Bureau. Longmans, London

Department for Education and Employment 1999 The Special Educational Needs Code of Practice. The Stationery Office, London

Department for Education and Employment (DfEE) 2001 Sure Start. A guide for fourth wave programmes. DfEE, Nottingham

Department for Education and Skills 2002a Accessible Schools: planning to increase access to schools for disabled pupils. The Stationery Office, London

Department for Education and Skills 2002b Inclusive Schooling: Children with special educational needs. The Stationery Office, London

Department for Education and Skills 2003 Every Child Matters. The Stationery Office, London

Department of Health 1998 Our healthier nation. The Stationery Office, London

Department of Health 2003 The National Service Framework: Emerging findings from the External Working Group on Disabled Children. The Stationery Office, London

Department of Health and Department for Education and Skills 2003 Together from the Start: Guidance for professionals working with families with young disabled children birth to three. The Stationery Office, London

Graham H 1999 Inequalities in health: patterns, pathways and policy. Community Practitioner 72(2)

Health Committee 1997 The House of Commons Health Select Committee. Health services for children and young people in the community: home and school. Third Report. The Stationery Office, London

Lenehan C & Carlin J 2003 Handbook on Risk
Management. National Children's Bureau, London

Robinson J 1999 Domiciliary health visiting: a systematic
review. Community Practitioner 72(2)

Russell P 1998 Having a Say? Partnership in decision-
making with disabled children. National Children's
Bureau, London

Russell P 1999 Disability and inequality. Council for
Disabled Children, London

Servian R, Jones V & Lenehan C 1998 Towards a healthy
future: multi-agency working in the management of
invasive and life-saving procedures for children in
family based services. Norah Fry Research Centre,
Bristol

Social Services Inspectorate Council for Disabled
Children 1998 Disabled children: directions for their
future care. Social Services Inspectorate/Department
of Health Publications, London

The Special Educational Needs and Disability Act 2001
The Stationery Office, London

Townsley R & Robinson C 1999 What rights for disabled
children? Home enteral tube feeding in the
community. Children and Society 13(1):48–60

Townsley R, Abbot D & Watson W 2003 Making a
difference? Exploring the impact of multi-agency
working on disabled children with complex health
care needs, their families and the professionals who
support them. The Policy Press, York

Chapter 8

Educating community children's nurses: a historical perspective

Mark Whiting

KEY ISSUES

- As the locus of care for children moves from hospital to community, it is essential that registered children's nurses undergo appropriate preparation for their role in community care.
- The history of the education of community nurses dates back over 100 years.
- It is only in the recent past that the specific learning needs of registered children's nurses in the community have been recognised.

INTRODUCTION

During the late 1980s, a research study focused on the development of community children's nursing services in England (Whiting 1988). Findings included:

- concern amongst many Community Children's Nurses (CCNs) on the educational preparation for their role in caring for children in community settings
- support of the need for a specific community education for children's nurses
- anxiety at what was perceived to be an increasing tendency to appoint CCNs who had received no formal community training
- a focus on district nursing education (the only community nursing training available to CCNs at that time)
- CCNs who had recently completed their district nursing courses commented favourably on the joint sessions held with health visitors during the common core elements of the courses, i.e. 'child development' and 'developmental psychology'.

It would be appropriate at this point to reflect back on the wider context of the provision of community nursing education and to consider the historical development of education provision in both district nursing and health visiting.

DISTRICT NURSING EDUCATION

The history of district nursing has been traced back to the visionary work of William Rathbone in Liverpool in the 1850s (Stocks 1960). Rathbone recognised from the outset the value of nurse training and he was not alone in seeking Florence Nightingale's advice on how to secure the services of trained nurses. Nor was he alone in receiving Miss Nightingale's cursory advice. If you want nurses then 'train them yourself' (Stocks 1960 p 25). With considerable support and advice from Miss Nightingale, William Rathbone established a training school in Liverpool and by May 1863 'six women had been trained as district nurses' (Stocks 1960 p 31).

In 1868, Rathbone became a Member of Parliament for Liverpool. As a politician he spent part of his time in London where, during the mid 1870s, he was actively involved in the establishment of the Metropolitan and National Nursing Association for the Provision of Trained Nurses for the Sick Poor (Baly et al 1987, Stocks 1960) which rapidly established the requirement for a training in district nursing of 6 months' duration.

In 1887 a donation of over £70 000 from Queen Victoria's Silver Jubilee appeal was made to extend the work of district nurses (DNs) through the UK and led to the establishment of the Queen Victoria's Silver Jubilee Institute for Nurses. Through a process of affiliation of a number of the existing training organisations, each of which had been established in different areas of the UK by this stage, the Queen's Nursing Institute as it is now known, rapidly became the national benchmark for district nursing education.

The introduction of state registration for all nurses by the Nurses Registration Act 1919 meant that registration with the new General Nursing Council became a prerequisite for entry to district nursing education. At the time of the Act however, and in order to facilitate initial establishment of the nurses' Register, it was not a requirement for registrants to have completed a formal training as a nurse (Abel-Smith 1960). This required only the production of:

'Evidence to the satisfaction of the Council that they are of good character, are of the prescribed age, are persons who were for at least three years before the first day of November 1919 bona fide *engaged in practice as nurses in attendance of the sick under conditions which appear to the Council to be satisfactory for the purposes of this provision and have adequate knowledge and experience of the nursing of the sick.'*

(Nurses Registration Act 1919 ch. 94 section 3(2)(c))

Before the Act, the number of DNs had grown considerably. Many had received no formal training either in general or district nursing. As a result of the Act these individuals were not only able to register as nurses, but the absence of any statutory requirement for training in district nursing meant that they were also able to continue to describe themselves as DNs. This situation persisted beyond the time of the establishment of the NHS in 1948. However, during the 1950s, increasing concerns about the number of 'untrained' DNs led to the establishment of the 'Working party on the training of district nurses' (Ministry of Health 1955), which reported in 1955 that less than half of the 9203 DNs then in employment were 'Queen's trained' (Baly et al 1987). In response to this finding the panel of Assessors for District Nurse Training was established in 1959.

In 1968 the Panel took over from the Queen's Nursing Institute the responsibility for training of DNs at a national level. One of the Panel's key functions was to advise the Ministry of Health (and subsequently the Department of Health) on matters pertaining to the education of DNs. One of its first actions was to approve a reduction in the length of training of the district nursing certificate from 6 to 4 months. Whilst there was a widespread acceptance within the profession of the need to increase the proportion of 'trained' DNs, Baly et al (1987) were amongst a number of commentators who perceived this as a retrograde step: 'the emphasis was on the numbers rather than the need to meet the future health needs of the community' (Baly et al 1987 p 338).

Indeed, the Panel of Assessors themselves saw this as only a short-term solution to the issue of training and in 1976 the Panel's 'Report on the education and training of district nurses' recommended that a nationally approved DN training should consist of a 6-month programme, of which two thirds should be theoretical training and one third practical experience, to be followed by 3 months' supervised practice (DoH and Social Security 1976). Although the 6-month training was accepted in 1978 the supervised practice component was not introduced until 1982. A new curriculum for DN training was introduced in 1978 (DoH and Social Security 1978) and in 1981 the district nursing certificate became a mandatory requirement to practice (Kratz 1982).

HEALTH VISITOR EDUCATION

In the 1850s the original sanitary visitors in Manchester were not required to undertake any specific preparation for their role, but by 1880 a short course of lectures was introduced for new visitors and by 1882 all the women attending the course were required to pass an examination set by a local doctor (Dowling 1973). A requirement for nurses to have previously undertaken nurse training was introduced in Manchester in 1881 at the same time that the title Health Visitor (HV) was first used (Owen 1983).

Owen (1983) observed that in 1909 London was the first authority to demand a professional qualification for HVs. In 1919, with the publication of a circular by the recently established Ministry of Health, this standard became generally accepted throughout the country. The Ministry of Health decreed that by 1928 all HVs should hold the certificate of the Royal Sanitary Institute (later the Royal Society of Health), the official examining body. At this time, for registered nurses (who were also required to be qualified as midwives), a course of study of 6 months' duration was required to train as an HV, although 'direct entry' into health visiting was achievable by completion of a 2-year programme. In 1938, midwifery training was separated into two elements (formally identified as Part 1 and Part 2), and possession of Part 1 only was required for prospective HVs (Owen 1982, 1983), a requirement that remained in place until 1989.

The formal educational requirements were reinforced in the NHS Act 1946 and in the NHS (Qualifications of Health Visitors and Tuberculosis Visitors) Regulations 1948, which reiterated the requirement for possession of the HV qualification for all practitioners. The School Health Service (Handicapped Pupils) Regulations 1945 outlined the responsibilities of the HV within the school health services in line with the Education Act 1945.

Owen (1982) reported that by 1950, 32 institutions were involved in the training of around 700 student HVs per year. Despite this there was a significant shortage of HVs (Hale et al 1968) and to address this a working party was established with Sir Wilson Jameson as chair. The report of the working party (Ministry of Health 1956) led directly to the publication of the Health Visiting and Social Work Training Act 1962 and ultimately to the establishment of a new training body for HVs, the Council for the Education and Training of Health Visitors (CETHV) (Wilkie 1979). In terms of this particular chapter perhaps the most important work of the CETHV related to developments in the syllabus of training for HVs and the incremental introduction during the 1960s and early 1970s of a full 1-year programme of training to include a minimum of 3 months of supervised practice.

NURSES, MIDWIVES AND HEALTH VISITORS ACT 1979 AND THE NEW STATUTORY BODIES

The Nurses, Midwives and Health Visitors Act 1979 led to the dissolution of both the Panel of Assessors in District Nursing and the CETHV. Their responsibilities for training provision were taken over by the new statutory bodies, the UK Central Council for Nursing, Midwifery and Health Visiting (UKCC) and the four National Boards. In England, a key element of the English National Board's (ENB) work focused on its responsibilities within the Act to 'have proper regard for the interests of all groups within the profession including those with minority representation' (The Nurses, Midwives and Health Visitors Act 1979, section 2(2)). In fulfilling this responsibility the Board established two key committees: the District Nursing Joint Committee and the Health Visiting Joint Committee (both of which worked closely with colleagues in the other three National Boards). One of the primary functions of the Board related to its responsibilities, inherited from the Panel of Assessors and the CETHV, for the approval and re-approval of education courses (The Nurses, Midwives and Health Visitors Act 1979, section 6(1)(a) and (b)).

As early as 1983, the District Nursing Joint Committee recommended to the Board that, where institutions offered both the district nursing and health visiting courses, approval visits should be undertaken on a joint basis. However, at this stage the Health Visiting Joint Committee considered that such changes should be 'implemented slowly' (ENB 1983). This reticence was short lived and within 4 years 'increasing numbers of joint course approval visits being made by members of the HV and DN joint committees' (ENB 1987 p 21). By this stage, it was clear that in many education institutions there was an increasing tendency towards the closer alignment of HV and DN courses in terms of an emerging 'common core' of content and in respect of the overall structure and length of the programmes.

TOWARDS A QUALIFICATION IN COMMUNITY CHILDREN'S NURSING

In the autumn of 1987, a small group of nurses came together and established a special interest group for paediatric community nurses (now referred to as community children's nurses) within the Royal College of Nursing (RCN). Within a year the group was formally recognised as a professional 'forum' within the RCN. One of the first issues to which the group turned its attention was that of educational provision for prospective (and in some instances already practising) CCNs. Contact was made with the ENB and in its annual report of 1988–1989 the District Nursing Joint Committee noted that 'the issue of community nursing services for sick children, highlighted as an area requiring attention, is being discussed by the Committee as a matter of urgency' (ENB 1989 p 10). In April 1989, a working group was established within the ENB consisting of members of the General and Paediatric Committee and the District Nursing Joint Committee in order to address 'how the longer term needs of paediatric community nurses might be met' (Langlands 1990 p 8).

In 1990, the District Nursing Joint Committee forwarded a paper to the Education Advisory Policy Committee of the UKCC in which it outlined a number of issues that it was hoped the UKCC might consider within its on-going deliberations on post-registration education. In addition, and in order to provide a short-term solution to the problems outlined in the opening section of this chapter, the ENB produced and circulated to all institutions offering the district nursing course, 'Modified Regulations and Guidelines' for what was described as the 'District nurse and paediatric community nursing course' (ENB 1990). These regulations provided a framework within which registered children's nurses (who must also be registered as a general nurse) might gain a period of experience of 'between four and six weeks caring for the sick/handicapped child' (ENB 1990 p 98) during the supervised practice element of the course and might also undertake some of the examined elements of the course with a focus upon the child. At this time the ENB formally elected to refer to all registered children's nurses practising in community settings as 'Community Children's Nurses' (Langlands 1990).

A number of institutions, including the Combined Buckinghamshire College (Whiting et al 1994), Southampton University (Gastrell 1993) and South Bank Polytechnic, sought formal approval from the ENB to provide these modified programmes during the early 1990s. In spite of the imaginative approaches to curriculum development within these programmes, it remained a fact that the qualification gained upon successful completion of the course was that of district nurse. As Godman observed: 'the time that was "wasted" in both academic and practical preparation of a paediatric nurse to care for adults in the community seems to be an inappropriate use of scarce resources' (Whiting et al 1994).

To provide further opportunities for registered children's nurses, the ENB also agreed to approve 'programmes generated by institutions specifically to prepare RSCNs and RNs (Child)' and leading to 'recordable qualifications on the UKCC professional register' relating to the community nursing care of children (Langlands & McDonagh 1995). Two institutions, the Oxford Brookes University and the Manchester Metropolitan University, gained approval for such courses in 'Paediatric community nursing/Diploma of Higher Education in Community Health Care for Nurses on Part 8 or 15 of the Professional Register (A50)'.

In 1991 the UKCC published the 'Report on proposals for the future of community education and practice'. This consultation document formally introduced the concept of 'community healthcare nursing'. In addition, it included a strong endorsement for the emerging 'modular approach to education, which gives flexibility and offers scope for multidisciplinary and interdisciplinary working' (UKCC 1991 para 26). The report clearly identified a range of nursing needs in the community, however it completely failed to recognise the specific needs of sick children and made no mention of the rapidly expanding discipline of community children's nursing. These concerns were voiced in a formal written response to the consultation report by the RCN, Action for Sick Children, the Association for British Paediatric Nurses, the British Association for Community Child Health, the Joint Committee of Professional Nursing, Midwifery and Health Visiting Associations (England) and the ENB (UKCC 1992).

The development of proposals by the UKCC for the reform of community nursing education was a major part of the Council's broader work within the Post-Registration Education and Practice Project (PREPP) (UKCC 1990). In 1993, the Council formally incorporated its work on community nursing education into PREPP in a consultation document (UKCC 1993), which commenced by stating that 'The Council has now concluded its work on the proposals arising from the Post Registration Education and Practice Project and the Report on Proposals for the future of Community Education and Practice' (p 1). Within this final consultation document the UKCC proposed six areas of practice in community nursing including, somewhat inexplicably, the 'general nursing care of children which relates to the practice of school nursing and paediatric nursing' (UKCC 1993 annexe 3 p 1). This proposal was greeted with understandable concern by both school nurses and CCNs and in 1994, when the final proposals for the reform of community nursing education were published (UKCC 1994), the two discrete disciplines of school nursing and community children's nursing were formally recognised as separate strands of the new discipline of 'specialist community health nursing'. CCNs would become one of a new breed of 'specialist practitioners' in community nursing.

For many CCNs who had been involved in extensive lobbying of the ENB and UKCC, in particular during the previous 4 years, a collective sigh of relief could now be breathed. The final proposals (UKCC 1994) created a route to specialist professional practice for CCNs within the framework of an equivalent educational pathway to each of the other seven community nursing disciplines. Early in 1995, the ENB published updated regulations and guidelines to educational institutions to allow implementation of the UKCC proposals (ENB 1995).

Box 8.1 Areas of community healthcare nursing practice (UKCC 1994)

- General practice nursing
- Community mental health nursing
- Community mental handicap nursing
- Community children's nursing
- Public health nursing – health visiting
- Occupational health nursing
- Nursing in the home – district nursing
- School nursing

A major problem however still remained. By the time the UKCC published its final proposals there were over 250 nurses employed within community children's nursing teams in the UK (Whiting & RCN 1994). At this time these nurses were employed in community children's nursing teams within over 80 NHS Trusts and health districts. Many of these nurses had previously gained qualifications in health visiting or district nursing, however this was far from universal. A survey at the end of 1995 in the Thames Regions found that over 70% of the 139 CCNs employed within 31 teams possessed no community qualification at all (Whiting 1997). This was not a problem that was unique to community children's nursing. The field of practice nursing was predominantly made up of nurses who did not possess a community qualification at all and practice nurse numbers had grown in the 10 years from 1984 to 1994 from 1920 to 9100 whole-time equivalent staff (NHS Executive 1996).

The UKCC recognised that this was a significant concern and, in order to address this, a series of 'transitional arrangements' was proposed to facilitate nurses in the attainment of 'specialist practitioner' status (UKCC 1994 section 10, UKCC 1996). These arrangements provided a series of pathways through which CCNs might gain accreditation of previous learning and experience (Langlands & McDonagh 1995, Myles 1997) in order to allow CCNs to become eligible to use the 'specialist practitioner' title. The 'transitional arrangements' expired in October 1998.

CONCLUSION This chapter has sought to review the historical development of educational provision for CCNs, including an examination of a range of community nursing educational programmes dating back to the 1860s. There can be little doubt however that the rapid growth in the number of community children's nursing services within the UK during the late 1980s and 1990s has been the single greatest influence upon educational development. Whilst district nursing, and to a lesser extent health visiting educational programmes, offered a 'stop gap' solution to the expressed educational needs of the growing number of registered children's nurses wishing to work in the community, such a solution was clearly unsustainable in the long term. As the number of CCNs grew, so did the need to provide an appropriate educational framework. This chapter has provided a historical review of the background to the introduction of a range of new education programmes and to the development of the specialist practitioner programme in community children's nursing.

REFERENCES

Abel-Smith B 1960 A history of the nursing profession. Heinemann, London

Baly M E, Robottom B & Clark J M 1987 District nursing, 2nd edn. Heinemann, London

Department of Health and Social Security: Panel of Assessors for District Nurse Training 1976 Report on the education and training of district nurses (SRN/RCN). HMSO, London.

Department of Health and Social Security: Panel of Assessors for District Nurse Training 1978 Curriculum in district nursing for State Registered Nurses and Registered General Nurses. HMSO, London

Dowling W C 1973 Health visiting – expansion. Health Visitor 46(11):371–372

English National Board for Nursing, Midwifery and Health Visiting (ENB) 1983 Annual report – 1983 ENB, London

English National Board for Nursing, Midwifery and Health Visiting (ENB)1987 Annual report – 1986/1987. ENB, London

English National Board for Nursing, Midwifery and Health Visiting (ENB) 1989 Annual report – 1988/1989. ENB, London

English National Board for Nursing, Midwifery and Health Visiting (ENB) 1990 Regulations and guidelines for the approval of institutions and courses 1990. ENB, London

English National Board for Nursing, Midwifery and Health Visiting (ENB) 1995 Regulations and guidelines relating to programmes of education leading to the qualification of specialist practitioner. Circular 1995/04/RLV. ENB, London

Gastrell P 1993 Diploma courses for PDNs. Paediatric Nursing 5(10):13–14

Hale R, Loveland M K & Owen G M 1968 The principles and practice of health visiting. Pergamon Press, London

Kratz C R 1982 District nursing. Cited in: Allen P & Jolley M (eds) Nursing, midwifery and health visiting since 1900. Faber and Faber, London, p 80

Langlands T 1990 Meeting future needs. Paediatric Nursing 2(3):8–9

Langlands T & McDonagh M 1995 The pathways to a specialism. Paediatric Nursing 7(8):6–7

Ministry of Health 1955 Report of the working party on the training of district nurses. HMSO, London

Ministry of Health 1956 An enquiry into health visiting: report of the working party on the field of work, training and recruitment of health visitors (chair, Sir W Jameson). HMSO, London

Myles A 1997 Desperately seeking 'specialist practitioner'? Paediatric Nursing 9(10):14

NHS Executive 1996 Primary care: the future. The Stationery Office, London

Owen G M 1982 Health visiting. In: Allen P & Jolley M (eds) Nursing, midwifery and health visiting since 1900. Faber and Faber, London, p 92

Owen G M 1983 The development of health visiting as a profession. In: Owen G M (ed) Health visiting, 2nd edn. Baillière Tindall, Eastbourne, p 1

Stocks M 1960 A hundred years of district nursing. Allen and Unwin, London

The Nurses, Midwives and Health Visitor's Act 1979 Registration Act, HMSO, London

UK Central Council for Nursing, Midwifery and Health Visiting (UKCC) 1990 The report of the Post-Registration Education and Practice Project (PREPP). UKCC, London

UK Central Council for Nursing, Midwifery and Health Visiting (UKCC) 1991 Report on proposals for the future of community education and practice. UKCC, London

UK Central Council for Nursing, Midwifery and Health Visiting (UKCC) 1992 Report on responses on the 'Report on proposals for the future of community education and practice'. UKCC, London

UK Central Council for Nursing, Midwifery and Health Visiting (UKCC) 1993 Consultation on the Council's proposed standards for post-registration education. UKCC, London

UK Central Council for Nursing, Midwifery and Health Visiting (UKCC) 1994 The future of professional practice – the Council's standards for education and practice following registration. UKCC, London

UK Central Council for Nursing, Midwifery and Health Visiting (UKCC) 1996 The Council's standards for education and practice following registration (PREP) transitional arrangements – specialist practitioner title/specialist qualification. Registrar's Letter 15/1996. UKCC, London

Whiting M 1988 Community paediatric nursing in England in 1988. MSc thesis, University of London

Whiting M 1997 Community children's nursing: a bright future. Paediatric Nursing 9(4):6–8

Whiting M & Royal College of Nursing (RCN) 1994 Directory of paediatric community nursing. RCN, London

Whiting M, Godman, L & Manly S 1994 Meeting needs: RSCNs in the community. Paediatric Nursing 6(1):9–11

Wilkie E 1979 The history of the Council for the Education and Training of Health Visitors. Allen and Unwin, London

Chapter 9

Setting the agenda for education

Christine Wint

KEY ISSUES

- Community specialist practitioner.
- Diversity of student need.
- Availability and range of community experience.
- Educational standards.

INTRODUCTION

As previous chapters have recognised, community children's nursing has been on the periphery of both children's nursing and community nursing for some time. In April 2002 the Nursing and Midwifery Council (NMC 2002a) published revised standards for education and practice following registration, which include standards for post-registration education programmes leading to the specialist practitioner qualification. Eight areas of specialist practice in the community are recognised (see Chapter 8, p 99). This publication continues to acknowledge community children's nursing as a discrete community specialist practitioner qualification, a precedent first established by the UK Central Council (UKCC) in 1994 (UKCC 1994). This precedent provided the opportunity to advance the development of children's nursing for not only did it recognise that the needs of children must be provided by a discrete community specialist, it also recognised that to be a Community Children's Nurse (CCN) it is not enough to simply practice outside the hospital setting. The UKCC (1994) and NMC (2002a) acknowledged the complexity of community children's nursing and the need for specialist nurses who are skilled and knowledgeable children's nurses. In addition, it established that CCNs not only have the clinical expertise to care for children but also have the ability to translate their experience within the complex and changing environment known as the community.

Since 1994 educationalists in higher education institutions have been working with their practice colleagues to produce courses that not only fit the variable needs for CCNs locally but also address the wider national context within the framework of the NMC's requirements. Given that the notion of the role of the CCN has not yet reached maturity or consensus, this has been a difficult task (Procter et al 1998). A further complication is the fact that over 20% of the country still does not have a community children's nursing service (Royal College of Nursing 2004). This chapter will identify ways of continuing the development of educational provision to address the current diversity within practice and in addition will explore the educational needs of the CCN as a community specialist practitioner. The wider areas of child health will be discussed and consideration for future developments will be made.

DEVELOPMENT IN EDUCATIONAL PROVISION

In the past there were mandatory community qualifications only for district nurses and health visitors and so, historically, CCNs have either undertaken health visiting or district nursing courses in order to achieve a community qualification (Whiting 1988). However, the relevance of health visiting and district nursing to community children's nursing has always been questionable as district nurse training is focused primarily on the adult population and health visiting develops the students' skills to appreciate the health issues of the population. Hence the UKCC, in 1994, set standards for specialist nursing practice which included community children's nursing. With the community specialist practitioner programme came a recordable qualification and professional recognition. The community specialist practitioner status gives recognition of the unique educational needs of community children's nursing and clearly identifies the importance of this role to other healthcare professionals (see Chapter 8).

DEVELOPMENT OF THE SPECIALIST PRACTITIONER

Each community nursing specialism constitutes a separate and distinct professional group, yet there are some common elements that run through all the groups. Hyde (1995) explains how this has led to some confusion and tension in understanding and appreciating the uniqueness of new areas of practice. The NMC recognises that some commonality exists between the specialisms and stipulates that common core areas must occupy a minimum of one third and a maximum of two thirds of the total community specialist practitioner programme. These similarities and differences can be categorised into three types (Hyde 1995):

1. Areas that are common to all specialisms.
2. Areas that are common to some specialisms but not to others.
3. Areas that are unique to one specialism.

Areas common to all specialisms include subjects such as health promotion, primary healthcare policy, research, caseload management, teamwork and collaboration, leadership, scope of professional practice, quality assurance and audit. Subjects such as child protection and child health

Table 9.1 Examples of similarities within course content

Specialism	Course content
All specialisms	Health promotion, policy, clinical governance, child protection, etc.
Health visitors/school nurses	Child development, working with families
Community children's nurses/school nurses/health visitors	Mental and emotional health issues, child-specific health promotion, eczema management, constipation management

are not significant for occupational health nurses but are of paramount importance to health visitors, school nurses, learning disabilities nurses and CCNs (Table 9.1).

Hyde (1995) further believes that all the specialist pathways have more common areas than they have differences. By comparing the subject areas it is evident that the scope of the CCN's practice runs close to areas within other community specialisms. Nonetheless, the uniqueness of the specialism must not be undervalued.

Within the classroom the opportunity of sharing knowledge and experience can be advantageous as this setting provides a forum for discussion and debate where the students from the various community specialisms can begin to appreciate their new professional roles. The potential problems lie within practice, as it is essential that students gain the most appropriate experience to ensure the development of a competent and confident CCN who has the skills and knowledge required to move practice forward in a creative, flexible and innovative way (Fradd 1994). The changing dynamics of child health have sought to blur professional boundaries (Porter 1996), providing an opportunity for the student and the educationalist to identify varied practice experiences that will help to prepare the student for the discrete role of a CCN within a placement that reflects the belief and values of the service.

The framework for the community specialist practitioner (community children's nursing) experience must embrace a holistic approach to the care of sick children through a family-centred approach (Porter 1996) and must equip students with the appropriate knowledge and skills to undertake their complex and challenging role (Whyte 1992, Procter et al 1998). The experience must recognise that, unlike children in the hospital setting who are recipients of care in an artificially controlled environment, children in the community are in a setting well known to themselves and over which they and their family usually have the majority of control. This sense of control and involvement in the care process must be fostered so that the child and family and the CCN work together. The uniqueness of each child and family must be recognised and accepted as fundamental to the provision of nursing care. It is therefore important that the preparation of CCNs ensures that students value their individuality within the context of the home environment.

With the recognition that community care expands beyond the boundaries of nursing to overlap with the work of other caring agencies, the student must be encouraged to recognise and embrace the valuable contribution of other workers and professionals in the health, education and social care field and to explore ways in which collaborative partnerships can be developed (Richardson 1996, Newbury et al 1997, Department for Education and Skills 2004). This approach should form the basis of teaching, learning and assessment in the practice environment and was clearly illustrated by the English National Board (ENB) (1995) (Box 9.1).

Box 9.1 ENB statement of fitness for purpose: community specialist practitioner

Practitioners who are skilled to meet changing healthcare needs should be (ENB 1995):

■ Innovative in their practice
■ Responsive to changing demand
■ Resourceful in their methods of working
■ Able to share good practice/knowledge
■ Adaptable to changing healthcare needs
■ Challenging and creative in their practice
■ Self-reliant in their way of working
■ Responsible and accountable for their work

This includes the identification and integration of:

1. The existing knowledge/skills of the prospective student
2. The knowledge/skills required by the potential practice
3. The learning outcomes identified by the NMC
4. The experiences available locally and identification of the potential alternative experiences available to complement the learning experience

---

To qualify as a specialist practitioner, the student must undertake a programme of study that meets the requirements set out by the NMC. Programmes of specialist education should contain four broad areas of practice:

● clinical practice
● care and programme management
● clinical practice development
● clinical practice leadership.

For the CCN, specific learning outcomes also include (NMC 2002a):

1. Clinical nursing practice
   ● assess, plan, provide and evaluate specialist clinical nursing care to meet care needs of acutely and chronically ill children at home
   ● assess, diagnose and treat specific diseases in accordance with agreed medical and nursing protocols

2. Care and programme management
   - initiate and contribute to strategies designed to promote and improve health and prevent disease in children, their families and the wider community
   - initiate action to identify and minimise risk to children and ensure child protection and safety
   - initiate management of potential and actual physical and psychological abuse of children and potentially violent situations and settings.

These areas of practice must be translated into practice competencies that the student has to achieve to gain professional recognition from the NMC within their area of specialist community practice. The specialist practitioner programme must:

- be at first degree level
- include common core, not less than one third and more than two thirds of the total programme
- be flexible and modular
- be a minimum of one academic year in length (32 weeks minimum)
- be 50% theory and 50% practice.

For community children's nursing there is the challenge of developing courses that address the many interpretations within practice delivery. This is further complicated by the fact that even in 2004 there are so few individuals who have the appropriate qualifications and/or appropriate practice experience to provide the course. Muir (1995) identified the potential challenge of addressing the possible diversity of students who may come from a wide variety of clinical backgrounds, all of whom have completely different individual learning needs (see Box 9.2). This requires careful consideration to ensure that all students have their learning needs met so that they can gain the most appropriate experience and achieve the professional competencies required to gain the community specialist practitioner (community children's nursing) qualification.

Box 9.2 Range of potential students (Muir 1995)

- Experienced CCNs with no community qualification
- Traditionally trained hospital-based children's nurses
- DipHE/RN(Child) nurses

It is recognised that all students need to acquire new skills and knowledge in order to fulfil the generic role of community specialist practitioner (Porter 1996). Although students will enter the programme with a wide range of experience, their status on entry must be considered as that of a relative novice, in that they are being prepared for a new role within the community that brings new responsibilities and a higher level of decision making. Benner (1984) describes a model of levels of learning from novice to expert professional practitioner that is concerned with levels of professional activity on theory and practice (Table 9.2).

Table 9.2 Levels of learning: Benner's model (1984)

Level	Description	Professional activity
Certificate	Novice	Competent professional practitioner who participates in professional activities safely and can discuss with confidence the theory and research that informs practice
Diploma	Competent	Proficient professional practitioner who responds flexibly to the needs of the individual, demonstrating the ability to analyse and evaluate quality of care critically
Degree	Proficient	Expert advanced professional practitioner who demonstrates expertise in a particular clinical or community setting by responding flexibly and creatively to situations in order to provide a quality personal service for clients and co-workers

The ability to reflect upon performance is an essential feature, particularly relevant in the search for new knowledge to push forward the boundaries of professional knowledge, skills and attitudes (Porter 1996). The transition from novice to expert should be facilitated through reflective practice, the art of reflection being viewed as a central process in bridging the theory–practice gap in nursing (Box 9.3).

Box 9.3 Mandatory skills required by community specialist practitioner (Reveley, unpublished work, 1997)

- Acts as team leader
- Manages resources effectively
- Manages a caseload
- Manages/supervises others
- Liaises/collaborates with other agencies
- An accountable decision maker
- Initiates/monitors patient/client care
- Uses evidence-based practice
- Develops/monitors standards of practice
- Develops clinical practice through research/experience
- Responds to clients'/carers' needs
- Promotes health where possible
- Empowers clients/carers
- Has highly developed clinical skills/uses these in an innovative manner

(These skills are linked directly to the NMC learning outcomes that the student must achieve through a competence profile.)

EDUCATION PROVISION

Pre-registration education is designed to equip practitioners with the knowledge, skills and attitudes needed to provide safe and effective care to children. However, pre-registration education alone does not prepare these practitioners adequately to meet the additional needs of specialist practice. Some practitioners are required to exercise higher levels of judgement and higher levels of clinical decision making in practice and will need to monitor and improve standards of care through supervising others. This will include undertaking clinical audit, skilled professional leadership and the development of practice through research, teaching and professional support of colleagues (NMC 2002b).

The community course must recognise that community healthcare nurses are:

- reflective practitioners
- independent in attending to their learning needs
- flexible in applying core principles to complex practical issues
- able to design solutions appropriate to meet individual needs.

Through the learning process it is important that students contribute not only to their individual learning needs but also to the learning of others. Each student will bring to the course a variety of experiences that, in being shared, will both contribute to the learning that takes place and help shape the specific experience of the course for each student.

THE STUDENT

It is essential that each student can achieve all the NMC learning outcomes and so be deemed competent within practice. As each student will be entering the pathway with a variety of experiences, the development of a personal profile enables students to reflect clearly on their own strengths and identify specific areas for development. For example, experienced hospital-based children's nurses may identify their specific needs as being the transfer of highly developed skills into the community setting, whereas the experienced community-based children's nurses may gain more by focusing on developing knowledge and skills by working with other members of the primary healthcare team.

To ensure that each student's needs are met within the educational standards of the specialist practitioner programme it is important that the pathway leader meets with the student and identifies:

- past nursing experience
- individual learning needs
- the learning opportunities available within the district.

The individual characteristics of each student must be taken into consideration in the placement selection process. A flexible approach is needed which takes into account the combination of:

- no single recognised model of community children's nursing within practice
- the potential variety of student experience on entering the programme.

The overall course experience must be developed to facilitate the diverse needs of each student. The educationalist must therefore negotiate with students to maintain a balance of recognising the individual needs of the student whilst incorporating the overall philosophy of community specialist practitioner education. It is essential that the integrity of the total educational experience is maintained. This further ensures that the student can gain the relevant experience to achieve the community specialist practitioner competencies for community children's nursing.

The experience for each student must be recognised as individual and dynamic. It is therefore essential that each student should identify their initial learning needs. The student and pathway leader will then be able to work together to plan the most appropriate clinical placement. At this point it is important that the needs of the service are borne in mind. It is expected that service managers will be involved in this discussion.

The initial needs assessment should result in an action plan. The student then maintains an ongoing personal 'needs analysis' (Neill & Muir 1997), a process that can be facilitated through the development of a personal profile (NMC 2002a). Students will demonstrate their needs and how these have been met through a learning contract that will incorporate an action plan and evidence of how objectives have been achieved. As Neill & Muir (1997) explain, the learning experience is a dynamic process and the student's needs will develop and change. To facilitate this process students maintain a reflective diary to help them identify their learning needs and specific areas of personal development. Learning contracts, a useful method of quantifying individual learning needs, can be used to inform the ongoing dialogue between student, pathway leader and community practice teacher and will facilitate the development of community specialist practitioner skills.

DEVELOPING EDUCATION PROVISION IN THE CLINICAL SETTING

Two key challenges that relate to the process of establishing and running a community children's specialist practitioner pathway are placements and supervision.

The placement

Placements can be a particularly challenging issue, especially where no community children's nursing service exists. Even where services do exist, the provision can be focused on a specialist area such as cystic fibrosis, diabetes or asthma. Equally the service may be very limited in the provision offered. To move forward it is essential that a flexible, creative and responsive approach is taken which allows the student to play an integral part in the whole experience. Students may identify their own areas for development that are not available to them within their current practice experience. Comparative practice can be utilised as a means of addressing these deficits. The length and type of experience will be dependent on the student's individual need. Trust managers must also be involved as students are guaranteed practical placements under the supervision of a community practice teacher or equivalent. The placement will form part of a tripartite agreement between employer, student and the educational institution. The seconding manager is deemed to be someone who is in a position to guarantee placements, and their involvement is essential. Planning between the course tutor and the student is therefore a crucial component. It is preferable that both supervised and taught practice placements are undertaken (i) in different community children's nursing services and (ii) away from a student's previous practice area if already employed in the community. Furthermore it is essential that, during both placements, students are supernumerary to existing CCN numbers.

The supervision

The UKCC (1995) recognised the need for flexibility within the supervisory process. It suggested that it 'does not advocate either a statutory or prescriptive approach nor a single model approach'. It also recognised that in some areas 'a colleague from another clinical profession may act as a clinical supervisor'. Some would argue that students should be supervised in practice only by a CCN, but situations may dictate the need for alternative approaches. Anecdotal experience suggests that where there is a need to utilise a clinical supervisor from a different discipline, this model of supervision is of less value to a student with no community experience than the student with previous community experience. Muir (1995) described this as the 'chicken and egg' scenario whereby specialist students require supervision on courses in areas with no existing community children's nursing service. These students will become the future supervisors in practice. An innovative approach to the practice experience must therefore be adopted by all involved. This anomaly, although less common, continues in the twenty-first century.

COMMUNITY PRACTICE TEACHERS

It is recognised and accepted that Community Practice Teachers (CPTs) or their equivalent will vary in their experience to meet the individual learning needs of students. However, it is important that the experience is facilitated by a skilled practitioner to ensure that:

- Concepts and principles of practice examined within the classroom are then applied in practice.
- The student is developing competently in their practice.

The tripartite model emerged to address the development of a more theory- and practice-based experience (Neill & Muir 1997) (Fig. 9.1).

This model serves the student well as it allows for the diverse dynamics within practice yet maintains the integrity of community children's nursing. The individual needs of students can be addressed as the student, pathway leader and CPT (or equivalent) are brought together to explore and develop the learning needs of each student. For this approach to work it is essential that pathway leaders have a clear understanding of community children's nursing practice. Ideally they should hold the community children's nursing specialist practitioner qualification and have experience of practice as a CCN. It is therefore essential that pathway leaders have at least a children's nursing qualification and a community nursing qualification. They play the pivotal role of linking theory and practice whilst maintaining the focus of community children's nursing practice between the student and the CPT (Neill & Muir 1997). Without this appreciation there is a danger that the student will emerge as some form of quasi-community nurse who has an interest

Fig. 9.1 An example of a tripartite approach used for community children's nursing: Community Children's Nurse (CCN) students, Health Visitor (HV), Registered Sick Children's Nurse (RSCN).

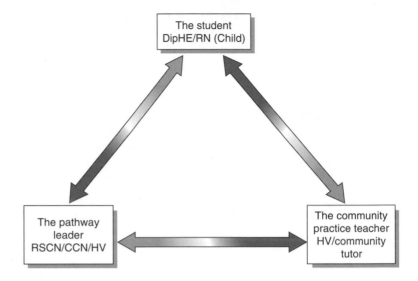

in the care of sick children. As Neill & Muir (1997) explain, the role of the pathway leader is thus 'essential for the immediate development of future practitioners and the longer-term development or extension of the service'.

The challenge of developing a caseload within the community setting provides a valuable opportunity to explore the political context of child-focused provision and to consider how theories debated in the classroom can be directly applied in practice. In addition, students visit other community children's nursing teams around the country and work with other community practitioners within the area.

FUNDING FOR COMMUNITY CHILDREN'S NURSING EDUCATION

Community children's nursing is a relatively young discipline. Problems lie in how the developments are recognised and valued within the various Trusts and Primary Care Trusts (PCT). This has a direct influence on how funding is made available for the educational development of children's nurses who seek to gain the community specialist qualification. Further problems arise with competition for funding between the traditional community nurses and the new areas of specialist practice. The allocation and arrangements for educational funding for community nurse education is decided within the Workforce Development arm of the local Strategic Health Authority in negotiation with the PCT and Trusts. They are required to produce evidence of workforce planning to support their applications for educational funding, which directly influences the maintenance and development of nursing services. These issues emphasise the need for educationalists and practitioners to work collaboratively with local PCT and Trust managers to raise awareness of the need to develop services for sick children within the community. Awareness needs to be raised at both a local and national level, clearly identifying and articulating the potential contribution of community children's nursing services to care for sick children at home (Neill & Muir 1997). The Health Committee (1997) report acknowledged these problems and recommended that the education of CCNs should be commissioned on the same basis as health visiting and district nursing education. The need for workforce planning is therefore central to the development. This requires evidence through detailed needs assessment. The hospital Trusts, together with the PCT (in England), need to identify clearly from this process the service that is required to address the health needs of children.

THE FUTURE

Community healthcare nursing is developing within a rapidly evolving health service alongside the changing pattern of child healthcare. Community children's nursing must be willing to embrace these changes. The recent development of Children's Trusts and National Service Frameworks for children will provide new opportunities for CCNs to develop new patterns of working, secure better integrated services and better outcomes for children (DoH 2002, 2003, Department for Education and Skills 2004). Hence, CCNs are strategically placed to develop services through their ability to be flexible, confident and competent in defining the needs of children and their families, and structuring their work to meet those needs. Although children's nurses have always striven to assert their role as advocates of children and their families, with ever-increasing demands and responsibilities being placed on families to care for their children, the need for intelligent, informed advocates for children and their families has never been stronger (Lock 1996). The community specialist practitioner programme provides the opportunity for education and practice to come together and inform the development of future practitioners to meet the challenges ahead.

CONCLUSION

This chapter has explored a range of issues that affect the educational provision for community specialist practitioners (community children's nursing). The situation is characterised by the changes in child health provision which is responding to the changing patterns of child health. The transfer of skills from hospital-based provision to community-focused care has led to the development of community children's nursing which seeks to serve the needs of children and their families within their home and community. No single model of provision is identified. It is therefore challenging for educationalists to develop community specialist practitioner courses that embrace the varied needs of potential students and practice. Innovative and flexible approaches, which include collaboration with professional colleagues, have allowed developments to move forward. Within education provision, the task is set to continue to embrace the ever-changing needs in practice within a framework that provides a flexible approach but does not compromise the maintenance and development of clinical excellence.

REFERENCES

Benner P 1984 From Novice to Expert: Excellence and Power in Clinical Nursing Practice. Addison-Wesley, Menlo Park, California

Department for Education and Skills (DfES) 2004 Every Child Matters: next steps. DfES, Nottingham

Department of Health 2002 Children's Trusts. The Stationery Office, London

Department of Health 2003 Getting the right start: National Service Framework for Children. Emerging Findings, The Stationery Office, London

English National Board for Nursing, Midwifery and Health Visiting (ENB) 1995 Creating lifelong learners. ENB, London

Fradd E 1994 A broader scope of practice. Professional development in paediatric nursing. Child Health, April/May:233–238

Health Committee 1997 House of Commons Select Committee. Health services for children and young people in the community: home and school. Third report. The Stationery Office, London

Hyde V 1995 Community nursing: a unified discipline? In: Cain P, Hyde V & Howkins E (eds) Community Nursing: Dimensions and Dilemmas. Arnold, London, p 17

Lock K 1996 The changing organization of health care: setting the scene. In: Twinn S, Roberts B & Andrews S (eds) Community Health Care Nursing. Principles and practice. Butterworth–Heinemann, Oxford, p 40

Muir J 1995 Community: the student perspective. Paediatric Nursing 7(8):8–10

Neill S J & Muir J 1997 Educating the new community children's nurses: challenges and opportunities. Nurse Education Today 17:7–15

Newbury J, Clarridge A & Skinner J 1997 Collaboration for care. In: Burley S, Mitchell E, Melling K, Smith M, Chilton S & Cromplin C (eds) Contemporary Community Nursing. Arnold, London, p 77

Nursing and Midwifery Council (NMC) 2002a Standards for Specialist Education and Practice. NMC, London

Nursing and Midwifery Council (NMC) 2002b Supporting Nurses and Midwives through Lifelong Learning. NMC, London

Porter E 1996 The child. In: Twinn S, Roberts B & Andrews S (eds) Community Health Care Nursing: Principles for Practice. Butterworth–Heinemann, Oxford, p 320

Procter S, Biott C, Campbell S, Edward S, Redpath N & Moran M 1998 Preparation for the Developing Role of the Community Children's Nurse. English National Board for Midwifery, Nursing and Health Visiting, London

Richardson J 1996 Shifting boundaries in paediatric community nursing. In: Gastrell P & Edwards J (eds) Community Health Nursing: Framework for Practice. Baillière Tindall, London, p 286

Royal College of Nursing (RCN) Community Children's Nursing Forum 2004 Directory of Community Children's Nursing Services. 16th edn. RCN, London

UK Central Council 1994 (UKCC) The Future of Professional Practice – The Council's Standards for Education and Practice Following Registration. UKCC, London

UK Central Council 1995 (UKCC) Position Statement on Clinical Supervision for Nursing and Health Visiting. UKCC, London

Whiting M 1988 Community Paediatric Nursing in England in 1988. MSc thesis, University of London

Whyte D A 1992 A family nursing approach to the care of the child with chronic illness. Journal of Advanced Nursing 17:326–327

The editors would like to acknowledge the contribution made by Patricia Livsey in the previous edition of this book, which has been used as a foundation for this chapter.

SECTION 2

Philosophical Issues Underpinning the Delivery of Community Children's Nursing Practice

SECTION CONTENTS

Philosophical principles should permeate practice and require careful consideration. A new chapter analysing the concepts of national identity and strategy provides a focus of thought for the remainder of the text. Legal and ethical frameworks are examined alongside more pervasive factors such as the need to deliver culturally sensitive care. This section also explores the everyday challenges of creating and maintaining the many complex relationships that develop in practice, including those between community children's nurses, children, their families and other professionals.

Chapter 10

A national strategy and corporate identity for community children's nursing?

Jackie Acornley

KEY ISSUES
- Service development.
- Corporate/national strategy and culture of community children's nursing.
- Corporate identity and image of community children's nurses.
- Professional identity of community children's nurses.
- The effect on training and education.

INTRODUCTION

District Nurses (DNs), Health Visitors (HVs), Community Psychiatric Nurses and School Nurses are well known to the public and medical and nursing professions. Their work role may not be fully understood but they have a framework in which they practice and are respected within the community. The funding and commissioning pathways for these nurses is well established. A national strategy and a corporate identity are evident to those involved with these services. In contrast, despite the evidence of a rapid growth of community children's nursing teams (see Chapter 2), many healthcare professionals are unaware of their existence. Even those concerned with the welfare of children lack both understanding of the service and insight into the role of the community children's nurse (CCN). A national strategy and a corporate identity are not evident to either practitioners or service users. This chapter will discuss the issues that have led to the poor recognition of CCNs and the services they provide and the impact this has on service development.

DEFINING CORPORATE STRATEGY AND CULTURE

Deal and Kennedy (1982) define corporate culture as encompassing how people in a company are likely to act in given situations both inside and outside the organisation. It includes a set of beliefs, a code of behaviour and minimum standards of performance and ethics. Based on evidence collected on 80 corporations in the United States Deal & Kennedy argue that organisations with strong and clearly identifiable cultures are likely to be more effective.

> **Box 10.1** Key features of a strong corporate culture
>
> - Characteristic/clear approach to the corporate environment, i.e. markets/clients/stakeholders, etc.
> - Shared values within organisation.
> - Heroes – people, who represent/communicate values/provide 'role models'.
> - Rites/rituals – systems/procedures people expected to follow.
> - Networks – informal communication/grapevine (Deal & Kennedy 1982. In: Winfield et al 2000 p 320).

Winfield et al (2000) define corporate strategy as the purpose, scope and long-term direction of an organisation. While some writers including Mintzberg et al (1998) and Glueck (1980) portray strategy as a master plan that directs and coordinates the activities of an organisation, other writers emphasise the business planning aspects (Kay 1996).

DEVELOPMENT OF CORPORATE IDENTITY WITHIN COMMUNITY CHILDREN'S NURSING

With the development of the first NHS community children's nursing service in Rotherham in 1949 in response to concerns about cross infection and infant mortality, the pattern of community children's nursing provision was formed as 'a response to local issue or need' (see p 21) (Gillet 1954). Without the provision of Government legislation, funding or a national strategy to guide development, community children's nursing has, in some areas, struggled to develop (Tatman & Woodroffe 1993). Some teams, established in areas where there is a regional children's centre, have continued to grow (Gow 1996). However, in some areas served by small district general hospitals, services are either non-existent or unable to expand (Health Committee 1997, Maunder 2003). Many community children's nursing teams have reputedly developed to provide whichever aspect of care has been identified within that area as 'a need'. Certainly the evaluations provided by some individual services demonstrated evidence of innovative and diverse service development in response to assessed need (Bergman et al 1965, Gow & Atwell 1980, Tatman et al 1992, Jennings 1994). In many areas the 'need' for a service has often been based on the availability of charitable funding or the individual priorities of trusts, rather than based on the real needs of children (Whiting et al 2001). As a consequence services have developed in a fragmented manner to bridge 'gaps' rather than as a planned strategic response to develop an integrated child health service to meet an identified need (Winter & Teare 1997).

One of the benefits of individual service development has been that, without clear boundaries or prescribed practices CCNs have been able to identify areas of need within service provision leading to innovative practice development. For example providing home traction (Clayton 1997) and the setting up of CCN-led clinics for the treatment of children with constipation or eczema (Muir 1999). 'The Department of Health has been reluctant to adopt a preferred service model recognising that there are already significant differences in local health provision and that a one model fits all approach would potentially stifle innovation' (Community Children's Nursing Forum 2002 p 4). Fragmented service development resulted in:

- A variety of services, many of which are providing the same elements of care, yet are marketed and identified in different ways, either as an extension of the acute service, a specialist nursing service or a community nursing service.
- Individual team functions dependent on locality, need, commitment, skills, resources and policies leading to inequitable provision of services.
- Many nurses and teams, for example outreach specialist nurses, community-based specialist nurses and generalist home care teams, who neither perceive themselves nor are perceived by other professionals as CCNs, are banded under the umbrella term of CCN. This contributes to confusion about the professional identity of their role and that of the generic CNN.
- Anecdotal evidence of inefficient, inappropriate or non-existent supervision of community practice by non-CCN managers who do not hold a qualification in community children's nursing supported by experienced practice in the speciality.
- Ad hoc development leading to community children's nursing as a divided service nationally, lacking both a corporate culture and a unified professional/corporate image.

Research based on individual service evaluations indicates that some larger services, for example Southampton, Nottingham and Croydon, have a strong corporate culture. Literature including Gow & Atwell (1980), Glasper et al (1989), Dryden (1994), Gow (1996) and Anderson (2000) shows these teams have:

1. Clear vision to market their services to clients and commissioners and clearly identifiable team roles.
2. Team members who have a strong commitment to providing care to children and their families in the community setting.
3. Strong management, i.e. CCNs providing role models and a clear marketing strategies.
4. Clear policies and guidelines.
5. Systems for networking with other teams that are highly valued.

Community children's nursing services collectively do not have a strong corporate culture. The numerous types of services listed in the directory of services (Royal College of Nursing 2004), and the confusion arising from the literature as to whether the services themselves consider they are community children's nursing services, typifies this.

Several examples listed in the directory are not perceived, by either the staff, managers or professional users of the service, as community children's nursing schemes or marketed as such. These include hospital at home schemes, children's home care teams and specialist outreach services.

One hospital at home scheme, according to Peter & Torr (1996), was comparable with many generic community children's nursing services. The service was responsible for the management of, for example, children with constipation, tracheostomies, those requiring follow up after day surgery and overnight oxygen saturation monitoring. However, rotating nurses from the ward staffed this scheme and there appeared no commitment to encourage staff to gain a community degree. The scheme was funded and staffed by the acute trust, as part of children's acute services, and it would appear it was marketed as an extension to the provision of acute services rather than a community service.

In contrast, a hospital at home service described by Jennings (1994), although funded by the acute service and set up in similar circumstances to the above scheme, was set up separately from the ward. This scheme was developed as a community children's nursing service, and appears to have been identified and marketed as such, with a commitment to encourage staff to undertake the CCN specialist degree.

Eaton (2001) and Whiting (p 34) identify specialist hospital outreach as one model of a community children's nursing service. Several of these services are listed in the services directory (Royal College of Nursing 2004), for example Paediatric Oncology Outreach Nurse Specialists who deal exclusively with children with cancer; nurses specialising in the care of children with diabetes or cystic fibrosis (CF). Many of the nurses are funded by charities such as the CF Trust or Macmillan Nursing fund. These nurses have a targeted client population and, as part of a national organisation, clear guidelines on audit, management and work role, provided, for example, by the CF Trust (2001). It would appear these services have a strong corporate culture within their specialities.

Anecdotal evidence and a study reported by Hunt (1999) however, suggest that both the nurses themselves and other professionals consider these services as a separate identity to community children's nursing services. This contrasts with specialist nurses who are members of a larger generic community children's nursing team and seen very much as part of the community children's nursing service and marketed as such (Fradd 1994, Gow 1996, Whyte et al 1998).

All organisations, in order to deliver a strategy (which advances its market position), require people to accept and believe in what the organisation is attempting to achieve (T Bottigliere, unpublished work, 1996). Whilst CCNs hold a strong belief in what their professional 'role and function' as a whole is attempting to achieve, between individual services numerous types of service models have led to individual marketing of each service and a lack of strategic direction and coordination. This may have weakened the organisation as a whole and led to confusion of (1) how community children's nursing is perceived and (2) why CCNs lack a professional or corporate image and identity.

CORPORATE IMAGE AND IDENTITY OF COMMUNITY CHILDREN'S NURSES

Large established community children's nursing services are able to achieve a corporate identity within their area and thus promote the service. This was reflected in a study undertaken by management following the expansion of the Southampton service (Gow 1996). The study had three main aims:

- to increase General Practitioner (GP) and consultant awareness of the service
- to evaluate GP and consultant views on the service and how they would like it to develop to effectively meet the needs of their practice population
- to develop a market strategy for community children's community nursing.

A high response rate to the survey was noted and Gow maintains that many of the responses reflected an unexpected understanding of the service.

Literature that looks at corporate identity within the health service often refers to bright hospital signs and logos. Internet searches reveal companies promoting identity by designs. One company defines corporate identity as not just a logo or name of a company, although these are the most visible of its components, but as what makes a company special and unique. They conclude that corporate identity expresses the company's approach to business, its values and business culture is reflected in everything from the quality of products, services, marketing strategies, communication media and working environment (Global Logo Designs 2002).

Conversely, Eaton (1993) believes corporate identity is only a small part of the marketing process, not about selling or promoting but rather understanding customer needs. According to Eaton a service cannot be promoted unless it has an identity, thus, to promote an identity the service has to understand:

- how it is perceived now
- what it wants in the future
- what key messages it wants to get across.

Payne (1993) asserts that corporate image is determined by the technical and functional quality of the service and that this, in turn, can influence the customers' (e.g. patients/Primary Care Trusts/Trusts) perceptions of service quality. Research to understand the factors influencing service quality was undertaken by Berry and Parasuraman in 1991 (cited in Payne 1993 p 221). Berry identified the following five key areas:

- tangibles – the physical facilities, equipment, appearance of personnel
- reliability – the ability to perform the desired service dependably, accurately and consistently
- responsiveness – willingness to provide prompt service and help customers
- assurance – employees' knowledge, courtesy and ability to convey trust and confidence
- empathy – caring, individualised attention to customers.

Within these key areas, community children's nursing services may lack some of the factors that influence quality, for example:

- The many types of services prevent the provision of one overall consistent and dependable national service.
- Services do not have equal facilities or provide the same equipment.
- The appearance of nursing staff differs in that uniforms, if worn, are not the same.
- Although willingness to provide a prompt service and help customers is valued by nursing staff, within the restrictions of many small services, this may be unachievable (Acornley 2002).

The successful and structured expansion of larger teams indicates they have achieved a corporate identity, are able to demonstrate quality, have a clear understanding of how they are perceived and are able to present key messages in the form of selling their services. Within smaller services however, managers with no understanding of community children's nursing can lack both vision and knowledge to take the service forward (Murphy 2001). These services fail to develop a corporate identity and are unable to sell their services and expand. The service manager should possess comprehensive understanding and experience of both children's and community nursing (Sidey 1995, Hughes 1997). Successful expanding teams with a strong corporate culture and professional identity have managers, preferably senior CCNs, who possess both qualities.

PROFESSIONAL IDENTITY OF COMMUNITY CHILDREN'S NURSES

The professional identity of nurses is often addressed in terms of related concepts including professionalism, perceptions of the nurse's role and the 'professional self' or 'self concept' of nurses (Fagermoen 1997, Ohlen & Segesten 1998). Fagermoen sees professionalism as:

- a framework used by professionals in identifying their work in a social role context
- professional identity, in terms of nurses' perception of the nurses' role, as focused on role content
- professional self concept as focused on the personal attributes brought to the role.

The lack of a readily identifiable professional image can affect collaboration with other professional groups due to the fact that there is no established stereotype (Hornby 1993). This was demonstrated in a study examining the relationships between CCNs and primary care nurses (Teare 2001). Expectations of the CCNs' roles were different for each professional group and how they would utilise the service was based on their perception of the role of the CCN in relationship to their own role. Thus small services with a poor identity have problems of acceptance by, and collaboration with, other services. Consequently they are unable to promote their service and attract funding for development.

Overall, community children's nursing services are unable to present unified technical and functional qualities to influence customers, that is stakeholders or commissioning trusts, and develop a corporate identity.

CCNs lack a readily identifiable professional image, which can ultimately affect the training and educational aspects of their role.

THE EFFECTS ON TRAINING AND EDUCATION

Larsen (1990) identified the central function of professions as that of 'organising the acquisition and certification of expertise in broad functional areas on the basis of formal educational qualifications held by individuals' (cited in Scott 1998 p 554). Larger community services have historically supported staff to undertake a community qualification and there is continued uptake of student places at the universities serving these teams (Moyse & Dryden 1999). The validation of courses in areas with limited or non-existent services would suggest an enthusiasm by educationalists and Trust managers to establish or extend provision of services with appropriately trained personnel (Neill & Muir 1997). This is not however reflected in the poor uptake of student places (Whiting 1997). The reasons identified in Box 10.2 reflect how both community children's nursing services and the role of the CCN are undervalued and poorly perceived by various Trusts. This ultimately has a direct influence on the availability of funding and workforce planning.

Box 10.2 Factors contributing to the poor uptake of CCN education (Burditt & Sidey 1999)

- Failure to obtain funding and/or secondment
- Failure of either non child or community managers to comprehend the value of the specialist course for CCNs
- Failure to comprehend that CCN education is funded in the same way as DN/HV education
- Difficulty in freeing up staff from understaffed existing community children's nursing services
- Lack of appropriate community placements and/or children's Community Practice Teachers
- Diversity of models of practice and content of courses/education in community children's nursing

---

Work force planning is only effective if a detailed needs assessment has taken place. DN and HV education have been established for many years and needs assessment has been viewed as part of their role (Cowley et al 1996) (see Chapter 17). The inability of CCNs to access training that includes community profiling and needs assessment may perpetuate the problems of recognition and development of community children's nursing. Without the appropriate skills to assess needs CCNs may not be able to affect workforce planning within their area, thus leading to a continuance of the cycle of problems pertaining to their education, recognition, development of services and development of a professional and corporate identity.

The diversity of service models may also affect the workforce planning and ultimate provision of education for CCNs. The perception of the service by the staff and management affects how those services view the need for CCN education (Marot 1993, Peter & Torr 1996, Hunt 1999). A hospital specialist outreach model may concentrate training on the particular disease, bypassing opportunities for community education. Specialist CCNs will benefit from dual qualifications in both community children's nursing and the disease in which they specialise. The results of an assessment of need for service provision and education may therefore be influenced by the views of the services already provided.

CONCLUSION

Community children's nursing services appear to have developed along two distinct pathways. Some teams, in particular those established within regional children's centres, have grown to provide a full range of care. They possess a strong corporate culture and professional image.

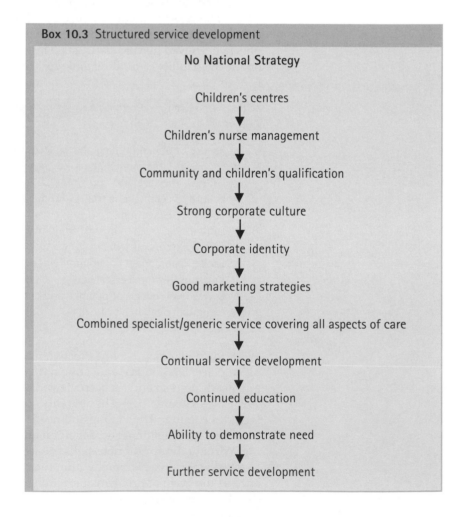

Box 10.3 Structured service development

No National Strategy

Children's centres
↓
Children's nurse management
↓
Community and children's qualification
↓
Strong corporate culture
↓
Corporate identity
↓
Good marketing strategies
↓
Combined specialist/generic service covering all aspects of care
↓
Continual service development
↓
Continued education
↓
Ability to demonstrate need
↓
Further service development

However, the development of teams in many areas is fragmented with patchy provision of care, mixed corporate cultures and mixed and often

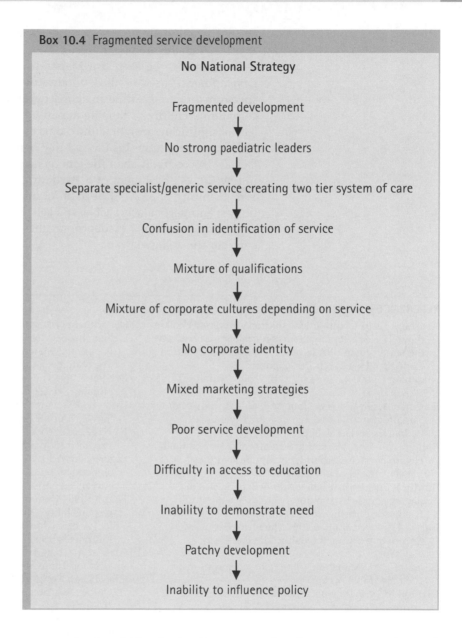

Box 10.4 Fragmented service development

No National Strategy

Fragmented development

↓

No strong paediatric leaders

↓

Separate specialist/generic service creating two tier system of care

↓

Confusion in identification of service

↓

Mixture of qualifications

↓

Mixture of corporate cultures depending on service

↓

No corporate identity

↓

Mixed marketing strategies

↓

Poor service development

↓

Difficulty in access to education

↓

Inability to demonstrate need

↓

Patchy development

↓

Inability to influence policy

poor professional identity leading to a cycle of events preventing real growth.

The children's National Service Framework aims to put into place national standards for children's services, built on the principle of collaborative work between agencies, focused on competencies and skills and not specific roles (DoH 2003, Maunder 2003). The benefit of this development may be lost in areas where community children's nursing does not enjoy a strong corporate and professional image as this principle may further weaken the identity of CCNs.

The money provided in memory of Diana, Princess of Wales was an opportunity to establish new community children's nursing teams and expand existing small services to provide care for children with life-limiting and -threatening illnesses.

It remains to be seen if a planned national strategy for all service development, based on those models of service able to provide the full spectrum of care, will be matched by clear and 'heroic' leadership of community children's nursing at national, regional and local levels. The lack of significant growth within some established teams could suggest a lack of power within this process that is mirrored within the RCN itself. Despite the recognition of the emergence of this field of children's nursing by the establishment of a Paediatric Community Nurses Forum in 1988 (Whiting et al 2001) Burr (in Chapter 4) maintains that children's nurses, and particularly CCNs, still lack a power base within the nursing profession. Anecdotal evidence suggests that a majority of CCNs also consider this to be so.

REFERENCES

Acornley J 2002 Community Children's Nurses. Who are they? The development of a corporate image could be the way forward. BA (Hons) Dissertation. Homerton College of Health Studies, Cambridge

Anderson P 2000 Taking care to the child. Nursing Times 17(33):51–53

Bergman A, Shrand H & Oppe M 1965 A pediatric home care program in London: ten years experience. Pediatrics 36(1):314–321

Bottigliere T 1996 Marketing Strategy and the National Health Service. Cambridge: Unpublished thesis. Master of Science in Management

Burditt J, Buckler K & Sidey A 1999 Experiences of a degree course in community children's nursing. Paediatric Nursing March 11(2):30–31

Bury L L & Parasuraman 1991 Marketing Services: Competing Through Quality. The Free Press, New York

Carnall C 1990 Managing Change in Organisations. Prentice Hall, London

Clayton M 1997 Traction at home: The Doncaster approach. Paediatric Nursing 9(2):21–23

Community Children's Nursing Forum 2002 Community Children's Nursing. Information for primary care organisations, strategic health authorities and all professional working with children in community settings. Royal College of Nursing, London

Cowley S, Bergen A, Young K & Kavanagh A 1996 Establishing a framework for research: the example of needs assessment. Journal of Clinical Nursing 5:53–61

Cystic Fibrosis Trust 2001 National Consensus Standards for the Nursing Management of Cystic Fibrosis. Cystic Fibrosis Trust, Bromley

Deal T E & Kennedy A A 1982 Corporate Cultures, the Rights of Corporate Life. Addison-Wesley, Reading, MA, USA

Department of Health 2003 Getting The Right Start: The National Service Framework for Children, Young People and Maternity Services – Emerging Findings. The Stationery Office, London

Dryden S 1994 The Nottingham Paediatric Community Nursing Service. Cascade 13:8–9

Eaton L 1993 More than just a pretty picture. Health Service Journal 12 August:29–30

Eaton N 2001 Models of community children's nursing. Paediatric Nursing February 13(1):32–36

Fagermoen M S 1997 Professional identity: values embedded in meaningful nursing practice. Journal of Advanced Nursing 25:434–441

Fradd E 1994 Community paediatric services: Whose responsibility? Nursing Times 90(6):34–37

Gillet J A 1954 Children's nursing unit. British Medical Journal 684:1954

Glasper A, Gow M & Yerrell P 1989 A family friend. Nursing Times 85(4):63–65

Global Logo Designs 2002 Creating a Corporate Identity. Online. Available: http://www.globallogodesigns.com 10 April 2004

Glueck W F 1980 Business policy and strategic management. McGraw-Hill, New York

Gow M 1996 Paediatric community nursing: doctors' views. Professional Nurse March 11(6):365–367

Gow M & Atwell J 1980 The role of the children's nurse in the community. Journal of Pediatric Surgery 15(1):26–30

Health Committee 1997 Third Report: Health Services for Children and Young People in the Community: Home and School. The Stationery Office, London

Hornby S 1993 Collaborative Care. Interprofessional, Interagency and Interpersonal. Oxford: Blackwell Scientific Publications

Hughes J 1997 Reflections on a community children's nursing service. Paediatric Nursing May 9(4):21–23

Hunt J 1999 A specialist nurse: an identified professional role or a personal agenda? Journal of Advanced Nursing 30(3):704–712

Jennings P 1994 Learning through experience: an evaluation of 'Hospital at Home' Journal of Advanced Nursing 19:905–911

Kay J 1996 The business of economics. Oxford University Press, Oxford

Larsen M S 1990 In the matter of experts and professionals, or how impossible it is to leave nothing unsaid. In: The Formation of Professions: Knowledge, State and Strategy. Torstendahl R & Burrage M (eds). Sage, London, pp 24–50

Marot F J 1993 A bridge from hospital to home: The role of the liaison neonatal nurse. Professional Nurse April:469–472

Maunder E Z 2003 Community children's nursing services: the need for development. Paediatric Nursing November 15(9):20–23

Mintzberg H, Quinn J B & Ghosal S 1998 The Strategy Process. Prentice Hall, London

Moyse K & Dryden S 1999 A degree in community children's nursing. Nursing Times 95(36):49–50

Muir J 1999 Advanced Practice in the Community. A nurse-led clinic for children with chronic constipation. Presented to the conference 'Advancing practice in children's nursing', Institute of Child Health, London, 19th February 1999

Murphy W 2001. Leadership and community children's nurses. Paediatric Nursing 13(10):36–40

Neill S & Muir J 1997 Educating the new Community Children's Nurses: challenges and opportunities? Nurse Education Today 17:7–15

Ohlen J & Segesten J 1998 The professional identity of the nurse: concept analysis and development. Journal of Advanced Nursing 28(4):720–727

Payne A 1993 The Essence of Service Marketing. Prentice Hall, London

Peter S & Torr G 1996 Paediatric Hospital at Home: the first year. Paediatric Nursing 8(5):20–24

Royal College of Nursing (RCN) 2004 Directory of Community Children's Nursing Services 16th edn. RCN, London

Scott C 1998 Specialist practice: advancing the profession? Journal of Advanced Nursing 28(3):554–562

Sidey A 1995 Competence for Community Health Care Nursing (Children). In: Sines D (ed.) Community Healthcare Nursing. London: Blackwell Science, Oxford

Tatman M & Woodroffe C 1993 Paediatric home care in the UK. Archives of Disease in Childhood 69:677–680

Tatman M, Woodroffe C, Kelly P & Harris R 1992 Paediatric home care in Tower Hamlets: a working partnership with parents. Quality in Health Care 1:98–103

Teare J 2001 Professional relationships: CCNs and primary care nurses. Journal of Child Health Care 5(2):60–64

Whiting M 1997 Community children's nursing: A bright future? Paediatric Nursing May 9(4):6–8

Whiting M, Greene A & Walker A 2001 Community Children's Nursing – Delivering on the 'Quality Agenda' In: Sines D, Appleby F & Raymond E (eds) Community Healthcare Nursing. 2nd edn. London: Blackwell Science, Oxford

Whyte D, Barton M E, Lamb A, Magennis C, Mallinson A, Marshall L, Oliver R, Reid P, Richardson H & Walford C 1998 Clinical effectiveness in community children's nursing. Clinical Effectiveness in Nursing 2:139–144

Winfield P, Bishop R & Porter K 2000 Core Management for HR Students and Practitioners. Butterworth-Heinemann, Oxford

Winter A & Teare J 1997 Construction and application of paediatric community nursing services. Journal of Child Health Care 1(1):24–27

Chapter 11

Nursing the family and supporting the nurse: exploring the nurse–patient relationship in community children's nursing

Brian Samwell

KEY ISSUES

- Value and dangers of intense relationships between the community children's nurse and clients in the context of chronic childhood illness.
- Family-centred care.
- Key factors in managing intense relationships with children and families, on both an individual and a team level.

INTRODUCTION

What is special about community children's nursing? As nurses we can focus on the increasing range of technical and practical care options that we can create in the community. As healthcare activists we can claim our role in redefining the nature of healthcare for children, moving the focus from hospital to community care. Yet many community children's nurses (CCNs) agree that their speciality is defined by the nature of the relationship they have with children and families. This chapter explores some aspects of that relationship and, in doing so, tries to define what is uniquely satisfying but also uniquely dangerous about the CCN's role. To do this, it focuses on the times when that relationship is most intense – when care is given to a child with a chronic or life-threatening illness or condition.

CARE OF THE CHILD WITH A CHRONIC ILLNESS

Care of the child with a chronic or serious illness presents a particular nursing challenge. While illness at any age is characterised by crisis and adaptation, in childhood this is superimposed on rapid physical, psychological and social growth. As the child grows, the manifestation and impact of the illness alters, and the psychological and social effects evolve. Such changes carry a potential for distress and psychological damage, often as great as the physical condition itself. This is highlighted by the fact that ill children show a higher incidence of behavioural problems and emotional difficulties than well children (Davis 1993).

The diagnosis of a serious childhood illness is also a crisis for parents. The illness threatens parents' ability to care for and protect their child and so becomes an attack on their own psychological integrity. They may grieve for the child and the anticipated future they have lost. Subsequent developments in diagnosis, condition or disability may compound and renew this sense of loss (Eiser 1993). Amidst this wholesale change in child and family expectations there is a demand to learn new skills: in nursing, in seeking information, and in dealing with a host of professional helpers. Family stress is inevitable, and both physical and psychological morbidity are a common consequence (Cairns 1992).

For the CCN to work effectively with these children and their carers, an understanding is needed of the problems and issues peculiar to care in this context. The nurse also needs a model of working which can sustain and make sense of a long-term supportive relationship rather than brief acute interventions. In the context of learning disability Madden noticed 'Parents are at the start of a life long journey they did not bargain for. They need to know professionals are going to be with them' (Madden 1995 p 91). A supportive relationship with the child and family, which engages with problems as defined and experienced by them, is a central part of the CCN's role (Procter et al 1998). It is also the medium through which long-term therapeutic goals of child and family health, self-efficacy and empowerment might be attained. CCNs need both to understand and to work with this relationship.

FAMILY-CENTRED CARE

The most commonly used conception of the relationship between nurse and client is that of family-centred care. It is a phrase that has become the touchstone for children's nursing practice in the UK. Indeed, community children's nursing owes its origins to a belief in the benefits of nursing children in the safe and familiar home environment (Royal College of Nursing 1994, 2000). The needs of the child are considered within the context of the family unit where family members are seen as the primary carers and effective care depends on negotiation and partnership. However the reality of social life stands in sharp contrast to any simple stereotype of the nuclear family. To work effectively within complex and varied family relationships can require quite exceptional insight and interpersonal skill (Muir & Sidey, 2003). A range of these skills is suggested in Shelton et al's (1987) framework for family-centred care (Box 11.1).

While family-centred care gives a welcome emphasis to the nursing relationship, in practice it has shortcomings. First, it tends to be stated as a service philosophy with little exploration of the very difficult professional, ethical and political issues raised by a comprehensive definition such as Shelton's. Second, it does not deal with the mutual effects of creating a relationship. CCNs often work in isolation within exceptionally

> **Box 11.1** A framework for family-centred care (Shelton et al 1987)
>
> - Recognition that the family is the constant in the child's life, whereas the service systems and personnel within those systems fluctuate
> - Facilitation of parent–professional collaboration at all levels of healthcare
> - Sharing of unbiased and complete information with parents about their child's care on an ongoing basis in an appropriate and supportive manner
> - Implementation of appropriate policies and programmes that are comprehensive and provide emotional and financial support to meet families' needs
> - Recognition of family strengths and individuality, and respect for different methods of coping
> - Understanding and incorporating the developmental and emotional needs of infants, children and adolescents, and their families into healthcare delivery systems
> - Encouragement and facilitation of parent to child support
> - Assurance that the design of healthcare delivery systems is flexible, accessible and responsive to family need

difficult situations. A nurse may need to work with 30–50 families, many of whom will be suffering extreme physical and emotional turmoil. The personal and practical implications of such care are the concern of the remainder of this chapter.

This chapter draws on the results of a pilot study which used the qualitative methodology of naturalistic inquiry to investigate the ways in which CCNs experience and manage long-term, intense relationships with families (Samwell 1999). The study involved interviews with four practising nurses drawn from community children's nursing teams in northern England. Their accounts were analysed to map out the phenomenon of their involvement with families. To make the accounts more personal yet maintain confidentiality, fictitious names have been given to the four nurses.

REWARDS AND DANGERS OF THE NURSE–CLIENT RELATIONSHIP

Like many healthcare workers, CCNs see their relationships with clients as one of the most satisfying parts of their work. All of the nurses in the study reported that their relationship with children and parents was intensely rewarding, often giving them a reason to 'keep going' in a difficult and demanding job. They found the relationships to be more intense and more productive than those experienced in hospital, so much so that two of the nurses said they would never consider moving out of community nursing.

While the client relationship in community children's nursing can give a uniquely rewarding work experience, it can also draw nurses into an ever-closer involvement with the families. Care in the home does not have the same inhibitions on involvement and intimacy as care in the busy hospital ward (May 1995, Totka 1996). Since most CCNs can ensure the continuity of their care, there is a greater potential to form personal bonds. Added to this, the nurse may identify closely with the family and the care situation, and find her nursing role confused by her personal roles of parent or protector (McAliley et al 1996). As a nurse in this study commented:

'You know how it feels not to have slept for the majority of the night and then to look after someone during the day, who is even more demanding than a normal healthy child. And how lucky I am to have two healthy kids really.'

In some circumstances close identification can lead the nurse to become a family friend or even to be seen as a part of the extended family. Yet such apparently simple human gestures can have dramatic personal effects. Participants described how their private time and emotional energy were absorbed by their personal commitment to families. As an example, the act of giving a home phone number could mean that the nurse was in effect never off duty:

'when I was at home I never felt as if I was off duty unless we went away. You couldn't have a drink, or I didn't feel I could have a drink at night just in case someone rang.'

Other examples of commitment included babysitting, visiting and socialising with families outside work hours, the giving of gifts, and helping families with all manner of personal favours. Jane described the temptation to try to organise everything for a family, to become a 'supernurse':

'You try to fill in all the forms for them [laughs], you know, sort the prescriptions out, take out the supplies and things like that, rather than sometimes saying "Look! This is how you go about it ... ".'

The participants described not just their own emotional difficulties in moving on from close relationships, but also the potential hurt for the family when the attachment was broken. Dependency could become both a professional and a personal problem, as Mary found:

'They know all about me and how do I separate, extricate myself from this?'

The challenge of managing this boundary between a personal and a professional involvement became the focus for this study. What follows are just two of the significant themes that summarise the experiences and concerns of this group of nurses. The themes highlight aspects of practice that either help or hinder the nurse who is struggling to maintain balance in her relationships with clients.

BEING FRIENDLY AND PROFESSIONAL

For nurses, conscious of the power and danger that lie within their relationships with families, there was a need consciously to regulate self-presentation, so as to prioritise their professional responsibilities. Sarah described this regulation as 'being friendly and professional'. While there was the potential to be seen as a friend, the nurses saw the inequality in that friendship: 'they see you as a friend but you don't necessarily see them as a friend'. Honesty in the relationship required the drawing of a line between being friendly and being a friend.

Being friendly was the use of interpersonal skills to communicate an interest and commitment: 'You give the smiles, you laugh and you might give some information away about your personal life'. It included being attentive to the needs of child and family, and pacing communication so as to establish confidence and trust. But it also required a certain distance and objectivity. As Jane described, when wrestling with this dilemma:

> 'I think … just a minute, it isn't acceptable to be there. I can't be objective. I can't be what I need to be for them if I'm too close, even though they want me to be that close.'

For Jane this objectivity was a necessary part of her professional standing: an ability to step back from the complexity of the family's problems in order to help them in their decision making, and to empower them rather than create dependence. The participants drew on their assessment skills and their experience in order to judge the fine line between commitment and over-involvement. Sarah described some of the guidelines she used:

> 'If I get drawn into conversations where families will say … "if you want to pop round for a drink or whatever?" … I will be quite firm about it and say no. I've learned to say now I don't mix business with pleasure really, which is not always easy.'

> 'Now one thing a colleague said to me … if she finds that she is getting into a situation where this is happening (becoming over-involved) she actually will mentally say to herself 'Who are you doing this for?' … if you at any point say you are not doing it for the family you're doing it for yourself, then you have gone too far.'

Such management requires sensitivity, emotional intelligence and skill. Jane noted the subtle signals that she might unwittingly give to a family by offering too much information about her personal life. The exchange of information had to be managed gently but firmly, to avoid signalling that a more personal friendship was possible or desirable. Such management required personal insight whereby the nurse could see the effect of her own needs, perhaps for affection or a 'need to be needed', which might drive her into a more intimate relationship.

THE LEARNING AND SHARING TEAM

The sharing of concern and commitment between nurse, child and family is clearly an aspect of personal practice. Yet the respondents in this study indicated the links between their personal practice and the wider world of team and health service organisation. Lack of resources was a key factor in forcing these nurses to over-commit themselves. Many families simply did not have the resources or continuity of support they needed so, driven by compassion and a sense of duty, the nurse was forced to give her personal time and commitment.

The history of community children's nursing has been marked by piecemeal investment with teams struggling to improve the quality and accessibility of their services (Health Committee 1997, Whiting 1997, see Chapters 2 and 10). All the respondents had experienced the danger and demoralisation of working in isolation either as a 'team' of one or within teams that had found no way of sharing the burdens of care. Yet these nurses also described how their teams had learned to respond to the private and personal demands of community children's nursing practice. These responses could be placed in two broad categories.

Creating a trusting and collaborative work environment

The ability of the team to share concerns and experiences was crucial. This did not mean that the team had to be a team of personal friends but rather that communication within the team was actively prioritised and managed. Such communication took place on many levels from the basic sharing of information, so that all the team had some awareness of the work and concerns of individuals, to a sharing of feelings and a sensitivity to the pressures on colleagues. Ann and Jane could seek help from team members when they found they had got themselves into difficult situations with particular families. Their trust in colleagues meant that they did not always have to be seen to be coping with the demands of the job but could ask for and expect both practical and emotional support.

All four nurses held their own caseloads yet their teams had found ways to overcome the natural territoriality that comes with deep involvement. They were able to share knowledge of children and families and, on occasions, share the practical involvement. Jane felt that this sharing gave her 'breathing space' in intense relationships that could at times seem unrelenting. For both Sarah and Jane it reduced dependence on them as individuals. The family could also benefit from the involvement of other team members who were less tied to the history and emotions in a situation. In addition, it gave the family access to the breadth of expertise of the whole nursing team. Such sharing could be powerful and enlightening:

> 'Well you just seem to be plodding along [with a care problem] and then, all of a sudden, it takes somebody else just to say "Perhaps you should have tried this".'

Team organisation

The participants had recognised the dangers of working in isolation and had developed practical ways of working collaboratively. Measures included a very basic commitment to sharing:

> 'Every day we go through all the patients that we have seen that morning and we discuss all the patients we have seen.' 'Not all the members of the team know all the children but as long … as two or three members of the team know the child then that way we do get some continuity for sickness, annual leave and all these sort of things.'

Team meetings were given a high priority and there was a willingness to discuss the interpersonal as well as the clinical dimensions of care. Ways were found for caseloads to be shared so that all the team members had some knowledge of the children on other caseloads. For one team it was a matter of principle that the named nurse would take the lead in establishing the relationship with a family but would then, over a period of weeks or months, gradually introduce the family to other team members. Families could come to see that care was not being delivered by one individual but by the whole team. For these nurses such very basic working practice was fundamental in helping them to cope with the stresses of their work. Perhaps such organisation appears exceptional only for nurses who had experienced the effect of its absence.

CONCLUSION

What does this exploratory study tell us about community children's nursing practice? First, it confirms the findings of studies by While (1991), Procter et al (1998) and others that the creation and maintenance of a supportive relationship with child and parent is an essential part of the CCN's role. Technical skills and clinical activity are vital but they do not define the work. Clearly a competence in interpersonal communication deserves much stronger emphasis in both the recruitment and training of CCNs. The management of relationships and relationship boundaries needs to be placed firmly on the educational agenda.

However, relationships are not determined solely by the ability or needs of the individual nurse. A nurse's skill or 'need to be needed' sit alongside other variables which may dictate the course of the relationship such as the family's lack of resources or the nurse's want of practical and emotional support. Managers, planners and politicians must share responsibility for the personal consequences of under-resourced services. We need to ensure that effective, responsive care can be provided without sacrificing the personal time and resources of individual nurses. Similarly, community children's nursing teams have to examine the effect of their team organisation on individual team members, recognising situations where territoriality or individualised working are unhealthy or indeed dangerous.

This study demonstrated that the creation and management of working relationships is complex and demanding. CCNs do have difficulty in identifying the boundaries between their personal and their professional involvement with families. These participants gave examples of crossing the line, of becoming too deeply involved, which were very similar to the behaviours described by Totka and others (Coffman 1995, Totka 1996). However, the study did not find any simple list of rules that might serve to define or limit the nursing relationship. As Sarah found, she had personal guidelines, gleaned from many years of experience, but these were not written in stone and did not give a recipe for managing her relationships with children and families. Complex situations demand flexible responses.

The participants in this pilot study revealed just the tip of an iceberg of 'situational knowledge' or 'know-how' which they had acquired over time as expert practitioners in their field (Rolfe 1997). The nature of such learning presents both personal and professional challenges to CCNs. We have to find ways to uncover and share experience and expertise. Reflective practice might help to translate this personal experience into the public knowledge necessary to inform the next generation of CCNs. Clinical supervision has an important role in opening up and sharing the personal aspects of work relationships. Clearly there is also an urgent need to continue an exploration of the theoretical basis of community children's nursing practice (see Introduction and Chapter 33).

Managing relationships with other people is central to the human experience. For CCNs it is also a crucial factor in effective therapeutic interventions with families exposed to the devastating effects of childhood illness and disability. Through exploring the nature of our relationships we can hope both to increase the power and influence of community children's nursing and to reduce the quite exceptional demands made on the nurses who give that care.

REFERENCES

Cairns I 1992 The health of mothers and fathers of a child with a disability. Health Visitor 65(7):238–239

Coffman S 1995 Crossing lines: parents' experiences with paediatric nurses in the home. Rehabilitation Nursing Research 4(4):136–143

Davis H 1993 Counselling Parents of Children with Chronic Illness and Disability. British Psychological Society, Leicester

Eiser C 1993 Growing up with a Chronic Disease. Kingsley, London

Health Committee 1997 House of Commons Health Select Committee. Health services for children and young people in the community: home and school. Third report. The Stationery Office, London

McAliley L, Ashenberg M, Lambert S & Dull S 1996 Therapeutic relations decision making: the Rainbow framework. Pediatric Nursing 22(3):199–203

Madden P 1995 Why parents: how parents. British Journal of Learning Disabilities 23:90–93

May C 1995 Patient autonomy and the politics of professional relationships. Journal of Advanced Nursing 21:83–87

Procter S, Biott C, Campbell S, Edward S, Redpath N & Moran M 1998 Preparation for the Developing Role of the Community Children's Nurse. English National Board, London

Rolfe G 1997 Beyond expertise: theory, practice and the reflexive practitioner. Journal of Clinical Nursing 6:93–97

Royal College of Nursing 1994 Wise Decisions: Developing Paediatric Home Care Teams. Royal College of Nursing, Paediatric Community Nurses Forum, London

Royal College of Nursing (RCN) 2000 Children's Community Nursing. Promoting effective team-working for children and their families. RCN, London

Samwell B 1999 Relationship Boundaries in Community Children's Nursing. MA dissertation, University of Sheffield

Shelton T, Jepson E & Johnson B 1987 Family Centred Care of Children with Special Health Care Needs. Association for the Care of Children's Health, Washington, DC

Totka J 1996 Exploring the boundaries of paediatric practice: nurse stories related to relationships. Pediatric Nursing 22(3):191–196

While A 1991 An evaluation of a paediatric home care scheme. Journal of Advanced Nursing 16:1413–1421

Whiting M 1997 Community children's nursing: a bright future? Paediatric Nursing 9(4):6–8

Whyte D 1992 A family nursing approach to the care of a child with a chronic illness. Journal of Advanced Nursing 17:326–327

Chapter 12

Legal aspects of the community care of the sick child

Bridgit Dimond

KEY ISSUES

- The law and guidance.
- Accountability.
- Accountability for negligent advice and instruction.
- Parental sharing in the care.
- Decision making and disputes with parents.
- Consent by the child: 16 and 17 years; under 16 years.
- Confidentiality.
- Children Act 1989; child protection issues.
- Parental rights and responsibilities.
- Education.
- Palliative and terminal care.
- Changing National Health Service structure: Primary Care Trusts, care trusts and children's trusts; clinical governance, National Institute of Clinical Excellence, Commission for Healthcare Audit and Inspection and Commission for Social Care Inspection.
- Role of the voluntary sector.

INTRODUCTION

This chapter provides the reader with the framework for the law that relates to the care of the sick child in the community (Dimond 2004). Further reading is offered for those who wish to study the law in more depth. The law relating to the care of sick children derives mainly from statutes (i.e. Acts of Parliament) and case law (otherwise known as common law or judge made law).

Increasingly there are international charters that set out the rights of the child. The United Nations Convention on the Rights of the Child was adopted on 20 November 1989. It is not directly enforceable in the courts

> **Box 12.1** Statutes relating to the care of sick children
>
> - Family Law Reform Act 1969, section 8
> - Children Act 1989
> - Education Act 1993
> - Education Act 1996
> - Health Services Act 1999
> - Health and Social Care Act 2000
> - Carers and Disabled Children Act 2000
> - Special Educational Needs and Disability Act 2001
> - NHS Reform and Health Care Professions Act 2002
> - Health and Social Care (Community Health and Standards) Act 2003

of England and Wales but observance of the convention principles is monitored on a biennial basis (HL Paper 117). The European Convention of Human Rights, to which this country was a signatory in 1951, has in the past been enforceable by application to the Court in Strasbourg. However, with the enactment of the Human Rights Act 1998, the articles of the convention have been directly enforceable in the courts of England and Wales from 2000 (in Scotland from devolution). For example, article 3 states that 'no person should be subjected to torture or to inhuman or degrading treatment or punishment'. It may be that some of the conditions in which sick children in the community are being kept are in breach of this article. Another important article for children is Article 8, which states that everyone has a right 'to respect for private and family life, his home and his correspondence'.

The child would have a right to take action in the courts of this country against any public organisation or organisation that performs public functions. Other charitable organisations have drawn up charters promoting standards in the care of children, but these, like the Patient's Charter (Department of Health 1992), are not directly enforceable in the courts of England and Wales. National Service Frameworks (NSFs) are being developed under the aegis of the DoH to establish standards for children's services (see Chapter 3 p 46). This was a recommendation of the Kennedy Report (Learning from Bristol 2001).

ACCOUNTABILITY

All professionals caring for sick children in the community are personally and professionally accountable for any harm that they cause or for any failure to follow an approved standard of care. Any person at fault could face criminal proceedings, civil proceedings, disciplinary proceedings brought by the employer and professional conduct proceedings by the registration body: Nursing and Midwifery Council (NMC), the General Medical Council (GMC) or the Health Professions Council (HPC).

Criminal proceedings

An unexpected death would be followed by an investigation by the coroner, who can order an autopsy to be performed and decide whether an inquest should be held. At any stage in the proceedings the coroner can adjourn the inquest for criminal proceedings to take place. Gross negligence or recklessness which led to the death of the child could be subject to criminal proceedings and a health professional could be liable for the death if his or her gross recklessness caused the death (R v Adomako 1994).

Civil proceedings

Health professionals owe a duty of care to the patient. Failure to provide a reasonable standard of care, which results in reasonably foreseeable harm, could lead to a civil action for compensation. The child's parents could sue on behalf of the child but if they fail to do so the child has 3 years from attaining the age of majority (i.e. 18 years) to sue on his or her own behalf for harm caused while a child. The action would be brought against the employer of the health professional, since the employer is vicariously liable for the negligence of an employee whilst acting in the course of employment. For example, a child might suffer from pressure sores as a result of failure to protect tissue viability. It may be that the community children's nurse (CCN) has failed to ensure that parents have been provided with a pressure-relieving mattress for their child or the CCN has failed to provide instruction on how to care for the child appropriately. The determination of whether there is a breach of the duty of care is based on what has become known as the Bolam Test, that is, what is the reasonable standard of care?

> '(A doctor) is not guilty of negligence if he has acted in accordance with a practice accepted as proper by a responsible body of medical men skilled in that particular art ... Putting it the other way round, a man is not negligent, if he acts in accordance with such a practice, merely because there is a body of opinion who would take a contrary view'
>
> (Bolam v Friern Hospital Management Committee 1957)

The House of Lords has emphasised that experts who give their opinion on what would be competent practice must ensure that such expert opinion flows logically, and reasonably, from the specific circumstances:

> 'The use of the adjectives "responsible, reasonable and respectable" (in the Bolam case) all showed that the court had to be satisfied that the exponents of the body of opinion relied upon could demonstrate that such opinion had a logical basis.'
>
> (Bolitho v City & Hackney Health Authority 1997)

In time, guidance given by the National Institute for Clinical Excellence (NICE), standards contained in the NSFs and recommendations made by NICE, Commission for Healthcare Audit and Inspection (CHAI) and Commission for Social Care Inspection may well be incorporated into the Bolam Test for reasonable practice. It would, however, always be possible for a health professional to argue that the particular circumstances of the patient required differences to standards set in local policies, procedures or protocols. Health professionals will always have to use their judgement over what is appropriate according to the individual circumstances of the patient.

Accountability for negligent advice and instruction

If a health professional were to give negligent advice to a patient or to the carers and, in reliance on that advice, harm was caused, then, if the advice was given knowing that it would be relied upon, the health professional or the employer could be held accountable and required to pay compensation. A physiotherapist might instruct parents on how to carry out percussion physiotherapy; if these instructions were negligent and the child suffered harm, the parents could sue the employer of the physiotherapist.

Disciplinary proceedings

Under the contract of employment, there are implied terms that require the employee to act with reasonable care and skill and to obey the reasonable instructions of the employer. Failure to comply with these implied terms could lead to disciplinary proceedings with the ultimate sanction of the employee being dismissed. The employee could bring an application for unfair dismissal to the employment tribunal, claiming compensation and reinstatement.

Professional conduct proceedings

A registered employee is subject to professional conduct proceedings by his or her own registration body. At present the NMC, GMC and HPC all have different definitions of the nature of misconduct that could lead to a striking off the register. A registered nurse could be guilty of professional misconduct if she has failed to follow the principles set out in the Code of Professional Conduct. A Council for the Regulation of Health Care Professions has been set up under the NHS Reform and Health Care Professions Act 2002 and its work will probably lead eventually to greater uniformity across the different health professions' regulatory bodies.

PARENTAL SHARING IN THE CARE; DECISION MAKING AND DISPUTES WITH PARENTS

Community care of the sick child is a partnership between the multi-agency, multiprofessional team and the family. Health professionals have a considerable responsibility to ensure that the family and other carers have the necessary instructions to enable the child to be safely cared for. For example, the role of a domiciliary physiotherapist in the treatment of children with cystic fibrosis was reviewed by Rogers and Goodchild (1996). They show that the provision of a domiciliary physiotherapy service for cystic fibrosis has been a major development, allowing patients and their families increased access to physiotherapy both in the clinic and at home. Compliance with physiotherapy has been improved by discussion and demonstration in the home. They conclude that there is room for improvement in the service, but more detailed feedback is required from patients and their families.

Sometimes parents are asked to sign an exemption form when they undertake treatments at home. Such notices would be invalid if they were relied upon to exempt the health professional from liability for negligence. For example, parents might agree that they will undertake intravenous administration of drugs at home for their child. They may be asked to sign a form, which states that they have had reasonable instruction and will not hold the Trust or its employees liable for any harm that occurs. If the nurse instructing the parents on how to carry out the intravenous injections fails to tell them about warning signs such as a rash or sudden change in temperature, for example, and the child were to suffer harm, the notice the parents signed would not prevent the Trust being held vicariously liable for the negligence of its staff. The Unfair Contract Terms Act 1977 prevents a person from relying on a notice or contract term to exempt him or her from negligence if personal injury or death is caused. A notice can be relied upon for exemption for negligence that leads to damage or loss of property, if such reliance is considered reasonable.

Good communication with parents would be considered to be part of the duty of care owed to the child, and health professionals should ensure that parents have easy contact with health professionals for advice and support.

CONSENT BY THE CHILD: 16 AND 17 YEARS; UNDER 16 YEARS

The Family Law Reform Act 1969 states that a child of 16 or 17 years has a statutory right to give consent to medical, surgical and dental treatment, and this includes diagnostic procedures and other ancillary procedures including anaesthetics. At 18 years the child becomes an adult and no person can then give consent on their behalf, including the parents. In the case of mental incapacity of an adult, others can act in the best interests of that person on the basis of the common law power to act out of necessity recognised by the House of Lords in the case of F v West Berkshire Health Authority (1989).

The parent can also give consent on behalf of a child up to the age of 18 years. Where a child of 16 or 17 years is refusing treatment that is in their best interests, the refusal of the child can, in exceptional circumstances, be over-ruled. This was the principle established by the Court of Appeal in the case of Re: W (1992), when it upheld the decision of the High Court judge to order a child of 16 years who was suffering from anorexia nervosa to undergo medical treatment against her will.

Jehovah's Witness parents of a boy aged 15 years, who was suffering from leukaemia, pleaded with the court that his refusal to have a blood transfusion should be upheld, but they were over-ruled on the grounds that the boy needed the transfusion as part of his treatment (Re: E, Family Division 1993).

A child below the age of 16 years does not have a statutory right to give consent to treatment, but the House of Lords has held that if the child is competent to understand the nature of the proposed treatment and its effects then he or she can give a valid consent to treatment (Gillick v West Norfolk and Wisbech Area Health Authority 1986). As a result of this case (which was brought by Mrs Gillick, who claimed that a DoH memorandum permitting doctors to give family planning advice to girls under 16 years without parental involvement was invalid), we now have the expression 'Gillick competent'. Where a child is refusing treatment which is in their best interests, parents could give consent to the treatment proceeding. However the older the child, the more preferable it is for an application to be made to court to determine whether the treatment should proceed in the child's best interests. Thus in the case of Re: M (1999) a girl of 15 years refused to have a heart transplant which was essential for her survival. The parents sought an injunction from the court that the transplant operation could proceed and this was granted in the best interests of the child.

CONFIDENTIALITY

General

There is a duty of care, originating in professional codes of conduct and also under the Data Protection Act 1998 (which applies to both computerised and manual records), to respect the confidentiality of information about the child and family. However, this is subject to many exceptions (Box 12.2).

Box 12.2 Exceptions to the duty of confidentiality

1. Consent of the parents (and of child if 'Gillick competent')
2. In the best interests of the patient
3. Order of court
4. Statutory exceptions (e.g. notification of infectious diseases)
5. Public interest

Information provided by the child

Where the child gives information to the health professional in the expectation that this will be kept secret, including from the parents, the health professional should warn the child that an absolute assurance of confidentiality can not be given. Clearly, the younger the child, the less likely it will be that information will be kept from the parents. If the child is reporting abuse of any kind, the health professional would have a duty to initiate appropriate steps in accordance with the procedures for the Area Child Protection Committee.

Under Data Protection legislation a child can access his or her own health records, if he or she has the competence to make the request and understand the information. The Gillick test of competency would probably be applied. Access can however be withheld if it would cause serious harm to the physical or mental health or condition of the applicant or another person, or reveal the identity of a third person (not being a health professional involved in the care of the child) if that person has asked not to be identified.

CHILDREN ACT 1989; CHILD PROTECTION ISSUES

The Children Act 1989 provides a clear framework for the lawful intervention in the care of the child and for reconciling disputes between parents (Box 12.3). The involvement of the child in the decision making is clearly emphasised. It sets out the principles that should underline the care of children. The over-riding principle is that 'The child's welfare shall be the court's paramount consideration'.

In May 2003 the DoH launched a 'single source' document for safeguarding children with the aim that all agencies will be working from the same succinct set of advice (DoH 2003). The publication is the result of one of the recommendations of the Laming Inquiry which investigated the circumstances surrounding the death of Victoria Climbie (Laming 2003). The Inquiry made over 100 recommendations for future practice by health

> **Box 12.3** Principles of the Children Act 1989
>
> 1. The welfare of the child is the paramount consideration in court proceedings.
> 2. Wherever possible, children should be brought up/cared for in their own families.
> 3. Courts should ensure that delay is avoided and may make an order only if to do so is better than making no order at all.
> 4. Children should be kept informed about what happens to them and should participate when decisions are made about their future.
> 5. Parents continue to have parental responsibility for their children, even when their children are no longer living with them. They should be kept informed about their children and participate when decisions are made about their children's future.
> 6. Parents with children in need should be helped to bring up their children themselves.
> 7. This help should be provided as a service to the child and the family, and should:
>   - be provided in partnership with parents
>   - meet each child's identified needs
>   - be appropriate to the child's race/culture/religion/language
>   - be open to effective independent representations/complaints procedures
>   - draw upon effective partnership between the local authority/other agencies/voluntary agencies.

and social services. Emerging from these a new 'single source' booklet 'What to do if you're worried a child is being abused' sets out:

- What people should do if they have concerns about children.
- What will happen once they have informed someone about those concerns.
- What further contribution they may be asked or expected to make to the process of assessment, planning and working with children, reviewing that work and how they should share that information (DoH 2003).

PARENTAL RIGHTS AND RESPONSIBILITIES

Even after parents are divorced, both still retain responsibilities in relation to the child. If disputes arise between parents over the care and treatment of their children, an application can be made to court for a prohibited steps order. This will prevent certain action being taken in respect of a child, unless the court's agreement is obtained.

EDUCATION

Those caring for sick children should ensure that every effort is made to support their continuing tuition so they do not suffer educationally as a result of the illness. The education authority has a statutory duty to provide home tuition but this is subject to different interpretations.

The Education Act 1993, section 298(1), which came into effect on 1 September 1994 (now consolidated in the Education Act 1996) placed a duty on local education authorities to provide suitable full-time or part-time education for children of compulsory school age who, by reason of illness, exclusion from school or otherwise, may not for any period receive suitable education unless such arrangements are made for them. Health professionals should liaise with the parents, school and education authority to ensure that this statutory duty is met.

The Special Educational Needs and Disability Act (SENDA) 2001 makes significant changes to the rights of the disabled child within the context of education. Schedules to the SENDA cover amendments to Statement of Special Educational Needs: the Procedure and Appeals; definitions of the responsible bodies for schools and for educational institutions; and amendments and modifications to the Disability Discrimination Act 1995 and to the Disability Rights Commission Act 1999 and other legislation (see Chapter 7).

The Carers and Disabled Children Act 2000 enables vouchers to be provided for the purchase of services for children and requires local authorities to take account of the needs of carers in assessing the services that should be provided to a child.

PALLIATIVE AND TERMINAL CARE

Pressure may sometimes be brought upon health professionals to assist in the speedy death of a terminally ill child. It would be a criminal offence for the health professional or the parent/carer to undertake such an action. The law recognises no right to accelerate the process of dying. Such an action would constitute murder or manslaughter. This does not mean, however, that medication for pain relief cannot be given if an unintended effect of that medication is that life is thereby shortened. This was the ruling in the case of Dr Bodkin Adams (Bedford 1961). The law also draws a distinction between killing and letting die. The former is a criminal offence; the latter may be part of the duty of care. The House of Lords recognised the distinction in the Tony Bland case, when it allowed artificial feeding of a patient in a persistent vegetative state to be discontinued (Airedale NHS Trust v Bland 1993). Annie Lindsell, who suffered from motor neuron disease, brought an action in court for a declaration that her doctor would be allowed to let her die peacefully and with dignity, but withdrew her action after an assurance that that would be the doctor's duty of care to her, even though administration of pain relief may inadvertently shorten her life (Wilkins 1997). Subsequently Diane Pretty lost her case to obtain an advanced pardon from an offence under the Suicide Act 1961 were her husband to assist her to die. She had claimed that the Suicide Act was contrary to her human rights as set out in the European Convention on Human Rights, but she failed in both the English Courts and before the European Court of Human Rights (ECHR) in Strasbourg (Pretty v UK ECHR 2002). Diane Pretty suffered from motor neuron disease and whilst she could have refused food and drink and medical treatment, she needed a person's help to die. In contrast Miss B was paraplegic and was placed on a ventilator against her will. She applied to court for a declaration that the ventilator should be switched off. The Court had to decide if she was mentally competent and when this was established the judge made a declaration that it was lawful to switch off the ventilator according to her wishes. As a mentally competent person she has the right to make decisions about her healthcare (Miss B 2002).

The Association for Children with Life-threatening or Terminal Conditions and their Families (ACT) & the Royal College of Paediatrics and Child Health (RCPCH) developed a charter for the care of children (ACT & RCPCH 1997, 2003). It emphasises the principle that every child shall be treated with dignity and respect and shall be afforded privacy whatever the child's physical or intellectual ability. Guidance has also been published by a working party that included the British Paediatric Association and the King's Fund on the care of dying children and their families (Thornes 1988).

The changing NHS structure

The white paper on the NHS (DoH 1997) envisaged major reorganisation and new organisations within the NHS. In April 1999 the internal market in healthcare and general practitioner fundholding was abolished. Primary Care Groups (PCGs) in England (Local Health Groups in Wales) were established to arrange provision of healthcare for patients in their catchment area, including the agreements with providers for secondary and tertiary services. These PCGs have now received Trust status. The effect is that the emphasis in healthcare is on primary care. This may, therefore, give an impetus to the provision of more day surgery and increasing community care of sick children. Community child health professionals should be part of the multiprofessional team employed by the Primary Care Trust to provide care at home. Care trusts have also been established under the Health and Social Care Act 2001 which combines social service and health care provision in the one organisation.

In addition, the establishment of the NICE and the former Commission for Health Improvement (since April 2004 CHAI) should ensure that research findings on clinically effective care are disseminated and that research-based practice is implemented. CHAI has powers of inspection and audit. There is a statutory duty upon primary care and NHS Trusts to put and keep in place arrangements for the purpose of monitoring and improving the quality of healthcare provided to individuals and the environment in which such services are provided. In the Health Services Act 1999 healthcare is defined as meaning 'services for or in connection with the prevention, diagnosis or treatment of illness'. NSFs are being published across the specialities to ensure high standards of provision. An NSF for the community care of the sick child should assist professionals in pressing for the necessary resources to ensure high standards of care for children being cared for at home.

The legal effect of these statutory changes is that, in future, parents who claim that their child has suffered harm as a result of a failure to provide a reasonable standard of care can point to published league tables and national evidence of research and standards which local providers have not implemented. In other words, the Bolam Test, when applied to a situation of alleged negligence, will be based on these national standards.

Even where harm has not occurred (so an action for negligence is not possible), parents are still able to use national evidence to draw attention to deficits in local standards as the basis for a complaint. This, potentially, could have a positive influence on the development of community children's nursing services. Currently there are great inequalities; for example 20% of the country has no access to such services (Royal College of Nursing 2004). National standards should ensure that such inequalities are highlighted and ended.

ROLE OF THE VOLUNTARY SECTOR

No analysis of the care provided in the community for sick children would be complete without a consideration of the role that is increasingly being played by the voluntary sector. All health professionals should be sure that they are aware of the local services provided for children by the many charities that care for children and provide specific advice on different disorders. The organisation Action for Sick Children has published a charter on the rights of the child. Other charities provide hospice care and Macmillan nurses. Support from these voluntary groups can assist families in carrying the burden of a sick child and provide them with essential respite (see Chapter 6).

CONCLUSION

The pressure on those who care for sick children in the community will continue to increase: shorter lengths of stay, day surgery and the preferred option to avoid hospitalisation for sick children are leading to more children being cared for at home with increasingly complex technological equipment and treatment regimens. Community staff must ensure that they are competent to practice in new areas of professional development. In addition, they must be aware of the publications from the new NHS institutions on best practice and national standards and ensure that their local services meet increasingly higher standards of care.

The establishment of Children's Trusts should bring together in one single organisation all those statutory services which are responsible for providing services to children: thus health, social services, education and other services for children may be placed under one roof. This could have enormous impact on the role of the CCN. Clearly much discussion needs to take place to ensure that any new statutory arrangements do bring benefits to the care and quality of life of the individual child.

REFERENCES

Association for Children with Life-threatening or Terminal Conditions and their Families (ACT) & the Royal College of Paediatrics and Child Health 1997 & 2003 A guide to the Development of Children's Palliative Care Services. ACT, London

Bedford S 1961 The Best We Can Do. Penguin Books, London

Department of Health 1992 The patient's charter. HMSO, London

Department of Health 1997 The new NHS. Modern, dependable. The Stationery Office, London

Department of Health 2003 What To Do If You're Worried A Child Is Being Abused. The Stationery Office, London

Dimond B 2004 The Legal Aspects of Nursing, 4th edn. Pearson Education, Harlow

Health Committee 1997 House of Commons select committee. Health services for children and young people in the community: home and school. Third report. The Stationery Office, London

HL Paper 117 (incorporating HL paper 98.i and ii of 2003) HC 81 (incorporating HC 1103-I of 2001–02 and 81-I of 2002–03). The Stationery Office, London

Laming 2003 The Victoria Climbie Enquiry. The Stationery Office, London

Learning from Bristol 2001 The report of the public inquiry into children's heart surgery at the Bristol Royal Infirmary 1984–1995. The Stationery Office, London

Rogers D & Goodchild M 1996 Role of a domiciliary physiotherapist in the treatment of children with cystic fibrosis. Physiotherapy 82(7):396–402

Royal College of Nursing (RCN) 2004 Directory of Community Children's Nursing Services 16th edn. Community Children's Nursing Forum. RCN, London

Thornes R 1988 The care of dying children and their families. National Association of Health Authorities, Birmingham

Wilkins E 1997 Dying woman granted wish for dignified death. The Times 29 October

Legal cases

Airedale NHS Trust v Bland, House of Lords [1993] 1 All ER 821

Bolam v Friern Hospital Management Committee [1957] 2 All ER 118

Bolitho v City & Hackney Health Authority [1997] 3 WLR 1151

B (re) (consent to treatment: capacity), Times Law Report 26 March 2002 [2002] 2 ALL ER 449

F v West Berkshire Health Authority and another [1989] 2 All ER 545

Gillick v West Norfolk and Wisbech Area Health Authority [1986] 1 AC 112

Pretty v UK European Court of Human Rights Current Law 380 June 2002

R v Adomako [1994] 2 All ER 79

Re: M (medical treatment: consent) [1999] 2FLR 1097

Re: W (a minor) (medical treatment) [1992] 4 All ER 627

Re: E (a minor) (wardship: medical treatment) Family Division [1993] 1 FLR 386

Chapter 13

Health promotion in community children's nursing

Lisa Whiting and Sue Miller

KEY ISSUES
- Health.
- Health education and health promotion.
- Child health promotion.
- Health promotion within community children's nursing.

INTRODUCTION

This chapter explores the role of the community children's nurse (CCN) in child health promotion. Tannahill's model (1996) is used as a framework to aid consideration of the potential diversity of the role, but in the first instance, the concepts of 'health' and 'health promotion' will be clarified. This will be followed by a brief overview of the value of community involvement in health promotion initiatives and the importance of promoting health to children and their families.

HEALTH

The critical examination of 'health' is fundamental to the practice of health promotion. Without an understanding of its many perspectives, there is a danger that professionals will 'continue to do what they have always done, because they know that they are right' (Seedhouse 1986 p 9). A great many authors have debated the concept of health, offering a range of definitions (World Health Organization 1984, Nutbeam 1986, Seedhouse 1986, King 1990, Downie et al 2002). These vary from a rather simplistic biomedical view in which it is argued that health is the absence of, or mirror image of, disease, to those that provide much broader approaches. Perhaps the most frequently quoted is that produced by the World Health Organization

(WHO) (1946, cited in Dines & Cribb 1993 p 5) which states that health is 'a complete state of physical, mental and emotional well-being and not merely the absence of disease or infirmity'. This definition has been heavily criticised as being unrealistic, idealistic and static (Dines & Cribb 1993, Ewles & Simnett 1995, Maben & Macleod Clark 1995). In addition, it has been argued that no one could claim to be healthy if this view is adhered to. It is important to remember that this description was written more than 50 years ago, since then more modern definitions and explanations have been offered (Nutbeam 1986, Seedhouse 1986, Downie et al 2002). For example, Seedhouse (1986 p 61) describes health as 'the state of the set of conditions which fulfil or enable a person to work to fulfil his or her realistic chosen and biological potentials'. The WHO has also given further consideration to its original work providing an updated definition. 'Health is therefore seen as a resource for everyday life, not the objective of living; it is a positive concept emphasising social, personal resources, as well as physical activities' (WHO 1984 p 5).

A number of authors have discussed the importance of enabling individuals to fulfil their potential so that quality and quantity of life can be enhanced (Seedhouse 1986, Tones 1990, Ewles & Simnett 1995). This is perhaps of particular relevance to the role of the CCN, who may have to acknowledge that return to complete health may not be feasible for every child. Antonovsky (1987 p 19) offers an additional insight within his model of health, which is based upon a 'sense of coherence'. This is defined as:

'a global orientation that expresses the extent to which one has a pervasive, enduring though dynamic feeling of confidence that (1) the stimuli deriving from one's internal and external environments in the course of living are structured, predictable, and explicable; (2) the resources are available to one to meet the demands posed by these stimuli; and (3) these demands are challenges, worthy of investment and engagement.'

He suggests that a sense of coherence is a major determinant of maintaining one's position on the health–disease continuum and of movement towards the healthy end. A sense of coherence is said to be made up of three central components: comprehensibility, manageability and meaningfulness.

Box 13.1 Central components of a sense of coherence (Antonovsky 1987)

- Comprehensibility – extent to which sense/order can be drawn from the situation, ability to process both familiar/unfamiliar stimuli.
- Manageability – extent to which people feel they have the resources to meet the demands that arise in their daily lives.
- Meaningfulness – extent to which one feels life makes sense emotionally, such that the problems/demands posed by living are worth investing energy in, including an ability to participate in processes shaping one's destiny.

A pronounced sense of coherence enables a person to respond flexibly to demands. According to Antonovsky (1987) the sense of coherence develops during childhood and youth, becoming more difficult to influence in adult life. The development of a weak or strong sense of coherence is largely dependent upon social circumstances and socialisation within the family. It can be concluded from this that it is important to create an environment in which children and adolescents experience consistency, can recover from stress and can participate in the decision-making process (Bengal et al 1999).

HEALTH PROMOTION

It is important to distinguish between the terms 'health education' and 'health promotion'. Although some authors, for example Dines and Cribb (1993), state that the two terms are frequently used synonymously, most theorists make clear distinctions in their definitions. There has been considerable debate about the role and purpose of both 'health education' and 'health promotion' (Catford & Nutbeam 1984, Seymour 1984, French 1985, Speller 1985, Tannahill 1985). Ewles and Simnett (1995) argue that this is because of the tremendous range of activities that are undertaken to facilitate optimum health. Health education has been defined as 'any planned activity which promotes health or illness-related learning, that is, some relatively permanent change in an individual's competence or disposition.' (Tones 1990 p 2). This view is reinforced by Tannahill (1985 p 167), who says it is concerned with 'enhancing well-being and preventing or diminishing ill-health'. According to Tones and Tilford (1994), health education may operate at a series of levels, which range from one-to-one interactions, to addressing large sections of the general population and utilising a whole array of resources.

It could be said that health education is just one aspect of health promotion. The literature concerning 'health promotion' is not so clear and concise. The WHO (1984 p 4) suggests that:

'Health promotion is the process of enabling people to increase control over, and to improve, their health.'

Bunton and Macdonald (1992 p 7) provide a broad description by stating that health promotion:

'represents at the very simplest level...a strategy for promoting, in some positive way, the health of whole populations.'

The view that individuals are not only able to make choices about their health needs but also able to take control of the decision-making process is widely accepted (Saan 1986, Whitehead 1989, Tones 1990, Dines & Cribb 1993, Downie et al 2002). It could be argued that the goals of health promotion are more challenging and include political, economic and social changes. Robertson and Minkler (1994 p 296) highlight key aspects of health promotion (Box 13.2).

It could be suggested that these definitions are based on a disease-orientated perspective, whereas Antonovsky (1987) poses an alternative approach, which he terms salutogenesis. His alternative view is further expanded within his river analogy (Box 13.3).

> **Box 13.2** Key aspects of health promotion
>
> - A broad definition of health and its determinants embracing social/economic contexts within which health or non health is produced
> - Movement beyond earlier emphasis on individual lifestyle strategies to broader social/political strategies
> - Embracement of the concept of empowerment, individual and collective, as a key health-promoting strategy
> - Advocating participation of communities in identifying health problems/development of strategies to address perceived problems

> **Box 13.3** The River Analogy (Antonovsky 1987)
>
> - Pathogenic approach: aimed at rescuing people at great expense from a raging river without looking upstream to enquire who or what is pushing people in.
> - Health education: tends to assume people jump into the river of their own volition while at the same time refusing to learn to swim.
> - Salutogenesis: the river is the stream of life. None walks the shores safely. The river is polluted and has forks that lead to gentle streams or to dangerous rapids and whirlpools. The important question to address is what helps people to swim well wherever they find themselves within the river?

If Antonovsky's (1987) view that health is a sense of coherence is recognised, then there is a 'necessity in asking "How can this person be helped to move toward greater health?" that must relate to all aspects of the person' (Antonovsky 1996).

There is no doubt that health promotion is open to interpretation but it is important for individual practitioners to clarify their role as a health promoter. There are no precise answers but personal values should be reflected upon and examined. It is not surprising, considering the differing views offered in relation to health promotion, that a range of approaches and frameworks have been developed. Naidoo and Wills (2000) suggest that there are five key approaches to health promotion:

- Medical or preventive: focuses upon strategies which reduce ill-health and early death.
- Behaviour change: encourages people to develop healthy lifestyles and behaviour.
- Educational: provides information so that individuals are able to make informed choices about their health and lifestyles.
- Empowerment: helps people identify their own health needs and develop abilities to mobilise the necessary resources.
- Social change: recognises the impact the socio-economic environment may have, aims to influence the factors within this environment that could affect health.

In addition to the above approaches, frameworks such as formulated by Caplan and Holland (1990); Beattie (1991) and Tones and Tilford (1994) have received much attention. A user-friendly tool is that produced by Tannahill (1996).

COMMUNITY PARTICIPATION AND HEALTH PROMOTION

The value of community participation within health promotion initiatives has been acknowledged (Ewles & Simnett 1995, Department of Health 1998a). The WHO (1986) emphasises the importance of empowering communities thereby enabling them to develop 'ownership' and gain control of their futures. In terms of community health promotion it is necessary to define the 'community'. Baric and Baric (1991 p 204) state that it is 'a large number of people living together and sharing certain values and interests as well as interacting for a certain purpose'. There appears to be consensus that the sharing of a goal is central to the ethos of a community. In terms of community children's nursing this may be a group of parents who have children with special needs campaigning for improved respite facilities. Alternatively, it may be a group of children with cystic fibrosis who are concerned about levels of air pollution in local built-up areas. This may lead to schools, councillors, local press and health professionals all working together to influence local policy.

The Government suggests that a healthier nation will be achieved only if everyone works together (DoH 1998a). Health Action Zones were instigated in England to target inequalities in health by bringing together a partnership that includes local authorities, community groups, the voluntary sector, local businesses and health professionals (see p 72). One area identified that may be particularly applicable to community children's nursing is the Healthy Schools initiative. This initiative aims to increase the awareness of children, teachers and families about a range of health issues including diet, exercise and environment, with the aim of improving the mental and physical health of children and young people. The high priority that the health of children and their families deserve is reiterated by the DoH (1998b). Health professionals have a central role in ensuring that health promotion is directed towards the younger population (Bagnall & Dilloway 1996, Hall 1996), however in reality this is not always overtly addressed within policy documents. CCNs are in an ideal position to facilitate child health promotion initiatives, but this must reflect a philosophy of family-centred care and include working in collaboration with a range of other personnel.

CHILD HEALTH PROMOTION

In the past a large proportion of child health promotion initiatives have either been directed towards the family and carers, rather than the children themselves, or problems have been identified by adults (Kalnins et al 1994). These initiatives were frequently linked with conditions that led to unnecessary mortality and morbidity (Kalnins et al 1994). Whilst the CCN should work in partnership with the parents promoting the health of the whole family, it is equally important to address the health of the child as an individual. Lee (1998) emphasises the importance of children having freedom to choose and Campbell (1994) suggests that, if the locus of control is with the child, a lifestyle change is more likely to occur. Certainly projects that have been initiated by children do appear to have some success. For example Treseder (1997) describes a programme developed by youngsters who have complex and multiple disabilities. The aim was to solve problems and share points of view about a range of issues including relationship difficulties and experiences of disability. Support was provided by staff and the commitment (and attendance) by the group members was evident throughout.

Kalnins et al (1994 p 195) state that 'children have to be seen as partners in health promotion rather than as a special group needing protection'. This view now appears to be widely accepted and has been reiterated by others (Seymour & Dean 1997, Lee 1998, Riley 1998). One of the prime conclusions was that not only are health visitors and nurses in an ideal position to coordinate projects between the school, family and community, but in addition they have a knowledge of how to influence policies (Seymour & Dean 1997).

Box 13.4 Key issues to be considered when promoting the health of children

- Local healthcare needs of children should be identified, taking into account age/development/culture/sociopolitical factors.
- A range of innovative health promotion strategies should be employed.
- The views of the children are essential.
- Appropriate health professionals are required to be available.
- Children should have the freedom to choose the 'way forward'/be given the locus of control where feasible.
- A philosophy of partnership between professional and child.
- Teamwork with a range of other personnel/community at large/other health professionals/schools/voluntary organisations.
- A strategy for evaluating the initiative.

Whilst current child health promotion projects are clearly valuable, there remain many opportunities for CCNs to explore additional areas. The Expert Patient (DoH 2001a) offers such an opportunity. This policy initiative aims to enable patients to have greater control over their lives, as they learn to manage their conditions more effectively, minimising its impact within their daily lives. Whilst current programmes mainly focus on adult patient groups there is much scope to apply the principles of such programmes to children and their families. This could be of great benefit to a variety of patient groups such as children suffering from asthma, diabetes or eczema. It could be argued that many of the features of Expert Patient programmes are already provided by CCNs, but user-led education programmes could facilitate empowerment of the child and his/her family to a greater extent. It is however important to note that whilst the Expert Patient initiative seems to support the notion of patients as partners, the content of programmes has largely been guided by professional opinion (Wilson 2002). In developing programmes for children and their families it would seem imperative to consult them regarding programme content and delivery, which could contribute to an increased 'sense of coherence' or enabling the family to 'swim well' as described by Antonovsky (1987).

The expansion of NHS Direct in order to support patients to become more empowered and better informed regarding health issues (DoH 2003a) is important in relation to CCN practice. It has the potential to offer health advice to young people in a medium with which they are familiar at a time convenient to them, but young people need to be aware that such services are available, and nurses will need to ensure that young people are accepted as true partners within the caring relationship. CCNs are in a key position to influence the future of child health promotion positively and to ensure a range of innovative and purposeful programmes are implemented.

ROLE OF THE COMMUNITY CHILDREN'S NURSE IN RELATION TO HEALTH PROMOTION

CCNs have always embraced a health-promoting role, however this may not have been overtly recognised by either practitioners themselves or the children and their families. The Government wants health promotion to assume a more central position than previously and for nurses to integrate it into their everyday practice (Miller et al 2001). The DoH and the Nursing and Midwifery Council (NMC) have reiterated this (DoH 1992, 1999, 2003b, NMC 2002) and stated that health promotion is an integral part of the nurse's role. It is still debatable how this should extend in the future. Government documents, such as the 'NHS Plan' (DoH 2001b) provide some direction by identifying ten key roles for nurses and placing an emphasis, within primary care, on 'prevention' and the bridging of inequalities in health. 'Liberating the Talents' (DoH 2002 p 8) highlights three core functions of Nurses, Midwives and Health Visitors, including 'public health/health protection and promotion programmes that improve health and reduce inequalities'.

The potential contribution of CCNs to health promotion has been recognised and should not be under-estimated (Gallagher & Rowe 2001). They are viewed as being in a unique position to influence people, especially mothers and children, at a critical time in their lives (Munday 1998). Authors such as Whitehead (1999) suggest that, despite the calls from nursing advisory and legislative bodies, there has been little action by the profession as a whole to become proactive in the development and implementation of the modern interpretation of health promotion. There is a need for individual CCNs to reflect upon their role and to consider the most beneficial 'way forward'. Tannahill's (1996) model will be explored as a framework to consider how the CCN may promote the health of children and their families (Fig. 13.1). It is composed of three overlapping circles: health education, prevention and health protection. The spheres encompass seven domains, each of which will now be described. The five approaches to health promotion highlighted by Naidoo and Wills (2000) will be integrated to demonstrate the flexibility and diversity such a model may offer.

Fig. 13.1 Tannahill's model (Tannahill 1996) (From 'Health Promotion: Models and Values' 2nd edn, by Downie RS et al (1996). By permission of Oxford University Press.)

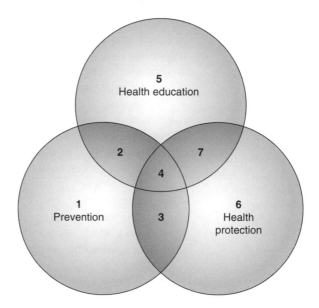

1. Preventive activities: The 'prevention' of disease and ill health links well with the medical approach identified by Naidoo and Wills (2000) and is often classified within three levels of intervention being commonly referred to as: primary, secondary and tertiary.
   - Primary prevention – aimed at disease prevention through education.
   - Secondary prevention – concerned with the early detection of a disease and preventing its progression. Insight into the family dynamics can be gained to enable emotional and practical support to be offered.
   - Tertiary prevention – involves the management of existing conditions to avoid or limit the development of complications. The CCN may have an extensive role in these situations, for example: (i) liaison with and possible referral to other professionals, (ii) it is important to gain insight into the family's understanding so that adherence to a programme of care can be enhanced, (iii) this may avoid hospitalisation and maintain a holistic and continuous approach to care, and (iv) spend time ascertaining the most appropriate way of managing the child's individual problems so that solutions can be identified.
2. Preventive health education: Tannahill (1996) suggests that this aspect of the model includes strategies that may influence lifestyle in the interests of preventing ill health. This domain could relate to the educational approach identified by Naidoo and Wills (2000). They state that the aim is to provide relevant 'knowledge and information' (p 8) so that individuals are able to make informed choices. It is anticipated that, as a result of advice, behavioural change will result. CCNs will underpin the strategy with a thorough understanding of child development to ensure information is delivered in a manner appropriate for the needs of the individual child and family.

3. Preventive health protection: This relates to policy commitment to provide preventive measures (Tannahill 1996) and could include professionals or organisations that run 'self-help' groups. If these services are unavailable, or the waiting list is so long as to make the help untimely, the CCN may consider lobbying for increased resources.

4. Health education for preventive health protection: This domain of the model advocates the education of policymakers (Tannahill 1996), an aspect of health promotion some CCNs may be less familiar with. For example, the importance of schools providing adequate drinking facilities and suitable toilets for children with constipation (Haines et al 2000, Croghan 2002). Alternatively, it could include liaising with local councillors to improve public toilets to make them more child-friendly.

5. Positive health education: This encompasses two categories: health education aimed at influencing behaviour on positive health grounds; that which seeks to help individuals and groups to develop positive health attributes (Tannahill 1996). The involvement of parents is central to community children's nursing (Procter et al 1998) and by working in partnership problems may be resolved with relative ease.

6. Positive health protection: This aims to make healthy choices easier choices. The social change approach (Naidoo & Wills 2000) would have some affiliation with this area of Tannahill's model (1996). One significant aspect is that it acknowledges other factors that influence health promotion, particularly socio-economic issues. A CCN may wish to identify policies regarding school meals and snacks available to pupils. This links well with the government's National School Fruit Scheme (DoH 2003c) that will entitle every child from nursery to 6 years of age to a portion of fruit each school day. A key issue is the concept of empowerment, a central tenet of health promotion and another approach identified by Naidoo and Wills (2000). This includes strategies that are child- and/or family-centred and increase the individual's control in the health promotion process. It is ideally suited to the community environment with the emphasis being on the family to identify their needs with the help and support of the CCN. Whilst this approach has many attributes it is time consuming. Everyone needs to have the opportunity to feel in control of their lives and young people are no exception. This is echoed by Antonovsky (1987) who stresses the importance of 'meaningfulness'. The CCN may have an advocacy role ensuring that the child's voice is heard. CCNs may also have a role in assisting families when limited finances make the purchase of fruit and vegetables difficult and they may require advice on claiming the benefits to which they are entitled.

7. Health education aimed at positive health promotion: This includes raising awareness of and seeking policy commitment to positive health education (Tannahill 1996). Asserting the need for more CCNs could be viewed as protective health education. An increase may enable more young people to receive help sooner thus minimising long-term difficulties. It may also enable children to receive care in their own homes rather than being admitted to hospital (which may affect the child's development).

CONCLUSION

Many of the activities undertaken by CCNs could be considered to be health promoting. The potential scope of the health-promoting role of the CCN could be further extended. However, all health-promoting activities are time consuming and can present nurses with difficulties in justifying the time required when the outcomes are not always tangible or measurable (Robinson & Hill 1998). If the health-promoting role of the CCN is extended other professionals may feel threatened. This could lead to conflict and defensiveness particularly in the light of the Health Committee recommendations (1997). Procter et al (1998) state that the roles of CCNs, Health Visitors and School Nurses have merged and that the need for a common knowledge base, which can be adapted for the professional caseload, is important. It could be argued that this will have the additional benefit of facilitating communication and enhancing campaign strategies in which professionals may be involved.

It is apparent that health promotion is an important and integral aspect of community children's nursing. However, it is for individual practitioners to clarify the meaning of health promotion and be accountable for their decisions in relation to these responsibilities. Many nurses have been taught within educational programmes based on a 'sickness' model and as a result health promotion did not receive the high profile it deserved. Whilst more recent nurse education programmes have explicitly addressed the concept of health promotion, integrating it into the curriculum, the practical application still presents some challenges. Nurses need to accept that health promotion is now fundamental to their role and cannot be avoided if true holistic and family-centred care is to be offered to all children and their families.

REFERENCES

Antonovsky A 1987 Unravelling the mystery of health. How people manage stress and stay well. Jossey-Bass Publishers, London

Antonovsky A 1996 The Salutogenic model as a theory to guide health promotion. Health Promotion International 11(1):11–18

Bagnall P & Dilloway M 1996 In a different light: school nurses and their role in meeting the needs of school-age children. Queens Nursing Institute and Department of Health, London

Baric L & Baric L F 1991 Health Promotion and Health Education, 2nd edn. Barns Publications, Altrincham

Beattie A 1991 Knowledge and control in health promotion: a test case for social policy and social theory. In: Gabe J, Calnan M & Bury M (eds) The Sociology of the Health Service. Routledge, London, pp 162–202

Bengal J, Strittmatter R & Willmann H 1999 What keeps people healthy? The current state of discussion and the relevance of Antonovsky's salutogenic model of health. Research and Practice of Health Promotion 4:14–104

Bunton R & Macdonald G 1992 Health Promotion: Disciplines and Diversity. Routledge, London

Campbell S 1994 The well and sick child. In: Webb P (ed) Health Promotion and Patient Education. A Professional's Guide. Chapman and Hall, London, pp 80–97

Caplan R & Holland R 1990 Rethinking health education theory. Health Education Journal 49:10–12

Catford J & Nutbeam D 1984 Towards a definition of health education and health promotion. Health Education Journal 43(2):38

Croghan E L 2002 A survey of drinking and toilet facilities in local state schools. British Journal of Nursing 7(2):76–79

Department of Health 1992 The Health of the Nation: A strategy for health in England. HMSO, London

Department of Health 1998a Our healthier nation. A contract for health. The Stationery Office, London

Department of Health 1998b Independent inquiry into inequalities in health report. (Chairman Sir Donald Acheson). The Stationery Office, London

Department of Health 1999 Saving lives: Our healthier nation. The Stationery Office, London

Department of Health 2001a The expert patient: A new approach to chronic disease management for the 21st century. The Stationery Office, London

Department of Health 2001b NHS plan – an action guide for nurses, midwives and health visitors. The Stationery Office, London

Department of Health 2002 Liberating the talents. The Stationery Office, London

Department of Health 2003a Developing NHS Direct. A strategy document for the next three years. The Stationery Office, London

Department of Health 2003b Getting the right start: National service framework for children, young people and maternity services – standard for hospital services. The Stationery Office, London

Department of Health 2003c Online. Available: http://www.dh.gov.uk/fiveaday/schoolfruit.htm 14 April 2004

Dines A & Cribb A (eds) 1993 Health Promotion: Concepts and Practice. Blackwell Scientific Publications, Oxford

Downie R S, Tannahill C & Tannahill A 2002 Health Promotion: Models and Values, 2nd edn. Oxford University Press, Oxford

Ewles L & Simnett I 1995 Promoting Health. A Practical Guide, 3rd edn. Scutari Press, London

French J 1985 To educate or promote health? Health Education Journal 44(3):115–116

Gallagher J & Rowe J 2001 Community nurses' contribution to oral health. British Journal of Nursing 6(10):526–534

Haines L, Rogers J & Dobson P 2000 A study of drinking facilities in schools. NTPLUS 96(10):2–4

Hall M B (ed) 1996 Health for all Children. 3rd edn. Oxford University Press, Oxford

Health Committee 1997 House of Commons Third Report of Session 1996–7 Health services for children and young people in the community: home and school. The Stationery Office, London

Kalnins I, McQueen D V, Backett K C, Curtice L & Currie C E 1994 Children, empowerment and health promotion: some new directions in research and practice. In: Gott M & Moloney B (eds) Child Health: A Reader. Radcliffe Medical Press, Oxford, pp 191–198

King M 1990 Health is a sustainable state. Lancet 336:664–667

Lee P 1998 Childhood accidents: how a health promotion model may help. Journal of Child Health Care 2(3):128–131

Maben J & Macleod Clark J 1995 Health promotion: a concept analysis. Journal of Advanced Nursing 22:1158–1165

Miller L, Arter K, High J, Fernando R, Prime N, Rosenfeld V, Harridge-March S, Mitchell L & Fletcher K 2001 Health promotion competence in nurses and occupational therapists. International Journal of Health Promotion and Education 39(2):44–51

Munday P 1998 Stategies for community oral health promotion. British Journal of Nursing 3(1):36–40

Naidoo J & Wills J 2000 Health Promotion. Foundations for Practice, 2nd edn. Baillière Tindall, London

Nursing and Midwifery Council (NMC) 2002 Guidelines for professional practice. NMC, London

Nutbeam D 1986 Health promotion glossary. Health Promotion 1(1):113–126

Procter S, Biott C, Campbell S, Edward S, Redpath N & Moran M 1998 Preparation for the developing role of the community children's nurse. English National Board, London

Riley R 1998 Foundations for a healthy future. Journal of Child Health Care 2(1):20–24

Robertson A & Minkler M 1994 New health promotion movement: a critical examination. Health Education Quarterly 21(3):295–312

Robinson S & Hill Y 1998 The health promoting nurse. Journal of Clinical Nursing 7:232–238

Saan H 1986 Health promotion and health education: living with a dominant concept. Health Promotion 1(3):253–255

Seedhouse D 1986 Health. The Foundations for Achievement. John Wiley, Chichester

Seymour H 1984 Health education versus health promotion – a practitioner's view. Health Education Journal 43(2):37–38

Seymour L & Dean A 1997 Adolescent smoking trends: a local investigation. Health Visitor 70(5):185–187

Speller V 1985 Defining health promotion: service implications. Health Education Journal 44(2):96

Tannahill A 1985 What is health promotion? Health Education Journal 44(4):167–168

Tannahill A 1996 A model of health promotion. In: Downie R S, Tannahill C & Tannahill A (eds) Health Promotion: Models and Values. Oxford University Press, Oxford, pp 50–75

Tones K 1990 Why theorise? Ideology in health education. Health Education Journal 49(1):2–6

Tones K & Tilford S 1994 Health Education: Effectiveness, Efficiency and Equity. Chapman and Hall, London

Treseder P 1997 Empowering children and young people – training manual. Save the Children, London

Whitehead D 1999 The nature of health promotion in acute and community settings. British Journal of Nursing 8(7):463–467

Whitehead M 1989 Swimming upstream: trends and prospects in education for health. King's Fund Institute, London

Wilson P M 2002 The expert patient: issues and implications for community nurses. British Journal of Community Nursing 7(10):514–519

World Health Organization (WHO) 1984 Health promotion. A discussion document on the concept and principles. WHO, Copenhagen

World Health Organization (WHO) 1986 Ottawa Charter for Health Promotion: an international conference on health promotion: the move towards a new public health. WHO, Copenhagen

Chapter 14

Cultural issues in community children's nursing

Paulajean Kelly and Saleha Uddin

KEY ISSUES

- Impact of culture on the care of sick children at home.
- Exploring definitions of culture.
- Health and ethnic minorities in the United Kingdom.
- Examination of practice examples highlighting the components of culture.
- Recommendations for practice developments in community children's nursing to achieve culturally sensitive care.

INTRODUCTION

This chapter will explore the impact of culture on the care of sick children in the home setting and the implications this has for the continued development of community children's nursing practice (Procter et al 1998). By exploring definitions of culture and how these relate to practice, issues of health for minority ethnic cultures in the UK will be considered. A number of practice examples will illustrate four key concepts:

1. How childhood is viewed
2. The home environment of care
3. Communication
4. Health beliefs.

Anthropological and sociological studies indicate that these concepts are not necessarily held in the same way by all cultures (James & Prout 1997). Since there are limited primary data to inform and guide nursing practice (Gates 1995, Scott 1998, Whiting 1999, Holland & Hogg 2001) the intention of this chapter is to stimulate debate rather than to present solutions or 'cultural checklists' (Galanti 2001). Through an ongoing examination of key issues Community Children's Nurses (CCNs) can develop dynamic models of care that respond effectively to the needs of children and their carers.

DEFINITIONS OF CULTURE

There are many ways in which culture can be defined and therefore explored (Helman 2000). Simplistic definitions, although attractive at first, can limit understanding (Richardson 1998). Kuper (1994) suggests two key variants within the overall concept of culture. First, culture may be seen as a tradition, learnt from generation to generation, that teaches how to behave and act. Second, specific actions and beliefs distinguish different human populations from one another. This may relate to religion, marriage practices, language and many other identifying behaviours. This concept highlights two important facets of culture: (1) all humans, all societies have culture, and (2) participation within a culture often gives a sense of identity and belonging. However, at the same time, culture can be excluding, in that it is what often marks us out as different from one another. This does not imply that within a culture there is homogeneity, whether the 'culture' in question is Jewish, black, nursing or childhood. All 'cultures' will have explicit and implicit divisions within them (Prout 1996). In some situations this leads to the emergence of a subculture; thus children's nursing could be seen as a subculture within the wider culture of nursing (Armitage 1998). Neither should we assume that a cultural perspective is static or unchanging. Baumann (1996), in examining the experiences of identity in multi-ethnic London, suggests that for young people in particular the notion of minority ethnic groups as static homogeneous communities is inaccurate and simplistic.

In addition to exposing the lack of homogeneity we must also consider the fact that culture does not exist within a political vacuum. Some groups within a society hold more power and their 'culture' may dominate; for example, within the healthcare profession, medical concerns may at times carry more weight than nursing concerns. For recipients of healthcare, cultural differences may have a negative effect when it comes to securing resources or communicating across cultures (University of Wales 1996, Webb 1996, Nazroo 2001, DoH 2003).

To comply with item 2.2 of the Nursing and Midwifery Council (NMC) 'Code of professional conduct' (2002) nurses need to apply modes of care that will effectively meet the needs of all cultural groups. In an effort to improve nursing practice and avoid the negative effects of 'cultural imposition', Leininger (1995) developed the concept of transcultural nursing. An understanding of cultural diversity is regarded as essential to the provision of safe and effective care (Canales & Bowers 2001). It could be argued that CCNs, operating outside the constraints imposed by hospital culture, are in a unique position to provide transcultural nursing. Furthermore, in the home setting the child and their carers may feel more able to assert their cultural needs.

HEALTH AND MINORITY CULTURES IN THE UK

In British healthcare literature the term culture, as discussed above, seems to be almost synonymous with ethnicity (Balarajan & Raleigh 1993). Although this is problematic a focus on ethnicity has served to highlight some of the key issues in meeting the cultural needs of recipients of healthcare (Madood 1997). There is considerable evidence of inequalities of access to, and delivery of, healthcare for minority ethnic communities (Fernando 1991, Heathley & Yip 1991, Slater 1993, Banatvala & Jayaratnam 1996, Kellerher & Hillier 1996, Cortis 1998, Gilthorpe et al 1998, Scott 1998, Bose 2000). Just one study relates directly to the needs of sick children from minority ethnic communities within a hospital setting (Slater 1993).

Caring at home for children with complex chronic or acute conditions is a continually developing area in children's nursing (Tatman & Woodruffe 1993, Parker et al 2003). As yet there are few published UK studies that focus on the impact of culture on care in the home setting (Menon et al 2001). Studies that evaluate service provision and examine the experience of children and families of ill health in childhood (Evans 1992, Tatman et al 1992, Bignold et al 1994, Wilson et al 1998) offer insight into the stress and burden of care faced by caregivers (usually mothers) and thus could be said to indicate the development of appropriate support services (Coyne 1997). These studies are problematic when considering the cultural needs of families as they regard the care both given and received as culturally neutral (Good 1994).

For CCNs to deliver culturally sensitive and therefore effective care, there is a need to recognize and reflect upon the implications of our personal and professional cultural backgrounds (Camphina-Bacote 1997) and to increase our knowledge of the cultural needs of individual children and families through assessment (Narayan 1997, Davidhizar et al 1999). The health circumstances of children from refugee families as highlighted by the Refugee Council demonstrates the importance of cultural issues being assessed in context by healthcare professionals (Dennison 2002, Heptinstall et al 2004).

CULTURAL CONSTRUCTION OF CHILDHOOD

Conceptualisations of 'childhood' are not universal (Prout 2000). This is evident in the historical review of the change in attitude towards child abuse in Britain (Jenks 1996). Similar variations exist, between social class and ethnic groups, in child-rearing practices (Ochs & Schieffelin 1984, Swanwick 1996, Whiting 1999, Mayall 2002). Examining parental perceptions in immigrant Chinese families of children with chronic illness, Elfert et al (1991) demonstrated that the illness was frequently described as having a global effect on many aspects of the child's present and future life. This was compared with Euro-Canadian parents who described the illness or disability as affecting only particular aspects of the child's life. Hillier and Rahman's (1996) study of Bangladeshi families in east London argued that, in child psychiatry, clinical care could be improved by: (i) setting the concerns of the family in a cultural context, (ii) exploring notions of child development held by parents. How a particular family conceptualises childhood will therefore affect their response to the illness and treatment, and how it is managed.

One way in which these responses can be seen as significant within the realms of community children's nursing is illustrated in Case study 14.1. Here, the notion of childhood as a time of freedom from responsibility was challenged by a sibling's involvement in nursing care.

> ### Case study 14.1
>
> Samera was the fifth child of Bangladeshi parents. Born at 28 weeks gestation she required mechanical ventilation for several weeks. She had a tracheostomy for subglottal stenosis. Before discharge her parents were taught all aspects of her nursing care by a CCN and ward staff. On a home visit, several weeks after discharge, the CCN was surprised to find Samera in the sole care of her 14-year-old sister. Her parents and the other children were visiting the General Practitioner at the time. The discharge teaching programme had failed to highlight that within this family it was expected that older daughters would have care responsibilities for younger children. This had potentially exposed both Samera and her older sibling to an unsafe situation. With help from the team's link worker, the expectations of care responsibilities for Samera were re-negotiated between the nursing team and the family. This process enabled the team to recognise that their own views on childhood were based within a particular legal, ethical and philosophical framework which was, in this case, challenged by a different conceptualisation of childhood.

ENVIRONMENT OF CARE

The home environment provides the physical structure within which care is managed in community nursing. The household is the area, where families manage the majority of their responsibilities, into which the many aspects of care for the sick child need to be incorporated. The home provides the context where the care actually takes place. Helman (2000) indicates that in healthcare, context has a considerable impact on the style and content of information giving by health professionals. Therefore CCNs need to consider how different areas of the house are managed, for example the use of reception rooms for visitors only or the separation and behaviour of ages and genders within household space. This physical environment can have tremendous implications for nursing practice, particularly for children with complex needs who may be technology-dependent (Case study 14.2).

> ### Case study 14.2
>
> A regional nurse specialist in nutrition referred John, aged 3 months, to a local CCN. Following interim surgery for a complex cardiac malformation John had failed to gain weight in the hospital or home setting. A trial of nasogastric feeding (before possible gastrostomy formation) was planned. John's family lived on a permanent site for travellers and expected to be there for a few months. Water was supplied from a standpipe and electricity from a generator during the day. The management of equipment in this setting was an initial concern for the CCNs. Their own expectations of a 'home' did not extend to a caravan. Visiting the family revealed that the way in which the space was used by the family to organise their day-to-day needs could safely incorporate an enteral feeding system. The caravan, spacious during the day when John would have bolus feeds, was adapted at night to accommodate the sleeping needs of

a large family in a confined but highly organised space. Together with the family the CCN decided to run the overnight feeding pump on batteries. John slept close to his parents, so problems during the night could be dealt with, causing minimal disruption for the rest of the family. The main difficulty arose with the delivery of feeding sets. The site was not recognised by the delivery service as an address. This was resolved by a local pharmacist receiving/storing supplies that the family collected on a regular basis. Both physical and political aspects of the household needed to be considered to achieve safe and appropriate care (Cleemput 2000).

COMMUNICATION

Child health nursing curricula devote considerable time for students to develop knowledge and communication skills with children of different developmental stages. As developmental age may be a barrier to communicating with children, so language may be a barrier for communicating with caregivers and children (Richardson 1998). Families for whom English is not the first language may receive a reduced quality of care because of communication difficulties (Slater 1993). It is acknowledged that the provision of skilled interpreters in the health service is inadequate (Audit Commission 1993, Cortis 1998). The cost of provision may seem prohibitive when the minority ethnic population is small or extremely diverse in terms of language needs. The use of relatives, especially children, or other health service staff, is usually problematic since they lack the skills required by a trained interpreter in addition to the conflicts of confidentiality. Where interpreters or link workers are available their effectiveness may be hampered by healthcare professionals' lack of experience in their use. The provision and use of skilled interpreters, by healthcare professionals, has received little attention in healthcare training (Heathley & Yip 1991). For CCNs visiting families in the home setting, other practical concerns arise concerning flexibility of visiting (if interpreting services have to be booked in advance) and maintaining continuity by visiting with the same interpreter (Twinn 1997) (Case study 14.3).

Case study 14.3

At 6 years of age, Ifat was diagnosed with acute lymphoblastic leukaemia. His parents were Turkish-speaking and he lived at home with them and his elder sister. During his hospital admission, interpreters had conveyed details of Ifat's diagnosis and planned medical treatment. The CCNs worked with a community-based Turkish interpreter to establish rapport with the family in their own home. Re-establishing home routines was an initial priority, in particular adapting the style of giving oral medication to a manner more suited to the family's needs. The seriousness of the diagnosis had led to a rigid interpretation of administering the medicines. As confidence in the CCN team developed, the family became more involved in the management of Ifat's central venous access line (CVL). The role of the interpreter was crucial in this and it was

case study continues

apparent that visiting without the interpreter meant halting the teaching programme despite the fact that both parents had some understanding and expression of English. A skilled experienced interpreter was essential to ensure that Ifat and his family received appropriate care. Concerns about his long-term prognosis and reintegration into school were raised by the family in an environment where they were able to communicate their needs. The CCNs were also able to give more detailed explanations because of the quality of the interpreting services. It was recognised that language was just one potential communication barrier. Styles of verbal and non-verbal communication also became a key aspect of care delivery. Written information on the care of the CVL was not available in the family's own language. The CCNs were able to have this information translated and supplemented by the team's own pictorial teaching tool (Sexton et al 1996, Smettem 1999). This not only helped to reinforce verbal information given but also provided access to information for other family members who were not always present on visits. This illustrates how a simplistic approach to culturally sensitive care could be problematic as both the gender and political views of the interpreter in this case were very important to the family, who were refugees. The use of specific dialect should also be considered in planning interpreting service needs.

HEALTH BELIEFS

The perceived neutrality of biomedical explanations of health and illness is problematic when considering the care needs of patients (Good 1994). Medical anthropologists suggest that, regardless of culture, most of us hold a range of explanations of health and illness (Helman 2000). Furthermore these explanations may be invoked to a greater or lesser extent depending on the context. Eade's (1997) review of beliefs and practices among Bangladeshis in Tower Hamlets indicates that, although 'experts' often demarcate the differences between medical, Islamic and folk models, 'ordinary people' operate with less-rigid boundaries.

Much of the literature on the response to illness in children from specific ethnic groups is comparative (Watson 1984, Pachter et al 1995, Leiser et al 1996). A comparative approach is problematic since it implies or explicitly sets the study group against a perceived standard of compliance or appropriate use by another population. This stance demonstrates the difficulties that Good (1994) outlined, in exposing the tendency for biomedical explanations to be regarded as facts and other models as beliefs. He suggests that medical anthropologists experience a tension between wishing to give weight to traditional explanations of ill health or misfortune and yet feeling an obligation to ensure access to 'biomedicine', therefore privileging that explanation. Nurses wishing to be culturally sensitive in their practice may experience the same tension. Weller (1994) advocates the use of an assessment framework, by nurses, to evaluate the impact of traditional health beliefs and practices on child and family health.

CONCLUSION

This chapter has illustrated some of the issues that may impact on the care of sick children in a community setting from a cultural perspective.

There are several implications for practice. Education programmes at pre- and post-registration level need to increase the opportunities for learning about culture (Gerrish et al 1996) and how differences in family structure may impact on the planning and delivery of nursing care. The work of Martinson et al (1997), on expectations of support for Chinese families caring for children with chronic illness, demonstrates the need for awareness of changing family structures. CCNs need to be mindful of the context for individual families and children. This may mean that a particular family will approach care through their previous experience, which may include immigration experiences, racism within or outside the health service, and a range of vulnerabilities and strengths.

The case studies focus predominantly on meeting the 'cultural' needs of carers. Ethnographers have demonstrated how children are active in constructing their own cultural identities (Briggs 1970, Bluebond-Langer 1978, Toren 1990, James 1993, Mayall et al 1996). Hall's (1995) study illustrated how fluid this cultural identity could be where British Sikh teenagers graded their behaviour more or less towards traditional expectations depending on the context. Practice models need to balance potential conflicting and changing interpretations of culture to meet the needs of children and carers. Assessments and evaluations of care need to incorporate an opportunity for cultural needs to be explored and the extent to which care given meets these needs (Chevannes 1997, Narayan 1997). Whyte's (1996) work on family nursing represents a framework that could be used.

There continues to be a need to develop research in this area that can inform and guide practice. Any investigation into the care needs of children and families in a community setting should address cultural needs. In addition, focused research on assessment and evaluation would be a valuable starting point in developing culturally sensitive care. How children construct their own cultural identities in sickness and health could provide a fruitful and fascinating area for collaborative research projects between health and social sciences.

REFERENCES

Armitage G 1998 Analysing childhood: a nursing perspective. Journal of Child Health Care 2(2):66–70

Audit Commission 1993 What seems to be the matter? Communication between hospitals and patients. HMSO, London

Balarajan R & Raleigh V S 1993 Ethnicity and health: a guide for the NHS. Department of Health, London

Banatvala N & Jayaratnam P 1996 The experiences of East London's minority ethnic community. Health in the East End: Annual Public Health Report 1995/6. Department of Public Health, East London and City Health Authority, London

Baumann G 1996 Contesting Culture: Discourses of Identity in Multi-ethnic London. Cambridge University Press, Cambridge

Bignold S, Ball S & Cribb A 1994 Nursing families of children with cancer: the work of the paediatric oncology outreach nurse specialists. Cancer Relief Macmillan Fund/Department of Health, King's College London

Bluebond-Langer M 1978 The Private World of Dying Children. Princeton Press, Newhaven, New Jersey

Bose R 2000 Families in transition. In: Lau A (ed) South Asian Children and Adolescents in Britain. Whurr Publishers, London

Briggs J 1970 Never in Anger. Harvard University Press, Cambridge, Massachusetts

Camphina-Bacote J 1997 Cultural competence: A critical factor in child health policy. Journal of Pediatric Nursing 12(4):260–262

Canales M K & Bowers B J 2001 Expanding conceptualizations of culturally competent care. Journal of Advanced Nursing 36(1):102–111

Chevannes M 1997 Nurses caring for families – issues in a multi racial society. Journal of Clinical Nursing 6(2):161–167

Cleemput P V 2000 Health care needs of travellers. Archives of Disease in Childhood 82:32–37

Cortis J D 1998 The experiences of nursing care received by Pakistani (Urdu speaking) patients in later life in Dewsbury, UK. Clinical Effectiveness in Nursing 2:131–138

Coyne I T 1997 Chronic illness: the importance of support for families caring for a child with cystic fibrosis. Journal of Clinical Nursing 6(2):121–129

Davidhizar R , Havens R & Bechtel G A 1999 Assessing culturally diverse pediatric clients Pediatric Nursing 25(4):371–376

Dennision J 2002 A case for change – how refugee children in England are missing out. London Refugee Council, London

Department of Health 2003 Quality Protects – Black and ethnic minority children and their families. Online. Available: www.dh.gov.uk/qualityprotects/work 16 July 2003

Eade J 1997 The power of the experts: the plurality of beliefs and practices concerning health and illness among Bangladeshis in contemporary Tower Hamlets, London. In: Marks L & Worboys M (eds) Migrants, Minorities and Health. Routledge, London

Elfert H, Anderson J M & Lai M 1991 Parents' perceptions of children with chronic illness: a study of immigrant Chinese families. Journal of Pediatric Nursing 6(2):114–120

Evans M 1992 An investigation into the feasibility of parental participation in the nursing care of their children. Journal of Advanced Nursing 29:477–482

Fernando S 1991 Mental Health: Race and Culture. Macmillan Press, Basingstoke

Galanti G 2001 An introduction to cultural differences. Western Journal of Medicine 172:335–336

Gates E 1995 Culture clash – the nursing care of dying children from cultural backgrounds that are different from the nurses. Nursing Times 91(7):42–43

Gerrish K, Husband C & Mackenzie J 1996 Nursing for a Multi Ethnic Society. Open University Press, Buckingham

Gilthorpe M S, Lay Yee T, Wilson R C, Walters S, Gryfiths R K & Bedi R 1998 Variations in hospitalisation rates for asthma among black and ethnic minority communities. Respiratory Medicine 92(4):642–648

Good B J 1994 Medicine Rationality and Experience: An Anthropological Perspective. Cambridge University Press, Cambridge

Hall K 1995 There's a time to act English and a time to act Indian: the politics of identity amongst British Sikh teenagers. In: Stephens S (ed.) Children and the Politics of Culture. Princeton University Press, Princeton

Heathley P T & Yip R Y W 1991 Analysis of general practice consultation rates among Asian patients. British Journal of General Practice 41:476

Helman C G 2000 Culture, Health and Illness, 4th edn. Butterworth Heinemann, Oxford

Heptinstall T, Kralj L & Lee G 2004 Asylum seekers: a health professional perspective. Nursing Standard 18(25):44–53

Hillier S & Rahman S 1996 Childhood development and behavioural and emotional problems as perceived by Bangladeshi parents in East London. In: Kellerher D & Hillier S (eds) Researching Cultural Differences in Health. Routledge, London

Holland K & Hogg C 2001 Cultural Awareness in Nursing and Health Care: An Introductory Text. Arnold, London

James A 1993 Childhood Identities: Self and Social Relationships in the Experience of the Child. Edinburgh University Press, Edinburgh

James A & Prout A 1997 Constructing and Reconstructing Childhood. Falmer Press, London

Jenks C 1996 Childhood. Routledge, London

Kellerher D & Hillier S (eds) 1996 Researching Cultural Differences in Health. Routledge, London

Kuper A 1994 Anthropological futures. In: Borofsky R (ed.) Assessing Cultural Anthropology. McGraw Hill, New York

Leininger M 1995 Transcultural Nursing: Concepts, Theories and Practices. John Wiley, New York

Leiser D, Doitsch E & Meyer J 1996 Mothers lay models of the causes and treatment of fever. Social Science & Medicine 43(3):379–387

Madood T 1997 Ethnic Minorities in Britain, Diversity and Disadvantage. PSI Press, London

Martinson I M, Armstrong V & Qiao J 1997 The experience of the family of children with chronic illness at home in China. Pediatric Nursing 23(4):371–375

Mayall B 2002 Towards a Sociology for Childhood-thinking from Children's Lives. Open University Press, Buckingham

Mayall B, Bendelow G, Barker S, Feltman M & Storey P 1996 Children's Health in Primary Schools. Falmer Press, London

Menon S, McKinlay I A & Faragher E B 2001 Knowledge and attitudes in multicultural healthcare. Child: Care, Health and Development 27(5):439–450

Narayan M C 1997 Cultural assessment in home health care. Home Health Care Nurse 15(10):663–670

Nazroo J Y 2001 Ethnicity, Class and Health. Policy Studies Institute, London

Nursing and Midwifery Council (NMC) 2002 Code of professional conduct. NMC, London

Ochs E & Schieffelin B 1984 Language acquisition and socialisation: three developmental stories and their implications. In: Shweder R A & Le Vine R A (eds) Culture Theory: Essays on Mind, Self and Emotion. Cambridge University Press, Cambridge, Massachusetts

Pachter L M, Cloutier M M & Bernstein B A 1995 Ethnomedical (folk) remedies for childhood asthma in a mainland Puerto Rican community. Archives of Paediatric Adolescent Medicine 149(9):982–988

Parker G, Bhakta P, Lovett C A, Paisley S, Olsen R, Turner D & Young B 2003 A systematic review of the costs and effectiveness of different models of paediatric home care. Health Technology Assessment 6:34

Procter S, Biott C, Campbell S, Edward S, Redpath N & Moran M 1998 Preparation for the developing role of the community children's nurse. English National Board for Nursing, Midwifery and Health Visiting, London

Prout A 1996 Families, cultural bias and health promotion, implications of an ethnographic study. Health Education Authority, London

Prout A 2000 The Body, Childhood and Society. Macmillan Press, London

Richardson J 1998 Culture and the child health ambulatory setting. In: Glasper E A & Lowson S (eds) Innovations in Paediatric Ambulatory Care: A Nursing Perspective. Macmillan, London

Scott P 1998 Lay beliefs and the management of disease amongst West Indians with diabetes. Health and Social Care in the Community 6(6):407–419

Sexton E, Paul L & Holden C 1996 A pictorial assisted teaching tool for families. Paediatric Nursing 8(5):24–26

Slater M 1993 Health for all our Children: Achieving Appropriate Health Care for Black and Minority Children and their Families. Action for Sick Children, London

Smettem S 1999 Welcome/Assalaam-u-alaikam: improving communications with ethnic minority families. Paediatric Nursing 11(2):33–35

Swanwick M 1996 Child rearing across cultures. Paediatric Nursing 8(7):13–17

Tatman M A & Woodruffe C 1993 Paediatric home care in the UK. Archives of Disease in Childhood 69:677–680

Tatman M A, Woodruffe C, Kelly P J & Harris R J 1992 Paediatric home care in Tower Hamlets: a working partnership with parents. Quality in Health Care 1:98–103

Toren C 1990 Making Sense of Hierarchy: Cognition as Social Process in Fiji. Athlone Press, London

Twinn S 1997 An exploratory study examining the influence of translation on the validity and reliability of qualitative data in nursing research. Journal of Advanced Nursing 26:418–423

University of Wales College of Medicine 1996 Equal Rights/Equal Access – Improving the care of minority ethnic children with disability or chronic illness. A training package. University of Wales. Department of Child Health

Watson E 1984 Health of infants and use of health services by mothers of different ethnic groups in East London. Community Medicine 6:127–135

Webb E 1996 Meeting the need of minority ethnic communities. Archives of Disease in Childhood 74 (3):264–267

Weller B 1994 Cultural aspects of children's health and illness. In: Lindsay B (ed.) The Child and Family: Contemporary Nursing Issues in Child Health and Care. Baillière Tindall, London

Whiting L S 1999 Caring for children of differing cultures. Journal of Child Health Care 3(4):33–38

Whyte D 1996 Explorations in Family Nursing. Routledge, London

Wilson S, Morse J M & Penrod J 1998 Absolute involvement: the experience of mothers of ventilator dependent children. Health and Social Care in the Community 6(4):224–233

SECTION 3

Dimensions of Community Children's Nursing Practice

SECTION CONTENTS

The ability of community children's nursing to be responsive and proactive is influenced by many factors. The aim of this section is not to provide a comprehensive review of clinical practice, but to offer the reader the opportunity to explore some of its diverse aspects. These include issues and skills for the Community Children's Nurse Manager to enable negotiation and representation of services within strategic and commissioning arenas. Team composition alongside organisational issues and information management are included alongside a new chapter on benchmarking. An examination of dependency measurement provides a necessary foundation to the increasing range of dependency encountered in practice. The fact that children and young people often act as carers is recognised and the broader implications of this for practitioners are explored.

Chapter 15

Strategic planning and commissioning of services

Suzanne Jones and Maybelle Tatman

KEY ISSUES

- Commissioning children's services and Local Delivery Plans.
- User involvement.
- Reconfiguration of children's services.
- Resourcing community children's nursing.
- Evaluation of service delivery.
- Economic evaluation.

INTRODUCTION

This is an exciting time for Community Children's Nurses (CCNs) to shape new patterns of local care and contribute to the processes by which healthcare funding decisions are made. There continues to be an urgent need for CCNs to be assisted by leadership programmes and degree courses in order to develop relevant knowledge and skills to enable them to articulate and influence the commissioning agenda and overcome the current constraints within children's services. This chapter describes the process of commissioning children's services and includes an overview of strategic planning. Issues surrounding the reconfiguration of children's services and establishment of ambulatory care as an alternative to inpatient care are presented. Methods for the evaluation of community children's nursing services are discussed together with aspects of user satisfaction and an introduction to economic evaluation.

COMMISSIONING CHILDREN'S SERVICES

Commissioning is the process of improving the health and meeting the health needs of the local community through planning and purchasing health services with the resources available. It is a broad strategic activity and individuals involved in the process bear a wide range of responsibilities (DoH 1994, 1996a). These include:

- assessment of health need
- development of local strategies
- targeting of resources
- working with providers, statutory and voluntary bodies
- seeking and responding to views of service users and the public
- improving the quality of care by setting standards and monitoring performances
- regular updated multi-agency assessment of need (including where little or no services exists).

Following the publication of the document 'Shifting the Balance of Power' (DoH 2001) Primary Care Trusts (PCTs) were made responsible for both providing primary health services and commissioning services for their local community, including children (Box 15.1). A plethora of guidance has since been made available on commissioning services for children to required clinical standards, including the children's National Service Framework (NSF).

Box 15.1 Key principles in strategic planning of children's services

- In all provision welfare of the child is paramount.
- Children's services should include all children between 0 and 19 years (inclusive) and services for the unborn child.
- All professionals dealing with children will have appropriate training and experience.
- Services should support family and carers/work in partnership with parents and children.
- All children to be cared for in a child-centred environment with due recognition of the needs of children of different ages.
- Care for children to be delivered as close to home as possible (including at home where appropriate).
- Access to services to take into account need/culture/disability/proximity/user friendliness/effectiveness, etc.
- Services to facilitate inter-disciplinary/multi-agency working.
- There should be a smooth transition at both ends of the service, i.e. from maternity care to children's services and on to adult services for children with long-term needs (see Chapter 32).
- Services should be seamless and unhampered by managerial and inter-disciplinary boundaries (Heywood 2002).

(Children Act 1989, Learning from Bristol 2001, Royal College of Paediatrics and Child Health 2001a, 2003, Laming 2003, Association for Children with Life-threatening or Terminal Conditions and their Families & Royal College of Paediatrics and Child Health 2003, DoH 2002a, 2003, National Association of Hospital Play Staff 2003)

The concept of a 'Strategic Partnership' has been developed to enable joint planning and commissioning of services between health and social care. Children's Trusts will increasingly take over the commissioning role from PCTs (see Chapter 3). Integration of services may occur to different degrees to include:

- better signposting and coordination of existing services
- jointly managed processes such as single assessments
- care pathways to structural integration of services within a single organisation (Department for Education and Skills 2003, Miller 2003).

A 'Children's and Young People's Strategic Partnership' must have appropriate membership to function effectively together with authority and reporting mechanisms to inform the Local Delivery Plan (LDP) and commissioning process. As well as commissioning services PCTs are major providers of children's services.

Local delivery plans

Strategic Health Authorities (SHAs) have replaced the former Health Authorities, forming a bridge between the DoH and local health services. Their primary role was defined as providing strategic leadership to ensure the delivery of improvements in local health services through quality assurance processes (DoH 2002a, 2002b). For example, as part of a capacity and planning process SHAs produce LDPs, in conjunction with PCTs, showing how any gaps in provision in meeting the NHS Plan can be overcome, and how the NHS Plan will be delivered in each locality from 2003 to 2006 (DoH 2000) (Box 15.2). LDPs are in two parts:

- A narrative to describe the strategic framework, the approach to key targets and the main risk management strategies.
- A series of 'output' schedules to show the planned trajectories towards achieving the main targets of the NHS Plan.

Box 15.2 Examples of generic requirements of LDPs applicable to children

- access to care
- emergency care
- inequalities
- children and young people's experience
- drug misuse
- workforce
- information technology
- recommendations of the NSF
- Public Inquiries
- infant mortality
- breast feeding/childhood nutrition/child obesity
- vulnerable children/improving life chances
- heath promotion
- Sure Start
- children's centres
- teenage pregnancy
- Child & Adolescent Mental Health Service (CAMHS)

NHS Trusts and PCTs will receive performance ratings to assess performance during the previous year. The 2003/04 Commission for Health Improvement (CHI) targets for the first time had two targets relating to children, CAMHS and child protection, which raised the profile of children's services within PCTs and NHS Trusts (CHI 2003/04).

Strategic planning

The underpinning strategy areas for children's services should cover a shared vision and set out a framework from which policies will be developed. Each family's needs are individual and change over time and therefore a spectrum of children's services are required to provide flexible care that complements the skills and contributions of families and those of their primary care team. Close cooperation between health, social services and education is essential for the planning and commissioning of children's services and LDPs should contain information on that collaboration. There will be many funding opportunities available to PCTs as part of this joint working agenda including:

- Sure Start
- Early Years Development
- Children's Fund
- Regeneration (including involvement in Local Strategic Partnerships)
- Connexions (13–19 years)
- Learning and Skills Councils (Workforce Development Issues).

Each PCT must genuinely commission services from the perspective of children rather than a service perspective and to do this they must ensure that the following requirements are met:

- A Children's Commissioner responsible for commissioning services from service providers in the public, private or voluntary sectors including commissioning regional specialties (DoH 2003).
- Determination of the current 'spend' of the PCT on health services for children in order to establish budgetary control and an ability to shift or re-commission services.
- Ensuring children's services are child-centred as a means of looking at the whole child rather than at a presenting illness or a problem (DoH 1996b, 2003).
- Patient Advice and Liaison Service/Advocacy sensitive to the needs of children of all ages (DoH 2003).
- Robust planning arrangements with the Local Authority (LA) and voluntary sector, including formal representation on cross-agency planning groups such as the Local Safe Guarding Children Boards, Children's Fund, Early Years, Connexions, etc.
- Voluntary sector providers consulted in the planning and commissioning process as major contributors particularly in children's palliative care and filling gaps in statutory provision (DoH 1991, Association for Children with Life-threatening or Terminal Conditions and their Families & Royal College of Paediatrics and Child Health 2003).
- Broader public health issues considered in planning children's services including teenage pregnancy, oral and dental health promotion,

substance abuse, issues of cultural/racial sensitivity, youth offending (DoH 2003).
- Consortium arrangements with other PCTs for commissioning or providing specialist services.
- Workforce planning to deliver the LDP (DoH 2002a, 2002c).
- Consideration given to cross referencing the workforce plans with the Trust's training commission.
- Reviewing arrangements for providing designated doctors and nurses for child protection in line with Lord Laming's recommendations (Laming 2003).
- Clear policies as to how care packages for children with continuing care needs are resourced and managed.

Continuing care strategy

Developing a continuing care strategy to facilitate effective care packages for children and families enables earlier discharge from hospital. Given the length of time to plan new services it is prudent for both Health and Social Services commissioners to develop contingency arrangements for caring for a child with complex healthcare needs. A clearly documented whole system approach is essential to ensure an individualised continuing care package that involves the child and parents as partners in care at all times. Key components of this strategy are improving information exchange, coordination between agencies and sharing implementation between neighbouring Trusts, together with dedicated teams to provide continuing care (Jardine et al 1999, Linter et al 2000). Investment in nurse training, education and leadership are required to develop integrated children's teams to provide the care and support (see Chapter 22).

USER INVOLVEMENT

There is evidence that children and young people can be involved in making choices about their local healthcare provision (Taylor 1996, Sheldon 1997, Vickers & Carlisle 2000, Children and Young Person's Unit 2001a). It is accepted that the effectiveness of services depends on listening and responding to users. Giving children and young people an active say in how these policies and services are developed, provided, evaluated and improved should ensure that policies and services more genuinely meet their needs. PCTs must have a visible commitment to involving children and young people and ensure that their involvement is valued, evaluated and improved (Taylor 1996, Sheldon 1997, Vickers & Carlisle 2000, Children's and Young Person's Unit 2001b).

Consumer satisfaction with services has become a key index of service quality (Ovretveit 1990, Association for Children with Life-threatening and Terminal Conditions and their Families & Royal College of Paediatrics and Child Health 2003). Seeking the views of those using services is not only respectful but may also offer insights about services that cannot be obtained from other sources. The outcomes of services for children and young people have previously been measured by seeking the opinions of parents (Stallard 1995). Children, as users, provide a perspective shaped by experiences of health issues and healthcare of which professionals may be unaware. Furthermore, they may contribute to making the wording of documentation, information sheets and reports understandable to children.

RECONFIGURATION OF CHILDREN'S SERVICES

It is widely accepted that there are advantages to caring for sick children and their families at home (Health Committee 1997). Thirty years ago the average admission to a children's ward was for 9 days. The majority of children now stay in hospital for less than 2 days and many for just a few hours. Replacing a child's inpatient service with an ambulatory form of children's medical care is a viable alternative accepted in some parts of the UK (British Paediatric Association 1996, Meates 1997, Cresswell 2000). It is supported by the Royal College of Paediatrics and Child Health (RCPCH) (Cresswell 2002). Both Meates and the RCPCH refer to community children's nursing teams contributing to the reduction in the length of inpatient stay and potentially preventing admission although the costs of an episode of community care can be equivalent to an inpatient episode (Whiting 2001). There is relatively little evidence on which to base decisions about the cost effectiveness of models of service delivery, however Trusts/PCTs should be explicit about the costs of proposed models and the impact on wider child health services of over-resourcing services in one area. Sometimes complete withdrawal of acute hospital-based services from the satellite location may be the correct answer.

- The economic evaluation of the Kidderminster service supported the view that an ambulatory service would be significantly cheaper than inpatient care but also noted that the Kidderminster model was over-resourced (Cresswell 2000).
- The evaluation of a Hospital at Home Service in central England found that the service was more costly than the transfer of all acute care to the nearby general hospital but cheaper than running a full inpatient service in the town in which it was based.
- Improving children's Accident & Emergency facilities is a priority in order to reduce long delays for children and carers waiting for simple treatments. The use of an 'outreach' CCN-staffed 'hospital at home' service may be a alternative solution (RCPCH 2001b, 2002).
- Eaton and Whiting (p 34) describe the service models within community children's nursing. Surveys of community nursing teams during the past 10 years demonstrate wide variation in availability of CCNs and service models (Tatman & Woodroffe 1993, Fraser et al 1997, Jardine et al 1999, Cramp et al 2003).

RESOURCING COMMUNITY CHILDREN'S NURSING

It can be difficult to secure funding for new or expanding services as there are many competing priorities. However, resources can become unexpectedly available. It is prudent to have a service bid prepared in advance, as presenting opportunities invariably have a tight deadline. These opportunities may include:

- Diversion of existing resources. Vacant posts within a directorate or the closure of a children's ward can fund a hospital-at-home service.

- Government initiatives. Pump priming money released into a specific area of healthcare, usually awarded on condition that the availability of ongoing local funding is proven once the initial grant has expired.
- Charity. The children's hospices are funded by the voluntary sector and some have established nursing outreach and respite care in the community (see Chapter 23). Some voluntary organisations have funded community children's oncology or respite nurses.
- Research grants. It is unusual for research grants to cover service costs except where funding comes from the pharmaceutical companies. Where posts are established they can only run for the life of the research project unless the funding is then taken over by an established source.
- Drug companies. For example within diabetes a number of posts have been initially funded by insulin manufacturers. Long-term funding has then been continued by the NHS Trust/PCT.

EVALUATION

Evaluation is defined as the formal determination of the effectiveness, efficiency and acceptability of a planned intervention in achieving stated objectives:

- Effectiveness is a measure of the technical outcome of health services in medical, social, and psychological terms: 'Does it work?'
- Efficiency is an economic concept relating the effect achieved to the cost (service costs, opportunity costs, costs to patients): 'Is it expensive?'
- Acceptability is the judgement of an intervention as professionally or socially satisfactory: 'Do we like it?'

Evaluation is considered an element of health services research: the integration of epidemiology, sociology, health economics and other analytical sciences in the study of health services. This form of research evidence differs from that obtained from a clinical trial which evaluates a new drug or intervention. Often qualitative methods are more important than quantitative methods in health services research, which is concerned with the relationships between need, demand, supply, use and outcome of health services. The information gained from this research enables organisational change (Jennings 1994).

A service evaluation is used as a reference and as a measure of work carried out over the previous years (see Chapter 18). It should consider:

- areas of unmet need identified in needs assessment
- stated aims and objectives of the service
- key questions which need to be answered about the service
- information already available as well as designing an efficient method for collecting any further information required
- involving the local audit and research and development departments to facilitate study design, registration and ethical approval (Tatman & Woodroffe 1993, Jennings 1994, Peter & Torr 1996).

The aims of an evaluation are to:

- explore the experiences of families using the community children's nursing service

- evaluate the satisfaction of children/parents/carers receiving the service
- obtain baseline data for future monitoring of user satisfaction
- identify key issues for future qualitative exploration.

Satisfaction studies have focused primarily on assessing satisfaction at one point in time. Families' experiences of services from qualitative interviews may help to determine what aspects are valued by families and why. Imaginative letter writing, for example about what it is like to be on a cancer ward, and story telling, can acknowledge children's feedback on the service (Whiting 2001, Cramp et al 2003).

Quality in the context of healthcare is a complex matter, compounded by the assertion that the consumer (the child and family) is the best judge of quality. However, as Redfern and Norman (1990) note, the expectations of consumers and their knowledge limitations may preclude them from a realistic appreciation of quality in terms of healthcare. The community children's nursing team leads and contributes to quality initiatives:

- Pre-action (control the setting of standards/goals of care).
- Concurrent (ongoing evaluation of care given).
- Feedback (evaluating of level of practice by consumers via narrative analysis or satisfaction surveys).

ECONOMIC EVALUATION

The main types of economic analysis are cost benefit, cost utility, cost minimisation and cost effectiveness:

- Cost benefit analysis measures both costs and benefits in monetary terms and may present results as a ratio of monetary gain versus loss.
- Cost utility analysis measures the outcomes of different types of care using scales such as quality-adjusted life years (QALYs) and may present results as relative costs per QALY.
- A cost minimisation analysis compares the costs of different ways of achieving the same health outcome and may present results as maximum outcome for a given level of resources.
- A cost effectiveness analysis measures the results of an intervention in terms of effect such as life years gained (Ungar & Santos 2004).

In community children's nursing cost comparisons need to include the costs to parents. They may give up work to look after the sick child, they may need to move house or adapt their home to meet the child's needs and they may have increased household expenses such as food, heating, laundry and replacing clothing and bedding. These costs can be hard to accurately measure but contribute to the total costs of care (Dobson & Middleton 1998). Evaluating the impact of a community children's nursing service on healthcare costs can be affected by other factors. Reduced bed occupancy on a hospital ward does not automatically cut costs as the running costs of the ward, such as staffing and maintenance, remain much the same. Closure of a unit will achieve a saving but often this cannot occur because of the need to provide core services to the local community.

There are no validated methods to measure outcomes in terms of life years gained in children who are naturally at the outset of their journey through life. Quality of life measures for adults do not compare with children's needs and aspirations. Consequently there are fewer economic evaluations published for children's services than for adult (Ungar & Santos 2004). West (2004) suggests that a factor may be the concentration of studies on chronic illness where costs of healthcare are high and the health outcomes may be marginal.

Published cost comparisons in community children's nursing have included: generalist community children's nursing (Atwell & Gow 1985, While 1991, Whiting 2001); home versus hospital chemotherapy (Close et al 1995); early discharge from a neonatal unit (Couriel & Davies 1988, Kotagal et al 1995); home management of newly diagnosed diabetes (Dougherty et al 1999).

CONCLUSION

Current health policy stresses the importance of partnership working. It is therefore important to look at new ways of working and approaches of managing care for sick children and their families in the community. Exploring creative solutions to care packages maximises the use of limited resources. These children are the responsibilities of many agencies not just the NHS. This chapter has discussed some of the barriers to working in partnership to improve services to children, young people and their families.

A realistically planned, monitored and evaluated service is attractive to purchasers. Appointing CCNs to leadership positions within PCTs and SHAs would result in appropriate identification of long-term funding to ensure the provision of comprehensive community care for children throughout the country.

REFERENCES

Association for Children with Life-threatening or Terminal Conditions and their Families (ACT) & The Royal College of Paediatrics and Child Health 2003a A Guide to the Development of Children's Palliative Care Services 2nd ed. ACT, Bristol

Association for Children with Life Threatening or Terminal Conditions and their Families (ACT) 2003b Voices for Change. Current Perception of services for children with palliative care needs and their families. ACT, Bristol

Atwell J D & Gow M A 1985 Paediatric trained district nurse in the community: expensive luxury or economic necessity? British Medical Journal 291:227–229

British Paediatric Association (BPA) 1996 Future Configuration of Paediatric Services. BPA, London

Children Act 1989 HMSO, London

Children and Young Person's Unit 2001a Building a strategy for children and young people. Consultation Document. Department for Education and Skills, London

Children and Young Person's Unit 2001b Learning to listen: Core principles for the involvement of children and young people. Online. Available: www.dfes.gov.uk/cypu 28 March 2003

Close P, Burkey E, Kazak A, Danz P & Lange B 1995 A prospective controlled evaluation of home chemotherapy for children with cancer. Pediatrics 95(6):896–900

Commission for Health Improvement (CHI) 2003/04. Online. Available: www.CHI.org 28 March 2003

Couriel J & Davies P 1988 Costs and benefits of a community special care baby service. British Medical Journal 296:1043–1046

Cramp C, Tripp S, Hughes N & Dale J 2003 Children's home nursing: results of a national survey. Paediatric Nursing 15(8):39–43

Cresswell T 2000 A review of recently developed models for acute child health services with ambulatory components. Commissioned by the Royal College of Paediatrics and Child Health, London

Cresswell T 2002 Old problems – new solutions. Royal College of Paediatrics and Child Health, London

Department for Education and Skills 2003 Every Child Matters. The Stationery Office, London

Department of Health 1991 Welfare of children and young people in hospital. HMSO, London

Department of Health 1994 Managing change. HMSO, London

Department of Health 1996a Children's Services Planning Guidance.The Stationery Office, London

Department of Health 1996b Child Health in the community: a guide to good practice. The Stationery Office, London

Department of Health 2000 The NHS Plan. The Stationery Office, London

Department of Health 2001 Shifting the balance of power within the NHS – securing delivery. The Stationery Office, London

Department of Health 2002a Securing delivery and next steps. The Stationery Office, London

Department of Health 2002b Improvement, Expansion and Reform: the next 3 years, Priorities and Planning Framework 2003–2006. The Stationery Office, London

Department of Health 2002c Keeping the NHS Local – a new direction of travel. The Stationery Office, London

Department of Health 2003 Getting the right start: National Service Framework for Children. Emerging Findings. The Stationery Office, London

Dobson B & Middleton S 1998 The Cost of Childhood Disability. Joseph Rowntree Foundation, York

Dougherty G, Schiffrin A, White D, Soderstrom L & Sufrategui M 1999 Home-based management can achieve intensification cost-effectively in type I diabetes. Pediatrics 103(1):122–128

Fraser J, Mok J & Tasker R 1997 Survey of occupancy of paediatric intensive care units by children who are dependent on ventilators. British Medical Journal 315:347–348

Health Committee 1997 House of Commons Health Select Committee. Health services for children and young people in the community: home and school. Third report. The Stationery Office, London

Heywood J 2002 Enhancing seamless care: a review. Paediatric Nursing. 14(5):18–20

Jardine E, Toole M, Payton J & Wallis C 1999 Current status of long-term ventilation of children in the United Kingdom: questionnaire survey. British Medical Journal 318:295–299

Jennings P 1994 Learning through experience: an evaluation of 'Hospital at Home'. Journal of Advanced Nursing 19:905–911

Kotagal U R, Perlstein P H, Gamblian V, Donovan E F & Atherton H D 1995 Description and evaluation of a program for the early discharge of infants from a neonatal intensive care unit. Pediatrics 127(2):285–290

Laming 2003 The Victoria Climbié Inquiry – Summary Report. The Stationery Office, London

Learning from Bristol 2001 The report of the public inquiry into children's heart surgery at the Bristol Royal Infirmary 1984–1995. The Stationery Office, London

Linter S, Perry M & Cherry D 2000 Continuing care: An integrated approach. Paediatric Nursing 12(8):17–18

Meates M 1997 Ambulatory paediatrics – making a difference. Archives of Disease in Childhood 76:468–473

Miller C 2003 The organisational implications of the Children's Services Green Paper. Office of Public Management, London

National Association of Hospital Play Staff 2003 Guidelines for Professional Practice. Online. Available: www.nahps.org.uk 16 April 2004

Ovretveit J 1990 What is quality in health services? Health Service Management. 8(3):132–133

Peter S & Torr G 1996 Paediatric hospital at home; the first year. Paediatric Nursing 8(5):20–23

Redfern S J & Norman I J 1990 Measuring the quality of nursing care: a consideration of different approaches. Journal of Advanced Nursing 15(11):1260–1271

Royal College of Paediatrics and Child Health (RCPCH) 2001a Paediatrics and Child Health: the next 10 years. RCPCH, London

Royal College of Paediatrics and Child Health (RCPCH) 2001b Joint inter-collegiate working party on A & E services for children. RCPCH, London

Royal College of Paediatrics and Child Health (RCPCH) 2002 Children's Attendance at a Minor Injury/Illness Service. Intercollegiate Group on A & E Medicine for Children. RCPCH, London

Royal College of Paediatrics and Child Health (RCPCH) 2003 Specialist health services for children and young people. A guide for Primary Care Organisations. RCPCH, London

Sheldon L M 1997 Making decisions: involving parents as partners in care. Journal of Child Health Care 1(4):172–177

Stallard S 1995 Parental satisfaction with intervention: differences between respondents and non-respondents to a postal questionnaire. British Journal of Clinical Psychology 34(Part 3)

Tatman M & Woodroffe C 1993 Paediatric home care in the UK. Archives of Disease in Childhood 69:677–680

Taylor B 1996 Parents as partners in care. Paediatric Nursing 8(4):24–27

Ungar W J & Santos T 2004 Trends in paediatric health economic evaluation: 1980 to 1999. Archives of Disease in Childhood 89(1):26–29

Vickers J L & Carlisle C 2000 Choices and control: parental experiences in pediatric terminal home care. Journal of Pediatric Oncology Nursing 17(1):12–21

West P 2004 Health economics in paediatrics. Archives of Disease in Childhood 89(1):2–3

While A 1991 An evaluation of a paediatric home care scheme. Journal of Advanced Nursing 16:1413–1421

Whiting M 2001 Community children's nursing – delivering on the quality agenda? In: Sines D, Appelby F & Raymond E (eds) Community Health Care Nursing. Blackwell Science, Oxford

Chapter 16

Issues for the composition of community children's nursing teams

Maybelle Tatman and Suzanne Jones

KEY ISSUES
- Clinical leadership.
- Supervision of practice.
- Clinical governance.
- Team competencies and specialism.
- Nurse Consultants.
- Workforce planning.
- Interagency working.
- Working with parents.

INTRODUCTION

This chapter considers the inter-related issues when planning or reviewing the structure of new or developing community children's nursing teams.

CLINICAL LEADERSHIP

Community children's nursing has developed diversely with patchy coverage often by small services, some generalist and some specialist, based either in acute units or in the community (Tatman & Woodroffe 1993). In recent years community children's nursing teams in the UK have increased in number, size and skill mix (Cramp et al 2003) (see Chapter 2). The increase in junior team members working under supervision reflects the maturity and development of community children's nursing practice, a requirement for service provision and the need for supervised placements of community children's nurses (CCNs) in training (see Chapter 9 p 111). Additionally the move to Children's Trusts (see Chapter 3) means that community children's nursing teams may incorporate colleagues from other disciplines both within and outside health, including social services, education and the voluntary sector.

Leadership for nurses has been lacking (Audit Commission 1993). There remains a clear need to strengthen leadership by placing nurses at the forefront of the process of improving and contributing to patient care (Royal College of Nursing 2003). Teams must, therefore, include a manager/clinical leader with the ability to plan and develop the service (Parkin 1998) and to manage the team, supervising and mentoring both junior and more experienced CCNs (see Conclusion). The manager will:

- ensure the service provides effective patient-focused care and responds to the differing needs of each child and family
- provide clinical supervision to the team
- coordinate and manage programmes of care, developing pathways for cooperation between teams
- develop and implement 'agreements of care' (see Chapter 22 p 255)
- establish clinical governance, including policies, standards and guidelines, comprehensive record keeping and caseload and service management, monitoring and audit systems
- control the service budget, negotiating and agreeing resources
- recruit, select and develop staff
- monitor Health and Safety regulations and undertake risk assessments

The personal leadership qualities required in community children's nursing may be summarised as (Murphy W 2001):

- vision and drive to set direction
- political acumen (see Chapter 4)
- role models at a local, regional and national level (see Chapter 10)
- innovation and creativity to provide new ways of working
- cognitive ability to have credibility
- empowerment of clients and team to maximise potential
- flexibility to adapt style to situation
- collaboration and networking to optimise input to clients
- awareness of environment
- ability to balance change and stability
- skills to teach both team and families
- thinking skills to problem solve and evaluate progress.

Reynolds & Rogers (2003) discussed adaptation of leadership style, balancing directiveness and supportiveness according to the situation and the levels of competence and commitment amongst staff. Leadership needs to work both 'upwards and downwards' influencing people at different places in the hierarchy or who belong to different organisations. A good leader facilitates leadership in those working around them.

SUPERVISION OF PRACTICE

Hickey (2000) surveyed newly qualified children's nurses and found that 98% chose not to work in the community on initial qualification, mostly due to feeling inadequately prepared to work in this setting. This could be considered to indicate deficiencies in pre-registration education, or that skills and experience were required to work in the community that could only be acquired through additional and post-qualification education and experience. By contrast 63% of student nurses surveyed by Cox et al (2003) were encouraged to work in the community by their placement experience.

Qualified nurses in their first community post will therefore lack grounding in community children's nursing even though they have consolidated their clinical skills in hospital practice. Preceptorship, formal support from a colleague with at least 1 year's relevant experience, is advocated for these nurses (Nursing and Midwifery Council 2002). The preceptor does not assume professional accountability for the practitioner's actions but acts as a resource to:

- facilitate the practitioner's professional development
- meet the practitioner's learning needs
- help the practitioner to apply knowledge to practice
- integrate into the new setting.

More experienced CCNs may be at risk of isolation by the nature of their work as usually they will be in a one-to-one situation with the families they visit. The service manager/team leader has a role in developing their boundary management. This means reviewing professional roles and caseload management and allocation and helping team members to work together to avoid professional isolation, over-involvement with clients and burnout (see Chapter 11). Team meetings to discuss cases, or debrief after a traumatic event such as a death are ways of achieving this.

On a more individual level, the manager has a role in establishing mentoring and appraisal arrangements for staff to promote reflective and evidence-based practice, and ensure appropriate clinical supervision (Sloan & Watson 2002). Appraisal involves private meetings between the appraiser and the appraisee at agreed intervals. The appraisee's performance and personal development are reviewed as are their responsibilities and job description. Targets are agreed which reflect the aims of the service and the role of the appraisee within it. The training, which the appraisee will require to achieve their targets, is identified. If there are concerns about an individual's performance then these may be alluded to during appraisal but specific concerns should be tackled as they arise with the individual and not left until the appraisal interview.

CLINICAL GOVERNANCE

The Royal College of Nursing (RCN) (2003) has stated that clinical governance is 'a framework which helps all clinicians, including nurses, to continuously improve quality and safeguard standards of care'. The key themes of clinical governance (underpinned by information on patient experience, resources, processes and outcomes) are:

- building blocks, which include leadership, consultation and patient involvement, service planning, performance review and health community partnerships
- supporting nurses in the workplace, including staffing and staff management, education, training and continuing professional development and team working
- quality improvement including risk management, incident reporting and complaints, research and effectiveness and audit

- placing the patient at the heart of healthcare, including the planning and organisation of care and the environment of care.

The benchmarking process can be used to improve the quality of the patient experience. The document 'Essence of Care' (DoH 2001) provides a guide to this process and a series of eight patient-focused benchmarks are identified as crucial to the patient experience. These include issues such as continence, hygiene, nutrition, privacy and dignity and record keeping (see Chapter 18).

Skill mix

There has been conflicting evidence on skill mix and quality of care. Some research has suggested that a highly qualified skill mix was expensive and unproductive and other studies have found the reverse (McKenna 1995). Many community children's nursing services have comprised one or two highly skilled nurses and have been too small to introduce skill mix (Tatman & Woodroffe 1993). Cramp et al (2003) in a national survey of community children's nursing identified that teams caring predominantly for children with chronic illnesses had more senior nurses (G grade) while predominantly acute teams had the greatest degree of skill mix and a high proportion of middle grade (E and F) nurses, with relatively few inexperienced staff (D grade or below) being employed.

European Working Time Directive (EWTD)

NHS Trusts must comply with the EWTD. This has challenged the working patterns and training of doctors and also the provision of out-of-hours emergency medical cover (DoH 2003). The core elements of the strategy for delivering compliance are:

- fewer out-of-hours rotas
- effective use of the skills of other staff
- team working and different ways of working and training
- continuing to increase the number of doctors working in the NHS.

For many nurses, however, this has proved a positive opportunity to develop their practice further and provide a more responsive service. The NHS Plan has recommended that nurse-led services should be set up with extended nursing roles in both clinical practice and clinical leadership and the establishment of new posts for Nurse Consultants (NC) (DoH 2000) (see p 188).

TEAM COMPETENCIES AND SPECIALISM

The competencies required by CCNs are shown in Box 16.1 Seven broad areas in which CCNs work are outlined in Chapter 2 (p 34). These areas include a number of sub-specialities such as oncology and cystic fibrosis care and no individual CCN could reasonably be expected to provide the same high level of competency in each. Some diagnosis-based specialisation is inevitable within teams if competencies are to be maintained across a wide range of diagnoses. This may have to be balanced with the need for the team members to:

- retain insight into one another's work
- cross cover for one another including out-of-hours cover where this is an aim of the team

> **Box 16.1** Skills and abilities required by CCNs
>
> - Work with a high level of independence in a child's home without immediate recourse to other clinicians
> - Assess complex needs of children requiring nursing in the community, and of their families
> - Formulate individual care plans
> - Teach and support families in carrying out their child's nursing care
> - Monitor the child's progress/solve problems/adapt the care plan accordingly
> - Manage time/workload to provide a reliable and responsive service (see Chapter 19)
> - Liaise with and teach other professionals and coordinate their input
> - Establish and audit service standards/policies/procedures
> - Teach/support other team members

- work in a geographical patch with the aim of improving liaison with primary care
- avoid practising in isolation.

There are two separate dimensions to specialisation:

- concentration of practice in a disorder specific sub-speciality
- increased level of expertise in the sense of advanced practice.

Benner's work (1984) encapsulated much of the early theory on advanced practice by explaining competencies in terms of five levels of practice from novice through to expert. The distinctions between these levels continues to be debated as nurses have examined the boundaries of advanced clinical practice. A survey of specialist and advanced nursing practice in England (McGee et al 1996) found a need to clarify the interface between these two roles and that of doctors. Maclaine (1998) suggested that the nurse practitioner had a more generalist range of practice than a nurse specialist and also used diagnostic skills including physical examination, but that many aspects of their roles were the same.

Hamric (1996) identified eight core competencies to define the advanced nurse practitioner role as expert clinical practice, expert guidance and coaching, consultation, research skills, clinical and professional leadership, collaboration, change agent skills and ethical decision making. Advanced practitioners are defined as 'Specially prepared nurses who are working in roles which demand a lot of nursing experience, education at master's degree level, and nursing skills that contribute to meeting the complex needs of vulnerable people and the need to be continuously questioning the fundamentals and boundaries of nursing' (Castledine 1996 pp 288–289) (see Chapter 30).

Procter et al (1998) described the relationship between generalist and specialist roles. They argued that the multiskilled generalists were advanced practitioners in community children's nursing. 'Generalist' may be used in the sense of 'not yet having acquired specialist expertise in a particular area' or in the sense of 'having moved beyond narrow specialisation into an expert role, capable of coping with a range of specialisms'. In the latter may lie the true meaning of 'advanced practice' (Procter et al 1998).

The Nursing and Midwifery Council (2001) defined specialist practice as the exercise of higher levels of judgement, discretion and decision making in four broad areas: clinical practice; care and programme management; clinical practice development; and clinical practice leadership (see Chapter 9). Standards for specialist community children's nursing were defined but no standards were set for advanced practice or for NCs.

NURSE CONSULTANTS IN COMMUNITY CHILDREN'S NURSING

Manley (1997) described the NC role as expert practitioner, educator, researcher, acting at clinical and strategic levels and as transformational, being able to lead change and empower staff. 'Making a Difference' stated that the objectives for NC posts were to:

- provide better outcomes for patients by improving the service and quality of care
- strengthen clinical leadership
- provide a career structure that would retain experienced nurses in clinical practice (DoH 1999).

There are four domains within the NC role:

- expert practice
- professional leadership and consultancy
- education, training and development
- practice and service development, research and evaluation (NHS Executive 1999).

These may vary depending on the context in which the NC works. The role may lean towards practice development, developing new services or facilitating care through multiprofessional teams. Practice is central to the NC role, but Reid and Dewing (2003) argued that NCs must never simply 'do' practice but also support others to 'do' practice and to explore their working environment. A culture change is required in teams and organisations that include an NC. Staff leadership can help to clarify values and overcome barriers to progress (Manley 2000a, 2000b). The outcomes expected of the NC relate to the modernisation and transformation of culture as much as to traditional healthcare outcomes (Jones 2002). Organisations need to consider how to facilitate the NC role as it challenges existing structures and needs high-level management support to succeed. Coady (2003) calls for role clarity within an organisation, realistic and achievable objectives, teamwork and peer support and realistic resourcing of administrative support, implementation of change and service development.

In children's services, NC appointments have been relatively low, 37 out of 400 (Linter 2003). At the time of writing, there were three NCs in community children's nursing in the UK. The first two were NCs for children with complex care needs and in 2003 an NC in community children's nursing was appointed.

Example of components of an NC role for children with complex care needs in the community

Expert practice

- Working at specialist hospital with child to gain a thorough understanding of needs and to update clinical skills.
- Working with CCNs to bring child home on visits.
- Working with carers when child first at home, to support carers and gain a deep understanding of how their role feels and works, check care plan and contingency plans in a real-life situation.
- Establishing support package, second on call to support CCNs taking on call role.
- Acting as key worker and case manager supporting CCNs to take over this role.

Professional leadership

- Acting as local expert adviser to children's commissioner and local PCT on the best package of care for child.
- Leading local multi-agency planning team for child.
- Using experience of child to work with local PCT to bid for continuing care.
- Working with referring hospital to celebrate strengths and learn lessons from the discharge.
- Working on NSF expert working group using experience to guide input.
- Working with ACT to develop a palliative care framework synthesising experience with research to formulate input.

Education, training and development

- Setting up carers' training and induction course.
- Developing carers' competencies for child.
- Using experience from working with child to teach undergraduate and postgraduate nurses.
- Developing a competency-based system for caring for children with complex needs with the multidisciplinary team and social services respite services.

Practice and service development

- Developing evidence-based risk assessment and care plan to support child in conjunction with CCNs.
- Supporting CCNs to audit child's care.
- Using lessons learnt from practice to support modernisation of continuing care process in local PCTs.
- Gathering and disseminating research and demonstrating research-based working.
- Using experience to formulate research questions for future research.

WORKFORCE PLANNING

Twenty-four-hour nursing support

Twenty-four-hour availability is seen by many parents, service providers and Government as a crucial feature of an effective community children's nursing service (Health Committee 1997, Forys 2001). This has been understandably slow to develop in many areas due to lack of resources, concerns about safety of staff and the intermittent need for 24-hour care. Anecdotal evidence suggests that 24-hour/7-day a week cover is regularly provided without realistic assessments of risks and available resources (see Chapter 31). The commonest reason for visits out of hours is terminal care. Uptake of 24-hour availability must be proactively planned and managed to ensure adequate staffing levels exist (Tatman et al 1994) and need is minimised. Evening visits by the nurses were identified as being the 'most important in allaying the worries and anxieties of the mothers, so that there have been very few emergency calls during the night' (Smellie 1956 p 256).

Staff safety

Violence against public sector employees has become more common in modern life. Community nurses are vulnerable because they frequently work alone and away from base. Recent research found there were more than one and a half million violent incidents against public sector staff in the UK every year, resulting in the loss of over 3.3 million working hours, and that many more incidents were not reported. The Government's zero-tolerance policy towards violence in the public sector and guidelines on lone-worker security have prompted employers to implement new levels of protection for staff working in more vulnerable environments. There are three important aspects to staff safety: spotting and dealing with aggressive behaviour; emergency call systems; systems for support after a violent incident (Royal College of Nursing 1998).

Following risk assessment, various options may be implemented to support lone workers. One option is an automated system, using standard telephones, either mobile or landline, that are available 24 hours a day, 7 days a week, across the UK. This offers two levels of response:

- Safety response. Staff ring a dedicated number before a visit, stating where they are and who they are visiting and keying in the expected length of the visit. If the visit over-runs a safety response is activated following a set telephone script customised to the community children's nursing team.
- Emergency response. If the user is in trouble, they hit a specific number on their phone. It automatically rings an emergency contact number and records the next 45 seconds of sound. The system will know who the member of staff is and what is happening, enabling help to be called.

Role of other disciplines

A dimension to skill mix exists beyond that of nursing competencies, it is the value of the different skills of others. Thornes described multidisciplinary teams set up within a pilot project programme for children with a life-threatening illness (NHS Executive 1998). Similar teams have been established, i.e. the Diana teams (Oliver 2000, Davies & Harding 2002) and others with New Opportunities Fund monies. The wide range of child and family need has led to a wide range of disciplines within teams:

- Social worker (SW): Role varied (may be 'named' generic SW from local services or part of a multidisciplinary team), includes: liaison between social services and health; multiprofessional assessments; social work advice to team members; individual work with children and families to offer support or to advocate for their needs; facilitation of parents groups; bereavement support; helping families to obtain financial assistance to meet the child's needs (see Chapter 23 p 266).

- Clinical psychologist: Role is to support the team in managing stress: enable debriefing for nurses and care staff either individually or on a group basis; complement the support already offered to families.
- Healthcare assistants and support workers: Provide respite care and practical help in the home such as domestic tasks related to the child's needs: trained by CCNs; provide a defined level of care with the overall responsibility for care retained by CCN (see Chapter 22 p 253).
- Clerical staff: Produce and distribute written information and referrals about children, help develop teaching packages and literature supporting the team.
- Nursery nurses: Collaborate with psychologist to tackle issues such as needle phobia through play, work with siblings, work with nursery nurses employed across health and social services (see Chapter 27).
- Bereavement carers or volunteers providing domestic help.

INTERAGENCY WORKING

Children with complex healthcare needs require the involvement of professionals from health, education and social care. For many years these professionals have been trying to ensure seamless services and easier access. Nurse-led services such as the Diana and children's Continuing Care teams have been set up to coordinate packages of care (Linter et al 2000, Oliver 2000, Davies & Harding 2002). Despite growth in multi-agency working many barriers have not been overcome. The 'Working Together' project explored the impact of multi-agency working on children with complex healthcare needs and their families (Watson et al 2002, Townsley et al 2003). It interviewed families, children and staff identified through six multi-agency services across the UK. Professionals viewed multi-agency working positively, citing improved communication and working relationships with other agencies and stating that they were making a positive difference to the lives of families. The families were satisfied with the support and education their children received together with the management of their complex healthcare needs.

Barriers to being at home and school had been removed but some gaps remained in the coordination of care. The services had differing arrangements for joint working and only one service shared resources at both strategic and operational level. Home adaptations, financial advice, respite care and social opportunities for parents and children were not provided in a coordinated way. Where key workers were provided, many families still felt that their care was uncoordinated and many were still experiencing multiple assessments. Families felt that the services focused on the child's healthcare needs at the expense of the family unit as a whole. The children and young people lacked opportunities for developing friendships and doing 'ordinary' things rather than specially designed activities. The Audit Commission (2003) identified that families of disabled children still encountered uncoordinated service planning and provision, poor multi-agency working around transitions such as hospital to home or children's to adult services (see Chapter 32), difficulties with eligibility criteria for services and poor continuity of care due to staff turnover.

Some barriers to interagency working may be due to the need to protect resources and limit caseloads. There is also the issue of organisational culture. Davies (2002a) identified different approaches to quality and to evidence-based care between health and social services. Professional identity, with its emphasis on the expertise of individual practitioners, can devalue others and undermine interdisciplinary working. The modern practitioner needs to respect the contributions of others in order to develop creative solutions (Davies 2002b). Heywood (2002) advocates multidisciplinary documentation, audit and reflective practice, supported by a shared vision of care and facilitated by managers willing to work across organisational boundaries.

Modernisation of the NHS has generated a new commitment to improving communication and working practices across professional and organisational boundaries, which harmonises with the holistic and patient-centred philosophy of nursing (Kenny 2002). Children's Trusts have been proposed to bring health, education and social services staff together in the same organisation, with the aim of joined-up working and information sharing and also a joining up of training, career pathways and terms and conditions of service (see Chapter 3 p 49). At the time of writing there were no published evaluations of Children's Trusts. The first combined Trust in England was formed in Somerset by the transfer of social services mental health staff to an NHS Trust. This was studied by Peck et al (2001). The first year of the new organisation was accompanied by a fall in staff job satisfaction and an increase in reported levels of emotional exhaustion, despite evidence of effective joint working. Staff clung to their professional identities and for nurses there was a debate on whether their professional role should continue to be developed by the national regulatory body or whether the national body (NMC) should merely reflect the changes taking place in the field. Staff and managers perceived a lack of identity for the Trust and a key problem was a clash of culture between health and social services. It appeared that the creation of a shared organisational culture will not follow automatically from the creation of a shared organisation, nor can it be manipulated or improved by managers in a top-down manner. Professional leadership and involvement of service users were felt to be more important drivers in cultural change. Manley (2000b) has highlighted the importance of leadership in achieving cultural change, in the context of the NC role.

WORKING WITH PARENTS

Parents are expected to be extensively involved in the care of their sick child in hospital and at home (Coyne 1995, Murphy G 2001a). The community setting enables parents to be more active participants in decision making about their child's care than is often the case in hospital (Taylor 2000). There has been lack of clarity among both nurses and parents about the boundaries of parental participation. Research has identified a high level of nursing tasks undertaken by families while key elements of the CCN's role were teaching and supporting the parental care of the child (While 1991, Tatman et al 1992, Procter et al 1998). A higher level of competency is required for the CCN to focus on the supportive role rather than on direct physical care (Procter et al 1998, Muir & Sidey 2003).

The process of discharge for a technology-dependent child may be complicated and lengthy (Jardine et al 1999). Linter et al (2000) identified that parents of technology-dependent children found discharge from hospital a difficult experience and often entered a grieving process for which support was required. Ground rules needed to be set out at an early stage. As parents developed trust in the continuing care team they gradually became able to deliver more care by themselves. The need for ongoing support for parents was described in the context of home ventilation by Boosfeld and O'Toole (2000) who identified issues including privacy and intrusion, alteration in parental roles, financial burdens and demands upon family members to provide care. Glendinning and Kirk (2000) found that parents assumed primary responsibility for their child's technical and nursing care, carrying out procedures which were often distressing for their children and hence for themselves. Their lives were dominated by the technology, their homes by medical equipment and their sleep disturbed. They developed a level of expertise that could be challenging to professionals. Difficulties were encountered in obtaining supplies and equipment and coordinating local services. CCNs need to fulfil a key worker role for these families, providing a point of contact and support and coordinating the care package (see Chapter 23 p 264).

Murphy G (2001a) reviewed costs to families, including the financial and social and emotional costs and the effects on siblings. She suggested that the development of community children's nursing has increased expectations that parents will care for technology-dependent children at home. She questioned whether an informed choice is genuinely offered to parents during the discharge planning process and recommended that frank discussion of the costs as well as the benefits should take place. Murphy G (2001b) also considered the respite needs of parents, who may feel trapped by caring for technology-dependent children in the home, with limited availability of suitable respite options. She argued that CCNs must advocate for the needs of the family as a whole and ensure a balance in discussions about discharge planning. Skill mix in community children's nursing teams should include appropriately trained and supported carers to incorporate respite into the service.

Packages of complex and respite care can be supported and strengthened by appropriate training for staff and adequate and realistic preparation for the child and parents.

Training for staff

- Defining roles/responsibilities of carers to reduce duplication.
- Establishing role boundaries/limits to avoid over involvement.
- Respecting parents' privacy/confidentiality/right to family life.
- Regular meetings between families/staff to address difficulties during the early stages/access to psychological support.
- Identification of lines of communication to key worker.
- Move staff around between them if there is more than one child in an area.

Preparation for child and family

- Care agreements (see Chapter 22).
- Impact on privacy and family life.
- Parental responsibilities.

- Identified lines of communication to a key worker.
- Psychological support for parents and siblings.
- Try to normalise the situation as much as possible.
- Parents involved in the recruitment process of staff.

CONCLUSION

Clinical and professional leadership is vital for the development of a team in which there is an appropriate skill mix, together with support and mentorship for junior members and close cooperation between senior members. Once this leadership is in place a team should maintain a service development plan based on ongoing review of caseload needs and adjustment of skill mix and team size accordingly. Multidisciplinary team working and involving parents in the development of the team should be part of team philosophy. 'Generalist' community children's nursing is a recognised specialisation in itself, necessitating a high level of competency within the nursing team. The key to change in nursing practice is the ability to improve the competencies of others.

Few families at the time of their child's diagnosis realise the extent to which chronic disease will change every aspect of their lives. Parents struggle with a long disease trajectory and looking after a child with complex needs. This makes prolonged and heavy demands upon families, affecting their health and wellbeing, relationships, family life and ability to cope. Improving service delivery together with access to services and resources for children in the community is the responsibility of many agencies. Current health policy stresses new ways of partnership working to develop creative solutions to care packages whilst maximising the use of resources.

REFERENCES

Audit Commission 1993 Children First: Study of Hospital Services. HMSO, London

Audit Commission 2003 Let me be me: A handbook for managers and staff working with disabled children and their families. Audit Commission, London

Benner P 1984 From Novice to Expert: Excellence and Power in Clinical Nursing Practice. Addison-Wesley, Menlo Park, California

Boosfeld B & O'Toole M 2000 Technology-dependent children: transition from hospital to home. Paediatric Nursing 12(6):20–22

Castledine G 1996 The role and criteria of an advanced nurse practitioner. British Journal of Nursing 5:288–289

Coady E 2003 Role models. Nursing Management 10(2):18–21

Cox S, Murrells T & Robinson S 2003 Careers in child health nursing: the influence of course experiences. Paediatric Nursing 15(10):36–41

Coyne I T 1995 Parental participation in care: a critical review of the literature. Journal of Advanced Nursing 21:716–722

Cramp C, Tripp S, Hughes N & Dale J 2003 Children's home nursing: results of a national survey. Paediatric Nursing 15 (8):39–43

Davies C 2002a Approaches to quality in health and social care. Nursing Management 9(4):34–37

Davies C 2002b Continuing to manage professional identities. Nursing Management 9(6):31–34

Davies R & Harding Y 2002 The first Diana Team in Wales: an update. Paediatric Nursing 14(2):24–25

Department of Health 1999 Making a difference: strengthening the nursing, midwifery and health visiting contribution to health and healthcare. The Stationery Office, London

Department of Health 2000 The NHS Plan – a plan for investment, a plan for reform. The Stationery Office, London

Department of Health 2001 Essence of Care. The Stationery Office, London

Department of Health 2003 Guidance on Implementing the European Working Time Directive for Doctors in Training. Health Service Circular 2003/001 Annex 1.

Online. Available: http://www.dh.gov.uk/ workingtime/ewtdguidance.pdf 26 January 2004

Forys J 2001 Do Community Children's Nurses offer 24 hour care? Primary Health Care 11(6):31–35

Glendinning C & Kirk S 2000 High-tech care: high-skilled parents. Paediatric Nursing 12(6):25–27

Hamric A B 1996 A definition of advanced nursing. In: Hamric A B, Spross J A & Hanson C M (eds) Advanced Nursing Practice: An Integrative Approach. W B Saunders, Philadelphia

Health Committee 1997 Health services for children and young people in the community: home and school. Third report. The Stationery Office, London

Heywood J 2002 Enhancing seamless care: a review. Paediatric Nursing 14(5):18–20

Hickey G 2000 Newly qualified and into the community? Paediatric Nursing 12(9):30–33

Jardine E, Toole M, Payton J & Wallis C 1999 Current status of long term ventilation of children in the United Kingdom: questionnaire survey. British Medical Journal 318:295–299

Jones S 2002 Consultant nurses and their potential impact upon health care delivery. Clinical Medicine 2(1):39–40

Kenny G 2002 Interprofessional working: opportunities and challenges. Nursing Standard 17(6):33–35

Linter S 2003 Consultant nurses in children's services. Nursing Management 10(8):16–18

Linter S, Perry M & Cherry D 2000 Continuing care: An integrated approach. Paediatric Nursing 12(8):17–18

McGee P, Castledine G & Brown R 1996 A survey of specialist and advanced nursing practice in England. British Journal of Nursing 5(11):682–686

McKenna H 1995 Nursing skill mix substitutions and quality of care: an exploration of assumptions from the research literature. Journal of Advanced Nursing 21:452–459

Maclaine K 1998 Clarifying higher level roles in nursing practice. Professional Nurse 14(3):159–163

Manley K 1997 Operationalising an advanced practice/consultant nurse role: an action research study. Journal of Clinical Nursing 6:179–190

Manley K 2000a Organisational culture and consultant nurse outcomes: part 1 Organisational culture. Nursing Standard 14(36):34–38

Manley K 2000b Organisational culture and consultant nurse outcomes: Part 2: Nurse outcomes. Nursing Standard 14(37):34–38

Muir J & Sidey A 2003 Community children's nursing. In: Watkins D, Edwards J & Gastrell P (eds) Community Health Nursing, 2nd edn. Baillière Tindall, Edinburgh, pp 271–279

Murphy G 2001a The technology dependent child at home. Part 1: In whose best interest? Paediatric Nursing 13(7):14–18

Murphy G 2001b The technology dependent child at home. Part 2: The need for respite. Paediatric Nursing 13(8):24–28

Murphy W 2001 Leadership and Community Children's Nurses. Paediatric Nursing 13(10):36–40

NHS Executive 1998 Evaluation of the pilot project programme for children with life threatening illnesses. The Stationery Office, London

NHS Executive 1999. Nurse, Midwife and Health Visitor Consultants: Establishing posts and making appointments HSC 1999/217 NHS Executive, Leeds

Nursing and Midwifery Council (NMC) 2001 Standards for specialist education and practice. NMC, London

Nursing and Midwifery Council (NMC) 2002 Supporting nurses and midwives through lifelong learning. NMC, London

Oliver H 2000 One year on: Cornwall's Diana Team. Paediatric Nursing 12(10):21–23

Parkin P 1998 An approach to management for community health professionals. British Journal of Community Nursing 3(8):374–381

Peck E, Towell D & Gulliver P 2001 The meanings of culture in health and social care: a study of the combined Trust in Somerset. Journal of Interprofessional Care 15(4) 319–327

Procter S, Biott C, Campbell S, Edward S, Redpath N & Moran M 1998 Preparation for the developing role of the community children's nurse. English National Board for Nursing, Midwifery and Health Visiting, London

Reid B & Dewing J 2003 A model for clinical practice within the nurse consultant role. Nursing Times 99:9

Reynolds J & Rogers A 2003 Leadership styles and situations. Nursing Management 9(10):27–30

Royal College of Nursing (RCN) 1998 Dealing with Violence Against Nursing Staff. RCN, London

Royal College of Nursing (RCN) 2003 Clinical Governance: an RCN resource guide. RCN, London

Sloan G & Watson H 2002 Clinical supervision models for nursing: structure, research and limitations. Nursing Standard 17(4):41–46

Smellie J M 1956 Domiciliary nursing service for infants and children. British Medical Journal i:256

Tatman M & Woodroffe C 1993 Paediatric home care in the UK. Archives of Disease in Childhood 69:677–680

Tatman M A, Woodroffe C, Kelly P J & Harris R J 1992 Paediatric home care in Tower Hamlets: a working partnership with parents. Quality in Health Care 1:98–103

Tatman M, Kelly P, Dryden S, Sappa M, Sidey A, Whiting M & Burr S 1994 Wise decisions: developing paediatric home care teams. Royal College of Nursing, London

Taylor J 2000 Partnership in the community and hospital: a comparison. Paediatric Nursing 12(5):28–30

Townsley R, Abbott D & Watson D 2003 Making a difference? Exploring the impact of multi-agency working on disabled children with complex health care needs, their families and the professionals who support them. Policy Press, Bristol

Watson D, Townsley R & Abbott D 2002 Exploring multi-agency working in services to disabled children with complex healthcare needs and their families. Journal of Clinical Nursing 11(3):367–375

While A 1991 An evaluation of a paediatric home care scheme. Journal of Advanced Nursing 16:1413–1421

Chapter 17

Needs analysis and profiling in community children's nursing

Julie Hughes, Anna Sidey and David Widdas

with a contribution from:

Suzanne Jones and Maybelle Tatman

KEY ISSUES

- Needs assessment.
- Profiling – defining the community in the context of community children's nursing.
- Needs analysis.
- Determining a need for a community children's nursing service.
- Producing a business plan to support service development.
- Promoting and marketing the service.

INTRODUCTION

During the past decade there has been a significant shift in healthcare policy and a drive to realign health services from the acute to the primary care setting (DoH 2000, 2001). This shift is significant for the role of the Community Children's Nurse (CCN) as the advocate for children and their families. Liaison, assessment and analysis provide evidence of the needs of their client group. These skills are components of a CCN's education. Profiling, needs assessment and analysis are key stages of service development and maintenance. Essential components of a business plan emerge from the retrospective evidence of service delivery and planned service activity. This chapter examines the skills required for each of these stages.

NEEDS ASSESSMENT

The principles of needs assessment are historically rooted within the health visiting profession (Tinson 1995) and should be applied to all specialist areas of community nursing. To facilitate this process a community children's nursing service will have established a philosophy, aims and objectiveness and clearly defined the geographical and referral boundaries.

What is need?

The concept of need takes on different meanings for different people. Three of the most functional theoretical frameworks have been developed by Bradshaw (1972), Orr (1985) and Hooper & Long (2002). Bradshaw (1972) identified need as:

- Normative – need based on professional perspective
- Felt – need identified by members of community
- Expressed – felt need progressed to demand for a service
- Comparative – need identified by comparison with another area.

In contrast Orr (1985) refers to need as:

- Social – need according to standards of communal life
- Relative – meaning of need will vary across people/society
- Evaluative – need based on value judgements.

Hooper and Long (2002), whilst acknowledging the perspective offered by Bradshaw, explore the concept of need in the NHS and define it as:

- Expressed – perception of the population
- Normative/epidemiological – severity and size of health issues/population characteristics
- Normative/corporate (national) – perceptions of service providers
- Normative/corporate (local) – perception of organisations commissioning/managing services within profiled community.

When developing a community children's nursing service the identification and assessment of unmet needs determines service priorities, clear understanding of the client group and the competencies and level of specialisation required. Assessment of needs helps:

- develop an accurate picture
- avoid operational conflicts/duplication of services already provided
- develop a business case
- create the basis for evaluation.

Assessment of needs may not necessitate specific population-based research on local health need (Box 17.1). On the development of children's palliative care services, for example, a number of research studies on need are cited by the Association for Children with Life-threatening or Terminal Conditions and their Families & Royal College of Paediatrics and Child Health (2003). They found that the same needs are duplicated throughout the country and research findings can be transferred to most local situations without requiring further local validation.

When defining the needs of the child and their family the CCN should explore need as expressed by the child and family and from a wide range of social and organisational perspectives. The recognition and incorporation of these broad and potentially conflicting needs is challenging. Robinson and Elkan (1996) argue that nurses are best placed to assess need as they have day-to-day contact with clients together with first-hand experience of the implications of healthcare policy on the user. Children and families may be helped to assess their needs through the use of patients' stories and focus groups (Kruger 1994).

Box 17.1 Objectives of a needs assessment in community children's nursing

- Define catchment population
- Review relevant published literature on community children's nursing
- Review NHS targets/priorities, identify those which enter the scope of the work
- Review local unpublished literature particularly small research projects/audit reports
- Capture local routine data on the population such as size/deprivation indices/geography/ patterns of hospital utilisation/education provision/primary care provision (including out of hours)
- Define/estimate need in target groups
- Review of and consultation with existing local services/voluntary organisations
- Consultation with service users
- In many areas Partnership Boards and Children's Trusts may exist to facilitate joint planning between health/education/social services, these will normally have representation from service users/voluntary organisations
- Visit CCNs elsewhere to experience different models of provision

What is the community?

The concept of a community is complex and diverse. Definitions of a community vary according to the context in which it is defined. For CCNs a much wider perspective of the community is required. The catchment area of a service will normally be determined by the organisational model within which they work. Despite an increase in the number of services available there remains no national strategic direction, corporate identity or models of service delivery (see Chapter 10). Consequently the community will be determined by the parameters of the local service model. Examples of the types of service delivery models are offered by Health Committee (1997), Winter & Teare (1997), Thomas (1997), Eaton (2001) and Whiting (p 34).

The geographical area covered may be vast and is likely to include urban and/or rural localities, neighbourhoods of wealth and deprivation and ethnic and cultural diversity (Box 17.2). The client group will be children and young people, aged 0–19 years, and their families. To determine the size of the potential client group, the CCN can obtain information on the numbers of children residing in their geographical area from the Office of Population Censuses and Surveys (2001) (Box 17.3).

Box 17.2 Sources of information about geographical area

- Strategic Health Authority
- Primary Care Trust
- Public Library
- Social Services Directorate
- Housing Department
- Local Education Authority

> **Box 17.3** Sources of information on the client group
>
> - Office of Population Censuses and Surveys
> - Hospital statistics, including patterns of admissions/length of stay/ regular clinics/wards attenders, etc.
> - Community Paediatricians
> - Caseload profiles of other community children's nursing teams
> - Charities

Having identified and defined the community in the context of a service, the next stage is to compile the data in the format of a profile.

Compiling a profile

The NHS and Community Care Act (DoH 1990) advocates the compilation of profiles for all community healthcare workers as a tool to identify healthcare need. Under the Act District Health Authorities and Local Authorities were required to assess need as a means of obtaining accurate and appropriate information on which to base policy and practice. Robinson and Elkan (1996) argued that nurses, midwives and health visitors are key workers in profiling and developing strategies to improve health and should therefore be actively involved throughout the process. Profiling is seen as a vital and specific skill that can empower nurses and services used to influence policy (Royal College of Nursing 1993, Tinson 1995, Cowley & Houston 2002).

A profile is a comprehensive picture of the population targeted by the service (Billings & Cowley 1995). A further definition suggests that 'profiling is a comprehensive description of the needs of the population that is defined or defines itself as a community and the resources that exist within that community carried out with active involvement of the community itself and for the purpose of developing an action plan or other means of improving the quality of life in the community' (Robotham & Sheldrake 2000 p 41). For the CCN a profile will include information on the community as a geographical area and on the children with a healthcare need residing in this area. Information gained will provide the foundation to the profile that will be compiled from demographic and epidemiological data. The service profile will also include data relating to the actual or potential client group.

Profiling is an ongoing process undertaken by the CCNs delivering the hands-on care and guided and supported by management (Burns 2003). The process of profiling assists in the targeting of resources. Factual data require assessment and analysis to provide a meaningful source of evidence (Audit Commission 1999). Hooper and Long (2002) offer a simple step model that allows for a pragmatic approach to the process of needs analysis and provides a useful framework:

1. STEP ONE: Getting started
   - Establish baseline
   - Collect relevant data

- Identify existing provision for children/families with health needs within local area.
2. STEP TWO: Identification of health priorities
   - Identify targets for the health of the local child population.
3. STEP THREE: Analysis and synthesis
   - Assess existing health provision
   - Identify gaps in service, e.g. respite care provision for children with disabilities.
4 STEP FOUR: Planning for health
   - Stakeholders meeting to identify how needs of children/families with a health need can best be met.
5. STEP FIVE: Evaluation
   - Regular evaluation of service delivery
   - Analysis/dissemination of results
   - Demonstrate ongoing need for service.

ASSESSING AND ANALYSING THE DATA

Only a small component of the child population will require the services of a CCN and it may be useful to consider the epidemiological factors within the identified and defined community. This will provide information on frequency, distribution and determinants of health and illness and the tracing of disease occurrence within the defined population (McMurray 1993). Having collated relevant data it is necessary to recognise the specific factual information that requires analysis in relation to children and families in the community. Tinson (1995) suggests that the knowledge level of the nurse will influence the quality of a needs analysis exercise. She recommends a literature search to ensure appropriate evidence is assimilated into the process. This evidence may be supported by political, environmental, sociological and technological data to provide a more comprehensive account of the findings (Buchan & Grey 1990) (Box 17.4).

Buchan and Grey (1990) argue that the analysis of need involves value judgements on the part of healthcare professionals and should therefore be balanced by the acquisition of qualitative data from children with healthcare needs and their families. User perspectives are a key driver for shaping healthcare policy and CCNs need to equip themselves with the appropriate skills for data collection. In addition, it is necessary to elicit views of other stakeholders. Hooper and Long (2002) recommend data should be collected from service providers and managers and from relevant local and national organisations. The Community Children's Nursing Forum within the Royal College of Nursing (RCN) has been influential in driving healthcare policy and practice for the profession since its inception in 1988 and is a useful source of national information for CCNs. Others could include specific charitable organisations such as Diabetes UK or more generic voluntary organisations such as Barnardo's.

An accurate and comprehensive needs analysis can raise awareness and identify the need for resources. It promotes a collaborative approach to care delivery as promoted by the Government (Blackie 1998). Cowley

---

Box 17.4 PEST analysis examples

- **Political:** Political influences that may affect the service from both local and national perspectives, e.g. CCN may incorporate recommendations from the Health Committee Report (1997) and National Service Framework (NSF) to provide arguments to support local service developments.
- **Environmental:** The urban or rural nature of service catchment area and the geographical spread. Variations in climate.
- **Sociological:** Sociological analysis is a well-researched component of community nursing. It is recognised that improvements in the overall health of a community have always come from changes in the social environment (Brown 1993, DoH 1998). Consideration should be given to areas such as undesirable living conditions, stress and poverty (Hall 1996).
- **Technological:** The number of technology-dependent children requiring support in the community has increased significantly over the last decade (Jardine et al 1999, Kirk & Glendinning 2000). Local hospital statistics may demonstrate that these children occupy a significant number of bed days. Combining this type of evidence with an economic evaluation may provide a sound argument for developing or expanding a community children's nursing service.

---

et al (2000) argue that profiling must be an essential component of the curriculum for specialist community practitioner education.

DETERMINING THE NEED TO DEVELOP THE COMMUNITY CHILDREN'S NURSING SERVICE

Having considered the components of needs assessment, profiling and needs analysis, the next stage is to demonstrate the need for developing a new or existing community children's nursing service. This should be in the form of an action and implementation plan and in order to demonstrate the need for service development to commissioners the data must be current, reliable and measurable. Analysing the statistics gathered from the hospital and community services and considering previous patterns of care for these children would be one way of demonstrating service gaps (RCN 1994). Ward attenders and hospital inpatient stays are measurable and could be costed against the provision of a community children's nursing service (Whiting 2001).

A SWOT (strengths, weaknesses, opportunities and threats) analysis can be used to present the data (Box 17.5). This is a strategic analysis of every aspect of an operation that enables objectives to be assessed and developed (Young 1986).

A SWOT analysis is a useful tool whether initiating or developing a service as it focuses on the issues that will be of importance to commissioners. However, objectives alluded to within the SWOT must be measurable or able to be demonstrated. It is essential that CCNs identify methods of collecting evidence from both qualitative and quantitative

---

Box 17.5 SWOT analysis examples

Strengths

- A well-established community children's nursing team to assess and plan nursing care
- A child development centre with children's therapy services on site
- Knowledge of the community from social/environmental/ political/economic/cultural perspectives
- Established links with social/ education/voluntary sectors
- Children/families key to strategic planning

Weaknesses

- Provision of fragmented package of health/social care
- Limited resources within community children's nursing team to introduce key worker roles/24-hour cover
- Limited resources for providing complete and comprehensive care packages to meet the needs of families, e.g. respite care/ sibling support/psychological support
- Social services under pressure to meet statutory obligations

Opportunities

- Provision of a key worker for all children and families with life-threatening/limiting illnesses
- Provision of coordinated/ collaborative package of care from health/social/ education/ voluntary sectors
- Development of supportive culture for staff from a variety of professional backgrounds
- Improved /communication across health/social/educational boundaries

Threats

- Difficulties convincing commissioners of need to invest in new services
- Moral/ethical implications of developing service with short-term investment
- Provision of 24-hour/7 day a week cover without sufficient number of CCNs to provide service/cover for leave/sickness/ professional and service development
- Emotional fatigue of team members
- Acknowledgement of service development in climate of organisational instability

---

perspectives. This could be through a variety of methods such as user satisfaction surveys, statistics of children visited against length of inpatient stay and focus groups. Whether the service is in its initial stages of development or well established it is likely that ongoing marketing and business planning will be processes that the CCN engages in on a regular basis. As advocates for community children's nursing, children and their families, and the professional with the expert knowledge, it is essential that CCNs undertake this activity.

COMPILING A BUSINESS PLAN

A business case forms the basis of any bid for funding. It needs to be compiled within the format set by the funding organisation. Normally the following issues will be covered:

- A summary of the findings of the needs assessment.
- A statement of the aims and objectives of the service.
- Estimates of the likely level of service activity and of the number of people likely to benefit.
- A discussion of alternative service models and whether there are other ways of doing the same thing.
- An estimate of costs to include staffing, accommodation, travelling, equipment and consumables. Staffing costs will need to take into account annual/study leave and training costs. The costs of implementation of a new team must include a lead-in time for appointment of a team leader/administrative and clerical staff/liaison with existing services to establish routes of referral/medical and nursing backup/appointment of other staff.
- A proposal for (1) service monitoring and evaluation based on the unmet needs found in the needs assessment and (2) determining the extent to which these needs are met by the new service.

Ongoing business plans should include retrospective and prospective achievements and evidence of service evaluation (Eaton & Thomas 1998). On review of the achievements, and in line with local Health Improvement Programmes and the children's NSF standards, an action plan should be drawn up which describes planned service developments. There is a dearth of literature relating to business planning for nurses which reflects its relatively recent assimilation into the profession, although it is interesting to note that the concept of 'planning' in nursing has been well researched for many years. Hyett (1988) indicates that planning will be undertaken on macro, meso and micro levels:

- The Trust plan
- The department plan
- The team plan.

It is important to consider the broader perspective when producing a business plan (Box 17.6) and to ensure that the service plan integrates with that of the employing Trusts.

Box 17.6 Proposed structure for a business plan

- Mission statement
- Service aims
- Existing service provision, e.g. location/facilities/human resources
- Analysis of activity
- Analysis of the community, e.g. PEST
- Analysis of service, e.g. SWOT
- Statement of need
- Proposal for meeting the need
- Action plan

MARKETING COMMUNITY CHILDREN'S NURSING SERVICES

The concept of marketing has become an implicit part of the culture of the NHS over the last decade. The NHS is made up of service providers and commissioners and as such has the nature of a market. Service managers and commissioners have been increasingly pressurised to review service delivery to ensure that they are meeting designated Government targets within a specified resource allocation. It is therefore essential to ensure that the service deliverer is able to demonstrate efficiency from a quality perspective alongside a value-for-money perspective.

CCNs need to clearly demonstrate a child and family focus while marrying qualitative and quantitative data with real-life child and family experiences (Kirk 1999). The ability to collect and present user views and related practice outcome data in a fluent and professional manner is paramount within the business culture of the NHS. This ability should focus on the process of the child's journey within their health experience and the contribution made by CCNs.

CONCLUSION

This chapter has outlined the complexities associated with profiling, needs assessment and analysis and the need for ongoing commitment to marketing and business planning. Acquiring these skills can enhance the autonomy of the profession and the CCNs ability to negotiate resources for service development (RCN 1998). The need to embrace these concepts is essential to ensure that a 'bottom-up' patient- and family-focused assessment of services informs developments rather than a 'top-down' approach (Tinson 1995, Hooper & Long 2002). Networking and sharing the relevant knowledge and skills may contribute to the ultimate aim of establishing an equitable service nationwide. Anecdotal evidence continues to indicate that a failure to clearly, realistically and accurately negotiate, define and assess available and finite resources, and to equitably and appropriately deliver them to those who need them most, can result in:

- comprehensive and inequitable provision to a few
- reactive and unsustainable services to many
- service delivery focused on inappropriate client groups
- unacceptable levels of practitioner stress and risk
- dependency-creating practice
- inappropriate professional boundaries
- dysfunctional team organisation.

Teams where service delivery is planned, as described within this chapter, demonstrate advocacy by ensuring the delivery of assessed and evaluated care to those who need the service most. Realistically this means delivering community children's nursing to a defined and limited population of sick children and ensuring an equally balanced equation exists between needs, as assessed by the CCN, and the identified available and finite resources. Ultimately it is better to embrace implicit and open rationing than the forced rationing that might be imposed by a failure to develop the required management, political and business acumen.

REFERENCES

Association for Children with Life-threatening or Terminal Conditions and their Families (ACT) & Royal College of Paediatrics and Child Health 2003 A Guide to the Development of Children's Palliative Care Services. ACT, Bristol

Audit Commission 1999 First Assessment: A Review of District Nursing Services in England and Wales. Audit Commission Publications, Abingdon

Billings J & Cowley S 1995 Approaches to community needs assessment: A literature review. Journal of Advanced Nursing 22:721–730

Blackie C 1998 Community Health Care Nursing. Churchill Livingstone, London

Bradshaw J 1972 The concept of social need. New Society 30:640–643

Brown V 1993 Health Care Policies, Health Policies or Policies for Health. In: Gardner H (ed) Health Policy Development, Implementation and Evaluation. Churchill Livingstone, Melbourne

Buchan H & Grey J A 1990 Needs assessment made simple. Health Service Journal 100:240–241

Burns S 2003 Caseload profiling: A district nurse perspective. Primary Health Care 8:36–38

Cowley S & Houston A M 2002 An empowerment approach to needs assessment in health visiting practice. Journal of Clinical Nursing 1(5):640–650

Cowley S, Bergen B, Young K & Kavannagh A 2000 Generalising to theory: the use of a multiple case study design to investigate needs assessment and quality of care. International Journal of Nursing Studies 37(3):219–228

Department of Health 1990 NHS and Community Care Act. HMSO, London

Department of Health 1998 The new NHS. Modern, dependable. The Stationery Office, London

Department of Health 2000 The NHS Plan: A plan for investment, a plan for reform. The Stationery Office, London

Department of Health 2001 Shifting the balance of power within the NHS: securing delivery. The Stationery Office, London

Eaton N 2001 Models of Community Children's Nursing. Paediatric Nursing 13(1):32–36

Eaton N & Thomas P 1998 Community children's nursing: An evaluative framework. Journal of Child Health Care 2(4):170–173

Hall D M B (ed) 1996 Health for all Children, 3rd edn. Oxford University Press, Oxford

Health Committee 1997 Third report. Health services for children and young people in the community: home and school. House of Commons Session 1996–97. The Stationery Office, London

Hooper J & Long P 2002 Health Needs Assessment workbook. NHS Development Agency, London

Hyett K 1988 Nursing Management Handbook. Churchill Livingstone, London

Jardine E, O'Toole M & Wallis C 1999 Current status of long-term ventilation of children in the United Kingdom: questionnaire survey. British Medical Journal 318:295–299

Kirk S 1999 Caring for children with specialized health care needs in the community: The challenges for primary care. Health and Social Care in the Community 7(5):350–357

Kirk S & Glendinning C 2000 High tech care: High skilled parents. Paediatric Nursing 12 (6):25–27

Kruger R 1994 Focus Groups, 2nd edn. A Practical Guide for Applied Research. Sage Publications, London

McMurray J W 1993 Community Health Nursing, 2nd edn. Churchill Livingstone, London

Office of Population, Censuses and Surveys 2001 General Household Survey. The Stationery Office, London

Orr J 1985 Individual and family needs. In: Luker K & Orr J (eds) Health Visiting. Blackwell Scientific, Oxford pp 67–120

Robinson J & Elkan R 1996 Health Needs Assessment: Theory and Practice. Churchill Livingstone, London

Robotham A & Sheldrake D 2000 Health Visiting Specialist and Higher Level Practice. Churchill Livingstone, London

Royal College of Nursing (RCN) 1993 The GP Practice Population Profile. RCN, London

Royal College of Nursing (RCN) 1994 Wise Decisions. Developing Paediatric Home Care Teams. RCN, London

Royal College of Nursing (RCN) 1998 Marketing Community and Specialist Nursing. RCN, London

Thomas E 1997 Community nursing profiles: their role in needs assessment. Nursing Standard 11(37):39–42

Tinson S 1995 Health needs assessment. In: Cain P, Hyde V & Howkins E (eds) Community Nursing: Dimensions and Dilemmas. Arnold, London, pp 144–166

Whiting M 2001 Community Children's Nursing – Delivering the 'Quality Agenda'. In: Sines D, Appelby F & Raymond E (eds) Community Health Care Nursing, 2nd edn. Blackwell Science. Oxford

Winter A & Teare J 1997 Construction and application of paediatric community nursing services. Journal of Child Health 1(1):24–29

Young A 1986 The Manager's Handbook. The Practical Guide to Successful Management. Sphere, London

Chapter 18

Benchmarking in community children's nursing – 'Essence of care'

Michael Bland

KEY ISSUES

- History of benchmarking.
- Process of benchmarking.
- A benchmark for community children's nursing.
- Children's palliative care benchmark.
- Future benchmarking.

INTRODUCTION

Benchmarking is a powerful tool, contributing to securing best practice and improved performance (Pantell 2001). The North West Clinical Practice Benchmarking Group (NWCPBG) was formed by seven children's departments in 1994 and rapidly expanded to over 32 Trusts delivering both primary and secondary children's nursing care (Ellis 1995). Additionally, the group benefited from contributions from six university faculties within the North of England. This benchmarking group has evolved over time and was instrumental in the development of the national benchmarking initiative 'Essence of Care' (DoH 2001), following the group's recognition as a quality improvement in Making a Difference (DoH 1999).

HISTORY OF BENCHMARKING

The principles of benchmarking have their origins in the United States and in the practices of privatised industries of the 1980s (Camp 1989). Companies used benchmarking in a competitive environment as a means of surpassing their competitors to lead world performance (Mears 1995). Benchmarking allowed these organisations to review and compare their own practice against the performance measures in both the internal and external setting. It enabled them to identify best practice and scrutinise their own performance in comparison with other members and to identify the actions required to attain it. The use of benchmarking in healthcare has grown since the early 1990s when the principles of private sector benchmarking were adapted to fit the needs and requirements of healthcare organisations. The data generated by organisational benchmarking activities tend to be quantitative and can be subjected to rigorous mathematical scrutiny. Such activities in the NHS have focused on data comparisons and concentrated on tangible measurements, particularly finance, cost and activity, with only limited regard to the process that produced the outcome (Philips 1995).

The driver for the NWCPBG revolved around the nursing care needs and requirements of children and their families rather than mechanical number crunching about service provision and cost (Bland 2001). The methodology has often created significant differences in both the methods of service provision and the range of services provided across the county. This was evident from the outset of the North West group and differences in practice emerged across the region's general and tertiary hospitals. Such variation makes formal auditing and comparative analysis extremely difficult and creates problems in determining the factors affecting best practice. Data generated from the NWCPBG is qualitative. This adds to the complexity of reliability and robustness in comparison to the quantitative data produced by organisational groups. However, it is the sharing of practice that is critical rather than the score determined by members.

The original group set the vision 'To nationally identify best paediatric practice, in order to facilitate the continuous improvement of paediatric care through comparison and sharing' (Ellis 2000) and this philosophy remains unchanged today. The tool developed by this group has been adopted extensively by other forums across the country, covering a wide range of specialties, although still predominately within neonatal and children's care, neurosciences (Warren 2000), community care (Stark et al 2002), accident and emergency (Greenidge 1998) or education and research (Feasey & Fox 2001). The NWCPBG itself is widely published (Ellis 1995, Ellis & Morris 1997, Ellis 2000, Bland 2000, 2001, 2002). Ellis established an internal benchmarking group within all directorates in a large teaching hospital in the North West. This formed a template for later work in the DoH national Essence of Care benchmarks (Ellis et al 2000a & 2000b).

PROCESS OF BENCHMARKING

The benchmarking tool was developed to apply the principles of best practice through comparison and sharing (Fig. 18.1).

The cyclical model allows for continuous quality improvement to develop over time through action planning and for the practice changes to be re-measured at a later given date.

Benchmark standards are determined within the NWCPBG and these standards are drawn from the expertise and consensus within the group as well as any supporting evidence base that enhances the academic

Fig. 18.1 Cyclical model to outline stages of a benchmarking tool

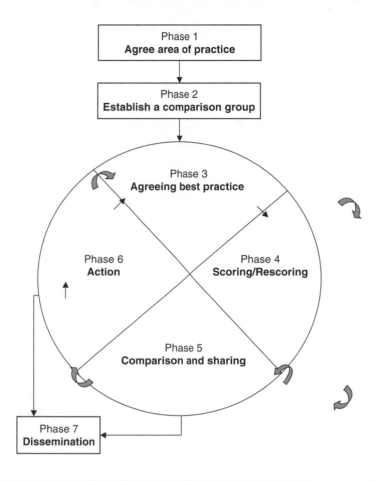

Fig. 18.2 Factor 1 – Specialist Qualification of Community Children's Nurse (CCN) Team Leader

Qualified nurses not children's trained	% Qualified staff children's trained <50% >50%	All qualified staff are children's trained	Team leader is a CCN (Degree level/Specialist Practitioner on NMC register)	
Score = 0	2 4	6	8 10	

standard of the benchmark. All the benchmarks developed by the group were until recently score based as seen in a continuum in Factor 1 (Fig. 18.2).

In this system practitioners have developed the best practice statements which are then returned to their practice environments. They determine the score of their own practice and present both a score and a justification for how that score had been generated. All the scores are returned to a central administrator who collates them and returns the completed scores to practice participants prior to the comparison meeting. This enables participants to review the practices of other participant members and be armed with potential challenges to examine how that practice has been developed and operates. All the participant members are then invited to attend the regional comparison group meetings, where everyone has the opportunity to share and compare practice.

Attendance at this meeting is open to all participant Trusts and any health professional who feels that they have a contribution to make.

COMMUNITY CHILDREN'S NURSING BENCHMARK

This benchmark was developed in the mid 1990s following the recognised need from the NWCPBG to consider the care of the child on discharge to community services. The pressure from within this group was instrumental in determining new service boundaries for children's nurses practising within the community sector. This is clearly reflected in the best practice statements within the benchmark: children's nursing qualification; specialist practice qualification and parental/child involvement.

At comparing and sharing meetings a series of best practices is shared and this illustrates significant improvements in both the establishment of children's nurses within community care and specialist practice for children and their families in the community. When practice is shared participants are encouraged to challenge and examine the practice

---

Box 18.1 Benchmark for community children's nursing

Key factors	Best practice statement
1 Specialist Qualification	All nursing team Children's Nurse (RSCN/RN Child)
2 Community Qualification	CCN (Degree level/ Specialist Practitioner Community Nursing)
3 Integrated/Seamless Child Health Service Provision	Child's package of care provided within a multi-agency framework
4 Hours/Service Availability	7-day/24-hour flexible nursing service
5 Risk Assessment for Equipment Used in the Community	All following issues have written protocols: ■ Training – competence, update ■ Maintenance/service ■ Monitoring – use, loan ■ Documentation in patients' records ■ Written information on correct use
6 Parental/Child Involvement in Record Keeping	Parents/child active in documentation process
7 Multidisciplinary Record Keeping/Documentation	Multidisciplinary/multi-agency (e.g. Social Services /Education) collaborative care planning/documentation
8 Equipment	Comprehensive range of standardised children's equipment available to the child/family when required
9 Consumables	Comprehensive range of standardised children's consumables available to the child/family when required
10 Discharge Plan	Child/family fully involved in ensuring a smooth transition between contexts of care

examples in more detail and reflect within the group how this practice may be developed within their own practice environments.

For participants of the regional group unable to attend the comparing and sharing meeting, the collated score acts as a prompt that identifies those members with 'best practice'. A condition of membership is being able to share information openly and permit its reproduction by other participating Trusts. Members make direct contacts between each other and work collaboratively in sharing practice and supporting developments across the organisations. As a concept, in the early 1990s, this was a radical move away from the lack of sharing across Trust boundaries brought about by the purchaser/provider systems. Organisations were in a position where sharing information relating to their organisation was not permitted as it may potentially have harmed their position in the healthcare marketplace. The central philosophy of the NWCPBG was clearly focused on enhancing children's care rather than becoming engaged in political competition.

CHILDREN'S PALLIATIVE CARE BENCHMARK

As with the community benchmark the palliative care benchmark was developed following a recognised need from within the group and in collaboration with national guidelines being developed by the DoH. In developing this benchmark, the first hurdle was to determine a working definition and categorise care groups to assist participants in developing both their score and practice.

The definition of palliative care was agreed as 'Palliative care for children and young people with life-limiting conditions is an active and total approach to care, embracing physical, emotional, social and spiritual elements' (Association for Children with Life-threatening and Terminal Conditions and their Families & Royal College of Paediatrics and Child Health 2003) (see Chapter 23) (Box 18.2).

Box 18.2 Example of best practice in benchmarking in palliative care

Key factors	Best practice statement
1 Agreed Service Provision	Multidisciplinary team (MDT) exists that provides children's palliative care led by a senior children's coordinator Link members: Children's nurse hospital and community/children's professional (not necessarily a medic)/Psychologist/Pharmacist/Occupational Therapist/Paediatrician/Complementary therapist/children's pain team/Clinical Nurse Specialists/bereavement services/Physiotherapy/Social Worker/Play therapist/spiritual input/teaching facilities
2 Strategic Policy	Policy exists that takes account of national guidelines and evidence-based practice and is implemented by a palliative care team
3 Referrals	Referral system for all children with a life-threatening illness which allows access to children's palliative care team

box continues

4 Respite Facilities	Local children's respite facilities available 24 hours. Working with children's palliative care teams/community teams linked to designated key worker
5 Training and Education of Staff	All staff are children's and community care trained/experienced/have further training in relevant courses: palliative care/specialist disease group, e.g. cystic fibrosis
6 Child and Family Support	Individualised, structured programme available for families and/or child to access all members of the MDT that is coordinated by a key worker
7 Funding of a Palliative Care Service	Designated funding of a multidisciplinary children's palliative care team service to meet the individual identified needs of the child/family

As with the community benchmark the comparing and sharing meetings illustrated significant developments in practice. It was evident that the leaders in practice within this benchmark were the children's hospices and the tertiary centres. Following 'comparing and sharing' meetings it was evident that the greatest developments within the District General Hospital (DGH) reflected improved communication between the hospice centres and collaborative care between the DGH and either the hospice or the tertiary centre.

FUTURE BENCHMARKING

The NWCPBG has undergone significant changes to reflect the changing climate of the NHS. Following an evaluation from an independent external auditor, the group strengthened its reporting and action planning strategy. In the light of clinical governance, participants are expected to map their action plan activity into their unit's clinical governance operations. This enhances the value of the work that members do within the benchmarking community and enables activity to be recognised and valued at the highest echelons of the organisation.

The greatest changes have been to alter the principles around scoring. As it moves into its tenth year (2004), the repetitive nature of the benchmark exercises has become apparent in the absence of the huge changes in practice evident in the early years (Ellis 2000, Bland 2001). A bold move to remove the scores was made, replacing the old score system with two key questions;

- What is it that you are doing that moves towards this best practice statement?
- What are the barriers that prevent you from moving towards these best practice statements?

The intention of this change was to discourage participants from being distracted into scoring their practice within the continuum and most importantly this would allow participants to demonstrate practice innovations they have made, even though generally the practice area may not be otherwise strong. The benchmarks themselves have been remodelled to reflect these changes and in particular the focus of the benchmark has altered. Historically, the group's experience has shown that benchmarks have been, in the main, led by nursing interventions. This may not accurately reflect the needs of the child and their family. Consequently, the group re-wrote the benchmarks to reflect the views of the child and the family's needs, the central philosophy being the 'child is central to all care'. This change is in line with DoH thinking around patient participation and involvement (Carter 2002), is reflected in the latest changes to the 'Essence of Care' initiative and enhances the original philosophy of the group. This change also permits the contribution of new partners (particularly children and their families) as well as other allied health professionals and patient advocacy liaison services with patient participation and involvement forums. These additional elements are part of the central message from within the National Service Framework for children.

CONCLUSION

Benchmarking is a powerful tool and contributes to securing best practice and improved performance. To be truly effective it must include the target group, children and their families. This ensures that benchmarking exercises are purposeful, current and meaningful (Bland 2001, Pantell 2001).

REFERENCES

Association for Children with Life-threatening or Terminal Conditions and their Families (ACT) & Royal College of Paediatrics and Child Health 2003 A guide to the development of children's palliative care services. ACT, Bristol

Bland M 2000 Producing benchmarks for clinical practice. Professional Nurse 15(12):767–770

Bland M 2001 North West Clinical Practice Benchmarking: principles, processes and evaluations. Nursing Times Research 6(2):581–593

Bland M 2002 Procedural restraint in children's nursing: using clinical benchmarks. Professional Nurse 17(12):712–715

Camp R C 1989 Benchmarking: The Search for the Industry Best Practice. ASQC, Associated Press, New York

Carter B 2002 Big elephants fighting whilst children's policy misses out? Journal of Child Health Care 6(3):154–157.

Department of Health 1999 Making a Difference. The Stationery Office, London

Department of Health 2001 Essence of Care: patient focused benchmarks for healthcare practitioners. The Stationery Office, London

Ellis J M 1995 Using benchmarks to improve practice. Nursing Standard 9:25–28.

Ellis J M 2000 Sharing the evidence: clinical practice benchmarking to improve continuously the quality of care. Journal of Advanced Nursing 32(1):215–225

Ellis J M & Morris A 1997 Paediatric benchmarking: a review of its development. Nursing Standard 12:43–46

Ellis J M, Cooper A, Davies D, Hadfield J, Oliver P, Onions J & Walmsley E 2000a Making a difference to practice: clinical practice benchmarking part 1. Nursing Standard 32:33–37

Ellis J M, Cooper A, Davies D, Hadfield J, Oliver P, Onions J & Walmsley E 2000b Making a difference to practice: clinical practice benchmarking part 2. Nursing Standard 33:35–39

Feasey S & Fox C 2001 Benchmarking evidenced base care. Paediatric Nursing 13(5):22–25

Greenidge P 1998 Benchmarking – from theory to practice. Emergency Nurse 5(9):22–27

Mears P 1995 Quality Improvement Tools and Techniques. McGraw-Hill, New York

Pantell J 2001 Benchmarking in healthcare. Nursing Times Research 6(2):568–580

Philips S 1995 Benchmarking: providing the direction for excellence. British Journal of Health Care Management 1(14):705–707

Stark S, MacHale A, Lennon E & Shaw L 2002 Benchmarking: implementing the process into practice. Nursing Standard 16(35):39–42

Warren A 2000 Paediatric coma scoring researched and benchmarked. Paediatric Nursing 12(3):14–18

Chapter 19

Dependency scoring in community children's nursing

Sue Facey

KEY ISSUES

- What is dependency scoring and why is it needed?
- Example of a dependency scoring tool.
- Elements of a community children's nurse's workload.
- Benefits of dependency scoring.

INTRODUCTION

Much has changed in the way sick children are nursed from the custodial style wards of years ago to, in many cases, the care of the sick child by parents, often in their own home. This shift has been accompanied by escalating productivity in the NHS (Royal College of Nursing 1994). In June 1994 the Secretary of State for Health reported that the output of NHS employees had risen by almost 30% between 1982 and 1991 (Royal College of Nursing 1994). The volume of work and the dependency of the patients have increased as the 'new' NHS strives, like all public sector organisations, to be more efficient and effective. Increased demands upon staff to be more productive require specific strategies to allocate work within teams as well as to ensure that resources match the work to be done. This will help to ensure high-quality care within a framework of good economic management, which should meet the requirements of clinical governance (DoH 1998).

DEPENDENCY SCORING

Dependency scoring is essential to avoid imbalances, which could have a detrimental effect on staff and patients, and provides an assessment of a patient's ability to care for themselves, i.e. feeding, personal hygiene, mobility. The measurement of nurse dependency should embrace the patient's total needs for nursing care including education, rehabilitation and psychological care (Audit Commission 1992). This identification of the patient's needs allows for appropriate allocation of nursing resources to either a ward of patients, a community nurse's caseload, or for individual patients.

Patient dependency and nursing workload are closely associated concepts and, without a dependency score, the allocation of resources is highly problematic. The Queensland Nurses Union (1999 p 1) asserts that 'patient dependency systems are the key to guide staffing levels to meet client needs'. The absence of such tools may lead to arbitrary and possibly mismatched staff utilisation and time management. The time required to provide care, the nursing skill mix, the quality of care and patient needs must all be considered if the equation of resources is to be in any way balanced (Charlesworth 1991).

Healthcare resources are not available on a demand basis and, to ameliorate inequities in delivery, staff should be required to offer evidence for resources and have tools to ensure their best use. Dependency scoring is one such tool. However it must be recognised that the dependency of patients is often measured by nursing activity which assumes that nurses are actually in touch with, and able to accurately identify, the patient's needs. Within community children's nursing this requirement is made more difficult as care is focused upon the needs of the whole family, rather than the individual child, and a child may be unable to articulate their own needs. This is further complicated by the significant change in the whole approach to the care of children from the almost custodial one to a child-centred approached and the impact this has on staffing.

Nurses in the Queensland Nurses' Union (1999) believe that they should be consulted when dependency systems are being implemented or changed given their ability to provide data which can influence skill mix, patient workload, nursing costs and rotas. Skill mix is the balance between different staff groups to provide a desired standard of service within the limits of the team's budget. Various approaches are used to determine skill mix, including task and activity analysis, professional judgement, reprofiling and patient dependency (World Health Organization/Organisation mondiale de Santé 2001). Community children's nursing teams have, in the past, consisted largely of senior, G Grade Community Children's Nurses (CCNs). More recently, however, teams increasingly utilise a degree of skill mix to include staff nurses and secretarial support to provide safe and effective care. Such developments offer staff the opportunity to work with families in their homes with little or no previous community experience or qualification. This may be contentious, however it is perhaps unrealistic to expect individuals to undertake degree courses without first experiencing work with children and families in the community setting.

Most of the work relating to dependency scoring in the UK has been based on acute-care settings and in particular in critical care (Royal College of Nursing 1995). Little about dependency scoring in the community, or in the area of community children's nursing, is available in this country. Nursing colleagues in health visiting, mental health and learning disability have made some inroads into non-acute-care dependency assessment (Frame & O'Donnell 1996). Dependency scoring systems and tools are also described as caseload management tools, which indicates their value, but within this chapter the term dependency scoring is used throughout.

WHEN TO BEGIN TO MEASURE DEPENDENCY

There is no right or wrong time to begin dependency scoring but the sooner the better. In a newly established team, where funding may be for a fixed period, dependency assessment may provide valuable evidence for repeat funding and skill requirements. In more established teams it will assist in ensuring efficiency and effectiveness, the latter being a key feature of the clinical governance agenda.

WHAT IS BEING MEASURED?

As a team, it is essential to consider what needs to be measured, for example to either:

- itemise each single nursing activity and the time it takes or
- aggregate the time spent with/for each patient regardless of the activity.

The former is clearly more accurate, but time consuming to collect, liable to collector error and needs complex and expensive information technology to analyse and interpret. The latter, whilst more of a guestimate of time per trained nurse per patient, is easier to use and more likely to be adopted by staff.

Box 19.1 Dependency scoring tool

Direct patient contact (DPC)	Indirect patient-related activity (IPA)	Non–patient-related activity
Calculated per week as follows: Visit frequency × length of visit	For example: Travel, record keeping, liaison, etc.	For example: Clinical supervision, professional development, team meetings, etc.
Method of scoring		
Frequency is scored: ×2 per day = 14 points ×1 per day = 7 points ×2 per week = 2 points ×1 per week = 1 point ×2 per month = 0.5 points Monthly or less = 0.25 points	Length of visit is calculated per 15 min: 15 min = 1 point 30 min = 2 points 45 min = 3 points 60 min = 4 points >60 min = 5 points	Record the amount of activity spent over several weeks in order to identify an average per week in hours. Transfer to a point scale by multiplying by 4 to match the direct patient contact score (i.e. per 15 min)

Example 1: A family requiring fortnightly visits, of 1 hour's duration, scores 2 points (0.5 × 4).

Example 2: A family requiring three visits per week, of 40 min each, scores 9 points (3 × 3).

Example of a dependency scoring tool

Frame and O'Donnell (1996) working in adult community nursing devised a method of scoring dependency based upon aggregation of time. The system has three main components calculated on a weekly basis (see Box 19.1):

- direct patient contact/related activity (DPC)
- indirect patient-related activity/contact (IPA)
- non-patient-related activity.

Sidey (A Sidey, unpublished work, 2003) suggests a ratio of approximately 25% patient-related activity and 75% non-patient-related activity for team leaders and 66–75% patient-related activity to 25–34% non-patient-related activity for team members, depending on grade, geography, area of expertise, etc. (Table 19.1). These ratios reflect the differing roles within the team, for example team leaders will have more management and service development responsibilities than other team members, whilst staff nurses would have a more clinical role. Sidey suggests that the ratios represent (DPC + IPA = total patient contact time):

- direct patient/family-related contact/activity time as the total of all activity involving direct patient/family contact (DPC)
- indirect patient-related activity/contact as all patient/family-related activity other than face-to-face contact (IPA).
- non-patient/family-related activity as (i) time allocated to individual caseload and service development and maintenance, (ii) individual professional development

Table 19.1 Ratio of time management of patient contact, caseload and service management and professional development (A Sidey, unpublished work, 2003)

Individual, service and caseload management	Direct patient contact time	Indirect patient contact time	Total patient contact time	Professional and service development time
1. Short term: a) New service b) Induction programme	0%	0%	0%	100%
2. Medium term: (for 3b, c & d below) Developing service/ caseload and/or practice/management	16% increasing to 44%	9% increasing to 22%	25% increasing to 66%	75% decreasing to 34%
3. Long term: a) Service manager b) Team leader c) Senior CCN with area/s of additional responsibility d) Junior CCNs (or students) depending on grade, geography, educational needs, area of expertise, etc.	16%–0% 44% 44% Between 44% and 50%	9%–0% 22% 22% Between 22% and 25%	25%–0% 66% 66% Between 66% and 75%	75%–100% 34% 34% Between 34% and 25%

Using the scores

1. Each team member is allocated a ceiling score based on the total number of hours worked per week, multiplied by 4 (to break the time into 15 min units). For example, a full-time CCN, working 37.5 hours per week, would have 150 points available; a part-time CCN, working 22.5 hours per week, would have 90 points available.
2. Deduct the score for non-patient-related activity. This will vary for each team member, depending on grade, study commitments, etc. and the developmental needs of the team at a particular time. The remaining score will indicate the points available for indirect and direct care for each team member.
3. Score direct and indirect activity and allocate work accordingly. For example, 22.5 hours of direct patient activity scores 90 points (22.5 × 4) and 10 hours of indirect patient-related activity scores 40 points, giving a total of 130 points. As new children are admitted to the caseload, their dependency score is calculated (Fig. 19.1). If the team does not have the capacity to take on new referrals, the child should remain in hospital where care can be provided and/or be placed on the team's waiting list.

Fig. 19.1 Example of a chart for recording dependency scores

Pt. ID no.	Direct			Indirect			Non-patient-related activity (15 min = 1 point)		
	Frequency × duration score			Duration (15 min = 1 point)					
	Visit frequency	(× by) duration	= no. of points	Activity	Time	Points	Activity	Time	Points

Total points [   ]   Total points [   ]   Total points [   ]

Points availabale [   ]   Total points recorded this sheet/week [   ]

4. It is possible to use this tool both retrospectively and prospectively. Comparison of the availability figures with the activity that the nurse is actually undertaking gives a clear indication as to the capacity for additional work or the need for assistance.

ELEMENTS OF THE COMMUNITY CHILDREN'S NURSE'S WORKLOAD

In calculating the direct and non-direct contact time it is important to recognise the scope of the CCN's role. Box 19.2 is by no means exhaustive or in order of priority, but provides some indication of the complexity and examples of the components of a CCN's workload. These components must be incorporated into a tool in order to represent the workload accurately. An element that is difficult to incorporate is the skill of the CCN undertaking the visit.

Box 19.2 Components of the CCN's workload

- Meetings (team, management, case conferences, discharge planning, etc.)
- Associated clinical visits (nursery, schools, outpatients, etc.)
- Professional resource
- Supervision
- Documentation
- Advice and support (carers, colleagues, students, etc.)
- Liaison (primary healthcare teams, voluntary and independent sectors, hospital staff)
- Management (time, team, caseload, etc.)
- Telephone triage
- Professional development
- Administration
- Equipment and supplies (organisation, ordering, maintenance)
- Teaching (students, families, colleagues)
- Direct care requirements
- Health promotion
- Emergencies
- Risk analysis
- Travel time (to take account of weather, geography, etc.)

HOW WILL DEPENDENCY SCORING HELP?

Dependency scoring may help nurses and nursing in a number of ways, as shown in Box 19.3. The application of this dependency scoring system demonstrates demand placed on the team and its members, and allows for better distribution of work amongst the team members. However, it is evident that the information can be used for a number of additional purposes.

Workload planning

An appropriate dependency tool will aid all team members to plan workload on a day-to-day basis. For example, this can help ensure that appointments are kept on time and families are not inconvenienced by having to wait in for the CCN to call. Procter et al (1998) noted that,

Box 19.3 Areas in which dependency scoring can help

- Workload planning
- Staff planning
- Staff development
- Report writing
- Business planning
- Cost-effectiveness and efficiency
- Comparisons and benchmarking
- Value
- Ensuring parity of workload within and between teams
- Providing an upper limit to caseload size

whilst families highly value the CCN, waiting when the nurse arrives late increases the stress in the family. The scores will also indicate to an extent the urgency of each visit, and how best to manage individual workloads, ensuring that team members' skills are used effectively.

Clinical care is undoubtedly a priority for nurses. However alongside clinical care nurses have a duty to provide evidence-based care, implement Government initiatives and evaluation of service delivery (Nursing and Midwifery Council 2002). It is all too easy to allow working time to be fully used in providing direct patient care. However the tool described effectively reserves time for non-patient duties, such as undertaking audits of care, networking with other teams, seeking information in the library or increasingly on the internet, or supervision of junior team members and self. Such activities contribute to provision of a quality service, safeguard high standards of care and are elements of the Clinical Governance agenda (DoH 1998, Norman & Brown 2003).

Cost-effectiveness and efficiency

Cost-effective care attempts to incorporate quality issues whilst making best use of available financial resources. Managers may require evidence in order to make judgements regarding the best use of resources in provision of quality service. Community children's nursing teams may be required to submit reports and evidence to demonstrate that they are providing a 'value for money' service. It is unlikely that the executive members of their Trust will have a good understanding of the role of the CCN. Therefore, a tool that gives some indication, and even a comparison, of the work will help to gain recognition along with continued if not extended funding. It could be suggested that even where such reports are not requested, it is worthwhile compiling an annual report to demonstrate development and raise the profile of the team within the organisation (see Chapter 17 p 204).

Comparisons and benchmarking

It would be ideal if a nationwide tool could be developed that would suit all community children's nursing services. This would enable benchmarking with other teams and perhaps go some way to ensure that children in the whole country received a similar service (see Chapter 18).

Value

It is essential that teams recognise the contribution made by individual nurses within the team and that individuals gain job satisfaction. A tool that encourages team members to reflect on the work undertaken will enhance an individual's sense of purpose and motivation. The production of an annual report will contribute to this.

Ensure fair workload within and between teams

It must be emphasised that caseload figures alone give no indication of the volume of work. Frame and O'Donnell (1996) described a district nursing team who were concerned that they were working under increased pressure. There was no change in the admission or discharge rate, or variance in the number of face-to-face contacts, but the increased pressure was due to the increased complexity of care needed by patients. This can be identified only if the dependency of patients is measured over a sustained time period.

Upper limit to caseload size

The Health Services Audit (2001) describes District Nursing Services as a service with no limitations. Botting (2003) also reports that one of the greatest difficulties for District Nurses (DNs) is that caseload boundaries are not static. This is a difficulty also faced by CCNs who may be expected to provide a safe and effective service for a large geographical area.

When the local children's ward is full, no more children are admitted to ensure that staffing levels are appropriate to meet the needs of those in their care. This is not the case in the community, where the caseload of the CCN can grow to unmanageable proportions unless evidence can be offered to indicate that capacity has been reached. It has been reported that DNs feel unable to control their work as they cannot influence entry to, or limit the size of their caseload (Queens Nursing Institute 2002). The Nursing and Midwifery Council Code of Conduct (2002, 8.1) states 'You must work with other members of the team to promote health care environments that are conducive to safe, therapeutic and ethical practice.' An audit tool to measure patient dependency will contribute to such safe patient care, by identifying critical ceiling levels for each nurse. Such levels will vary, according to grade, individuals' roles and caseload. The ability to provide evidence that the current staffing offers a specified amount of care delivery time, and the current workload demands more than that, will strengthen discussions relating to workload planning and caseload size. Decisions regarding the safety of taking on new patients can be made on the basis of facts rather than the general 'feeling' that the team is too busy. It also gives tangible evidence to managers that work has outgrown the team and funding is required for team expansion.

KEYS TO SUCCESS

- Involvement of all team members at the outset. As with any change in management, success is more likely with the cooperation of all those involved (Ottaway 1976). It is unreasonable to expect team members to complete long and complicated forms on a daily basis if they have no understanding of the need for gathering such data and what they will be used for.
- Information needs to be accurate and complete. It is therefore essential that each team member interprets and uses the tool in the same way.

- The information gained must be analysed from the outset and used to inform activity and planning to ensure the exercise has meaning to the team.
- Reductionist approaches to dependency analysis, which itemise all aspects of care, are time consuming to collect and collate and require extensive information technology support.

CONCLUSION

Only one example of a patient dependency tool has been offered here, chosen in part for its simplicity. Others are available, although not published in detail, which have taken teams many years to develop and which are expensive to buy and far more complicated to use. The time has come for all teams to calculate dependency scores of patients to ensure appropriate resource use. It is also essential, with the increasing trend towards community care, to ensure that the needs of the child and family can be safely met. Every children's nurse is aware that the primary place to care for a sick child is in the child's own home but only if the support required by the family is available. If it is not available, the child and family may actually be better placed in hospital. Currently children may be discharged into the community without careful consideration of whether or not the community children's nursing team can accommodate the family on to the caseload, perhaps with an assumption that where a team exists, so does the nursing time. In reality, this may not be the case. Many CCNs who do not use a patient dependency tool may be placing the families on the caseload in an unsafe position, by accepting them into a community children's nursing 'ward', which is already full. This will put pressure on community nursing staff, and may in turn lead to increased sickness levels as well as a potentially unsafe environment for the child and family. This important aspect of caseload management demands much more consideration.

REFERENCES

Audit Commission 1992 Caring Systems: A Handbook for Managers and Nursing Project Managers. HMSO, London

Botting L 2003 Referral criteria – the way forward for district nursing services. Primary Health Care 13(6):12–15

Charlesworth M 1991 Using Information in Managing the Nursing Resource–Workload. Mersey Regional Health Authority, Huddersfield

Department of Health 1998 The New NHS – Working Together: securing a quality workforce for the new NHS. The Stationery Office, London

Frame G & O'Donnell P 1996 Weight-lifters. Health Service Journal 10:30–31

Health Services Audit 2001 District Nursing Services in Northern Ireland. Health Services Audit, Belfast

Norman A & Brown J 2003 Quality in Health Care. In: Hinchcliff S, Norman S & Schober J (eds) Nursing Practice and Health Care. Arnold, London

Nursing and Midwifery Council (NMC) 2002 Code of Professional Conduct. NMC, London

Ottaway R N 1976 A change strategy to implement new norms, new styles and new environment in the work organisation. Personnel Review 5(1):13–18

Procter S, Biott C, Campbell S, Edward S, Redpath N & Moran M 1998 Preparation for the developing role of community children's nurse. English National Board for Nursing, Midwifery and Health Visiting, London

Queensland Nurses Union 1999 Patient Dependency Systems – an essential support system for nursing management. Online. Available: www.qnu.org.au/pds.htm 26 April 2004

Queens Nursing Institute 2002 The Invisible Workforce. The Queens Nursing Institute, London

Royal College of Nursing (RCN) 1994 Nurses and NHS productivity. RCN, London

Royal College of Nursing (RCN) 1995 Dependency scoring systems: guidelines for nurses. RCN, London

World Health Organization/Organisation Mondiale de Santé (WHO/OMS) 2001 Tool Kit for Planning, Training and Management: Approaches to determining skill mix. WHO/OMS, Geneva

Chapter 20

Information management

Anne Casey

KEY ISSUES

- Effective management of information improves care of children and families.
- Record keeping is one aspect of information management that requires development in order to ensure effective communication and continuity of care.
- Department of Health and professional guidance on information governance and record keeping supports good standards of information management.
- The community children's nursing team requires a range of tools and methods to manage information effectively.
- Information and e-health initiatives across the NHS need to take account of the context for care delivery such as the child's home and patient care philosophies such as child and family-centred care and parent/child-held records.

INTRODUCTION

Information management is about ensuring that relevant information is in the hands of those who need it, at the time they need it, and in a format they can understand and use. In healthcare, information is needed by patients and carers, clinical staff, managers and administrators so they can:

- make sense of the situation
- make decisions about what to do.

The right format for the information may be a laboratory report, a set of statistics, a video, a referral letter, or any of the range of methods available for presenting facts, opinions and concepts. Making the information relevant to the person receiving it and providing it at the right time can be more challenging, particularly in stressful situations.

Information management can be viewed as a number of processes in which information from different sources is collected, used, communicated and sometimes recorded. Unfortunately, the skills required for effective use of information are not well integrated into the training of health professionals, despite government and statutory body recommendations (English National Board 1997, NHS Information Policy Unit 1999), and despite the fact that every year the main criticisms made by the health ombudsman relate to inadequate communication and poor record keeping.

This chapter begins with a brief overview of some principles of information management and information governance. It then addresses three aspects of information management for Community Children's Nurses (CCNs):

1. Meeting the information needs of children and families.
2. Information management for care delivery, including record keeping.
3. Management of aggregated information for purposes such as auditing and improving care, and for costing and planning services.

In today's NHS, this last item is assuming greater importance for nurses and other clinical professionals as they take responsibility for the development of evidence-based care and contribute to clinical governance (Royal College of Nursing 2003). The aims of this chapter are to emphasise the importance of information as a resource and to demonstrate how effective information management can improve care and make life easier for the CCN.

PRINCIPLES OF INFORMATION MANAGEMENT

The first step towards effective information management is to identify information requirements. This exercise should always begin with the people who are to receive and use the information. CCNs often receive standard referral letters from other professionals, but how many of these letters were designed by the CCNs themselves to include the information that is important to them? Those giving the information usually decide what they think the other party needs to know, rather than asking what information they would like.

There are a number of methods for systematically identifying information requirements. These include modelling patient pathways and clinical workflows, and looking at information flows for common processes such as referring a patient, prescribing medication or telephone consultation (Craddock 2003). These approaches are much more likely to result in information systems that support patient care and the work of the CCN than simply computerising existing paper records.

Analysis of clinical information requirements begins with the patient pathway, a model used in the development of the National Service Framework for children's services in England (DoH 2003a). As the child progresses through an illness episode, or through daily life with a chronic condition, the points at which they interact with different healthcare agencies and professionals becomes apparent, as do the points at which information of different kinds is needed. For example, when a mother becomes concerned about her child's soiling, what routes might she take to address her concerns? She may seek direct answers from her General Practitioner (GP) or Health Visitor, refer to a childcare book, phone a national help line such as NHS Direct or NHS 24, or look for information on the internet. When an adolescent with diabetes is admitted in a coma, what information is immediately necessary and how can it be acquired rapidly to support care decisions? As the young person recovers, what kinds of information delivered through what media will be most helpful in addressing non-compliant behaviours in this age group?

Alongside patient pathways that provide the child-centred information view, models of nursing workflow begin to illustrate where access to the range of information tools and technologies can be of benefit. A 'typical working day' for the CCN may not exist but patterns of workflow will emerge that can inform a specification of requirements for information and technology support. Clinic-based work presents different requirements than home visits. Phone calls from parents or to other professionals about patients, case conferences, teaching sessions, referring children to other agencies, etc., all have requirements that can be met in different ways.

Many elements of the care process such as assessing patient needs or planning discharge are common to all professionals and lend themselves to common solutions. However, below the high-level description of the process, the detail of what is being done, by whom and where makes all the difference: one solution does not fit all.

Consideration of the working context is the most important, and most neglected, principle of information management in healthcare. Nurses do not work at desks, yet many information solutions in the health service rely on desk-top computers (Cowley 1994). Mobile technology is now sufficiently well advanced and affordable that access to patient records, email, electronic diaries, the internet, etc., can be truly 'independent of location': PDA (personal digital assistant) devices will revolutionise information management in community nursing in the next few years. The context of care also includes prevailing philosophies and practices. Some information solutions do not fit with the view that the parents and child should have full access to the clinical record and use it to record their own care. If the context of information use is considered, meeting information requirements can be simple and effective, and may often involve continued use of pen and paper rather than computers.

One way of ensuring sensible, practical solutions is to focus on another key information principle: 'fitness for purpose'. Do the information tools you use, including your nursing records, do the job that you require of them? If the answer is no or not very well, then you need to make changes, bearing in mind local and national developments and with an eye to the future direction of community children's nursing services. The future direction of children's health services is being driven by national frameworks (DoH 2003a, Scottish Executive 2003) and evidence-based clinical standards. A major support for these 'modernisation' initiatives is the national 'e-health' strategies being implemented across the UK. An 'integrated care record service' for the NHS in England will ensure that records are 'integrated across all health and social care settings, designed around the patient, and not around individual institutions and are therefore able to support the implementation of care pathways as part of National Service Frameworks' (NHS Information Policy Unit 2002). The Scottish e-health strategy identifies six priority areas including clinical information systems to support national care priorities, the protection of patient confidentiality and the provision of information for patients, the public and staff (NHS Scotland 2003).

Integration of records and sharing information across agencies and between professionals are all recognised as essential for the provision of safe, equitable and seamless services to children (Department for Education and Skills 2003). Although current information and e-health initiatives seek to address this requirement, the practicalities of information sharing are complex, particularly in relation to confidentiality. However, guidance is available, based on legislation, the views of the different services and importantly on the views of the public, including children and young people (Children and Young People's Unit 2003).

INFORMATION GOVERNANCE

Information governance provides a quality framework for how the NHS works with patient information. Bringing together the legislation and guidance that exists around record keeping, storage, access to records, data quality, etc., information governance initiatives seek to assure patients and the public that personal information is being handled according to 'appropriate ethical and quality standards' (NHS Information Authority 2003). A focus on standards and monitoring of practice 'aims to improve outcomes by ensuring that information processing is subject to continuous improvement' (Walker & Greenfield 2001).

The key principles of information governance are that information is:

- held securely and confidentially
- obtained fairly and efficiently
- recorded accurately and reliably
- used effectively and ethically
- shared appropriately and lawfully (Walker & Greenfield 2001).

Professional practice in relation to record keeping, disclosure of patient information and use of patient information for purposes other than direct clinical care (for example for research or audit), all come under the heading of information governance. There has been much debate about whether explicit consent should be obtained each time information in the patient's record is used for research, audit or other purposes. Professional guidance is clear on this point: 'the information contained in the record is confidential and should only be released, even to someone within the organisation, with the consent of the patient or client' (Nursing and Midwifery Council 2002a). The nurse is required to ensure that children, young people and carers are informed of what is recorded about them and who has access to that information so that they can choose whether to restrict access or withhold information that they do not wish to be shared. Although child/parent-held records are fairly widely used in the community, it is expected in the future that more children, young people and their families will have improved access to their own records in all settings.

INFORMATION FOR CHILDREN AND FAMILIES

In many situations the child and family will not know what information will be of use to them. However, they will usually have questions that indicate what they believe are their information needs. These questions are the starting point for the provision of meaningful information which can then be expanded to include what the nurse believes will be helpful to them in making sense of the situation and in deciding what to do. As with any other aspect of individualised care, no assumptions can be made about what the child already knows, what he should or should not be told, and what he is capable of understanding. In much the same way that a child's physical condition is regularly assessed so too should information requirements be identified: What does the child know? Has anything changed? What is likely to happen that the child needs to know about? And, with the goal of promoting independence, how can children be helped to access appropriate information themselves?

Everything from the telephone helpline through to the computer game and the internet can be drawn upon to provide information tailored for the individual's needs and preferences. These advances can be looked at in two ways: as a threat to the authority and control of the health professional, or as an opportunity for patients and public to be better informed and participate more in their healthcare (Cross 1998).

Health information on the internet is 'changing the balance of power between healthcare organisations and individual patients' (Cross 1998 p 22). There are many excellent websites for children, young people and families to access health-related information, from the award winning Contact a Family site (www.cafamily.org.uk) covering rare conditions, to interactive educational sites aimed at children and adolescents with specific conditions. A useful route into available resources can be found at www.lifebytes.gov.uk – a website maintained by the Health Development Agency, primarily for young people aged 11–14 years.

Nurses have two main roles in relation to health information on the internet: assuring the quality of information and supporting children and families to access and use appropriate information. Because anyone can set up an internet website the quality of information can be questionable and it would be poor practice to recommend a site unless you are confident of its quality. Some of the same criteria that apply when appraising published articles also apply here: the qualifications and place of work of the authors, date of publication, what kinds of reviews or quality checks the site owners undertake, etc. Some sites only include material that has been rigorously reviewed and is frequently updated, for example NHS Direct Online (www.nhsdirect.nhs.uk). Simple checks such as the site address will give you important information for appraising quality: is this a commercial site with advertising information (.com) or is it a professional or academic organisation (.org or .ac)? An international group, the Health on the Net Foundation, has published a code of conduct (HONcode) for health websites (Health on the Net Foundation 2003). The HONcode defines a set of rules for website developers covering basic ethical standards in the presentation of information to help ensure that readers always know the source and the purpose of what they are reading.

Not all children and parents can access the internet and almost all will require information that is tailored to local practices and their individual needs. Word processing and publishing software can be used to produce professional-looking and easily updatable information, with cartoons and pictures added to bring the information alive for the child. Guidance on producing good-quality patient information is available from many sources. The Centre for Health Information Quality provides practical guidelines for both reviewing and producing health information for patients and the public, based on three core principles: accuracy, clarity and relevance.

There are software packages available to check your information material for jargon, giving it a 'plain English' rating. Many organisations now employ information officers and involve children and families in the production of information materials, ensuring that content is at an appropriate level for different age groups. Hopefully the badly photocopied sheet of paper listing instructions in nursing and medical language is a thing of the past.

Although the provision of information must be individualised, there is a place for standardised material and, as the Audit Commission (1997) suggested, this could be produced more efficiently if there were more coordination. It is wasteful for each community children's nursing team to produce and update its own material on managing febrile convulsions, when to call the doctor, storing drugs in the home, etc. With the UK-wide network provided by the Royal College of Nursing Community Children's Nursing Forum, it should be possible to share and re-use well-developed material to save others the time and expense of development.

The growth of information technology to support clinical practice brings with it the requirement for a new set of skills for nurses. Not least of these will be the skills of working with highly informed individuals who may question your advice or clinical judgement. How comfortable will you be negotiating with an 8-year-old who questions her medical treatment by referring to details obtained from other patients on the internet?

INFORMATION MANAGEMENT FOR CLINICAL PRACTICE

To care for the child and family effectively, the community team manages two distinct types of information. First, clinical and contextual information about each child and his or her family is obtained, used, recorded and communicated – managing information about the patient. Second, general information from professional literature, local policies, guidelines, drug manuals and so on is used to inform decisions about the most effective approaches to the child's care – decision-support.

Managing information about the patient

The child's clinical record is the main tool for managing this information. The information principle of 'fitness for purpose' can be used to assist development of new records or to evaluate the structure, content and location of existing records, whether on paper or computer. In deciding what information to record, in what format and where the information should be held, there is one key question to answer: what is the purpose of the record? Every professional who comes in contact with the patient needs to be able to make timely decisions about what care is needed and how best to deliver that care. If it is to be an effective information tool, the record should support this process of clinical decision making. A key purpose of records is communication between disciplines, which suggests that moves towards a single record, used by all professionals and possibly held by the child or parent, will help to achieve 'fitness for purpose'.

One review of information management in the community identified a number of problems around the collection and recording of individual patient data, particularly the inefficient duplication of records by different professionals and the lack of standards for what information should be recorded (Audit Commission 1997). In the Audit Commission study, over 25% of the district nurses who were surveyed reported problems in obtaining details of the patient's care to date. The report concluded that 'critical decisions on patient care can be based on incomplete or unchecked data' (Audit Commission 1997 p 17).

Nursing and Midwifery Council (NMC) guidance on record keeping is at a very general level, stating only that the record should 'identify problems that have arisen and action taken to rectify them' and 'provide clear evidence of the care planned, the decisions made, the care delivered and the information shared' (NMC 2002a pp 8–9). The Essence of Care benchmark for record keeping, now part of the clinical governance framework for the NHS in England, states that 'all records must be legible, accurate, signed with designation stated, dated, timed, contemporaneous, be able to provide a chronology of events and use only agreed abbreviations' (NHS Modernisation Agency 2003). These 'patient-focused benchmarks' set standards for progress towards single, life-long, patient-held records that are secure and support high-quality, evidence-based care.

As yet there is no national standard for the content of children's health records but the next few years will see specification of standard content for core summaries held about all NHS patients available in a national data repository (with appropriate access controls). Because of the need to communicate patient data electronically and to provide standardised data for quality and performance monitoring, there will be standard 'datasets' specifying content for different patient groups and clinical conditions. These datasets will form the basis of the integrated records that will soon replace the many different records held about an individual patient. It is essential that these developments build on work already undertaken by professional groups to define record or dataset content, for example the Personal Child Health Record (Health for all Children 2003) and the Essential Core Dataset for Child Health (Child Health Informatics Consortium 2003a). A nationally agreed care record for children and young people would need to include space for information related to community children's nursing.

Decision support

As the evidence base for practice grows, so will the need to provide easily accessible and up-to-date knowledge to the practitioner at the bedside or in the patient's home. Practice guidelines, easy-reference texts and pocket-sized reminders are just some of the ways that nurses currently access knowledge in a timely way. But with new evidence and knowledge being produced at such a rapid pace, paper-based decision support tools soon become out of date. 'Online help' is a common feature of many non-clinical systems and the same technology can provide useful reference material when requested by the user. In one hospital system the nurse can click on a diagnosis, for example of 'RSV' (respiratory syncytial virus) bronchiolitis and choose from a list of help topics such as 'RSV investigations', 'RSV precautions' and 'RSV parent information'. The way such material is presented, who checks and updates it and how frequently are all questions that need to be addressed as part of the local information strategy. Many nurses already use computerised decision-support, particularly in primary care systems, which provide warnings on drug incompatibilities, remind the nurse to check the patient's blood pressure or weight, or prompt particular assessment questions depending on information already held about the patient. Decision algorithms form the basis of triage systems such as those used by nurses at NHS Direct and NHS 24 to focus questioning and arrive at a decision during a telephone call (O'Cathain et al 2003). Prompts or reminders on a monitor or computer screen are useful provided there are not so many of them that they irritate the user and are switched off or ignored. Clinical decision making is a skill that is developed over time: more junior staff rely on rules of thumb, rather than weighing up available evidence and assessing whether it is valid in the given clinical situation. Blanket application of guidance without consideration of the individual patient context can result in poor or unsafe practice (Hall 2003). The introduction of decision support systems and evidence-based guidelines or protocols needs to go hand in hand with further education in clinical reasoning.

One of the most promising approaches to getting evidence into practice is the use of care pathways (Clark 2003). Rather like standard care plans, these are standard approaches to the management of patients with particular problems developed from evidence or guidelines. They include progress and outcome measures as well as options for different interventions, depending on how the patient is progressing. By analysing variances in different patients who started with the same pathway, improvements can be made in the pathway for future patients. There are some published examples of care pathways relevant to community children's nursing (Powell & Austin 1998, Gordon et al 2002) and the National Electronic Library for Health has a care pathways index (www.nelh.nhs.uk). Because of the complexity of the evidence, the many different decision pathways that could be followed and the need for data collection and analysis, it is better to implement care pathways as part of a clinical information system (de Luc & Todd 2003).

Future developments

To manage the information required to support the care of child and family, the nurse can draw on all the information tools available: spoken and written words, electronic equipment, computers, telephone, etc. Each has its place but the electronic and computer tools will become more useful once NHS networks and systems are better developed. Clinical systems that support the work of community nurses (as distinct from administrative systems) need to be thought of in different terms than merely computerising existing paper records. Where community teams are integrated with primary care organisations, there is a temptation to simply expand the GP computer system to include recording of community information. This may be a useful first step but systems will need to be flexible enough to adapt as nurses become more aware of the potential that properly designed information technology could deliver. The biggest challenge continues to be to ensure that systems meet information needs in ways that are appropriate to the community setting and that do not compromise fundamental principles such as child and family involvement (Cowley 1994).

The most useful contribution that individual nurses and teams can make is to be very sure about what information they need to do their jobs effectively. Each team could have someone who leads on information and records, so that, as local developments are being planned, there will be someone who can contribute the community children's nursing team's perspective. Nationally agreed information requirements such as those developed by the Child Health Informatics Consortium (CHIC) (CHIC 2003b) are a useful starting point for anyone taking on the role of clinical information lead in any child health setting.

MANAGEMENT OF AGGREGATED INFORMATION

Data to support audit, research, costing and planning can be obtained directly from patient records or collected using specific data-collection tools. One of the benefits of computerising records is that these will provide structured data that can be easily aggregated and analysed. There will still be a need for other forms of data collection, for example the patient record won't tell you how many staff were available on a particular day or which nurses have specialist qualifications. However, data that are recorded in a structured way, for example from coded picking lists of clinical terms, will be re-useable for activity reports, quality reports, ad hoc queries, etc. Information governance issues need to be considered in the management of aggregated patient information, specifically:

1. Confidentiality and security
2. Data quality
3. Uses and ownership of the aggregated information.

The NMC code of conduct states that the nurse is personally accountable for protecting the patient's confidential information (NMC 2002b). If you believe that any patient information that you have obtained may be used by others in a way that could potentially identify the child and family, you are responsible for preventing that use. Implementing information governance standards and procedures helps to ensure compliance with confidentiality and security regulations. CCNs need to develop new skills for informing patients and families about the potential uses of information that is held about them, obtaining their consent for its use and helping them decide whether they wish certain pieces of information to be withheld or stored separately. An NHS code of practice for confidentiality

(DoH 2003b) provides useful material for those responsible for teaching or implementing information standards.

Whether on paper or computer, patient information needs to be accurate and meaningful. The responsibility for how information is gathered, checked to ensure it is recorded in a way that retains the original meaning, how it is stored and then retrieved for analysis is shared between the clinician and the information specialist. The nurse cannot know whether, for example, the power failure backup system is sufficient to prevent data loss, but they are responsible for the accuracy of what is recorded. There are several reasons why nurses themselves should manage the data they record about their patients and control how that information is used and by whom. First, because nurses collect the data, they know how accurately it reflects the real situation. A statement that the child is 'much improved' can have a huge range of meanings. It may mean that the child is terminally ill but that pain relief is more effective. How would a distant administrator interpret the same statement? Second, the results from analysing aggregated patient data are most useful in the hands of those providing patient care. You cannot improve care or plan your service more efficiently if you do not have data to show you how you are doing. If you know what your own management goals are, you will be able to identify the information requirements for achieving those goals. One of your quality goals might be to ensure that all day cases are contacted within 24 hours of discharge. You could set up a method of collecting a list of day cases from the day unit and comparing it with the calls logged by the team over the same period.

A management goal might be to persuade the Trust Board to fund another full-time post. The information requirement to support this goal might include the data you collect routinely on the activity of the team, your data on parent satisfaction with the service, and some form of economic evaluation study presented graphically alongside reminders of NHS policy. With paper or computer systems in place to collect management data quickly and simply as part of nurses' routine work, you would have this information available when and where you needed it. This is the goal of effective information management.

CONCLUSION

Information management in healthcare is moving away from an emphasis on computerisation to a broader understanding of the total information picture. Effective solutions for meeting the information needs of patients and carers, clinical staff, managers and administrators will be those that:

- identify the requirements of the users of the information
- consider the working environment and context
- focus on 'fitness for purpose' of tools and methods.

Many of these solutions will not include computers, but where computers are a practical and sensible option they can bring significant benefits for patients and staff. One of the main benefits will be in the use of aggregated data about clinical practice to obtain visible evidence about what works and what could be improved. If CCNs across the UK could agree on some common assessment formats, outcome measures and intervention categories, it would be possible to undertake comparative studies of the effectiveness of interventions and of different services. But the collection, analysis and interpretation of UK-wide data and the dissemination of results need to be owned by the nurses and used by them to manage and develop their own services. Information is a powerful and important resource for CCNs. Its proper management is central to safe, effective practice and to the future of community children's nursing services as they spread throughout the UK.

REFERENCES

Audit Commission 1997 Comparing notes: a study of information management in community trusts. Audit Commission, London

Child Health Informatics Consortium 2003a. Essential Core Dataset for Child Health. Online. Available: http://www.chiconsortium.org.uk 21 April 2004

Child Health Informatics Consortium 2003b. Functional specification for child health. Online. Available: http://www.chiconsortium.org.uk 21 April 2004

Children and Young People's Unit 2003. IRT: Information sharing to improve services for children: guidance on information sharing. Online. Available: http://www.dfes.gov.uk/publications/key.shtml 21 April 2004

Clark A 2003 Protocol-based care: 1. How integrated care pathways work. Professional Nurse 18(12):694–697

Cowley S 1994 Counting practice: the impact of information systems on community nursing. Journal of Nursing Management 1(6):273–278

Craddock M 2003 Building a computerised care pathway; practical lessons. In: de Luc K, Todd J (eds) e-Pathways: Computers and the Patient's Journey through Care. Radcliffe, Oxford pp 81–105

Cross M 1998 All tangled on the web. Health Service Journal 19:22–23

de Luc K & Todd J (eds) 2003 e-Pathways: Computers and the Patient's Journey through Care. Radcliffe, Oxford

Department for Education and Skills 2003 Every Child Matters. Online. Available: http://www.dfes.gov.uk/everychildmatters 21 April 2004

Department of Health 2003a Getting the right start: National Service Framework for Children, Young People and Maternity Services. Online. Available: http://www.dh.gov.uk/nsf/children/gettingtherightstart.htm January 2003

Department of Health 2003b Confidentiality: NHS Code of Practice. Online. Available: http://www.dh.gov.uk/ipu/confiden January 2004

English National Board for Nursing, Midwifery and Health Visiting (ENB) 1997 Information for caring: integrating informatics into learning programmes for nurses, midwives and health visitors. ENB, London

Gordon J, Reid P & Thompson C 2002 Idiopathic constipation management pathway. Nursing Times 98(43):48–50

Hall K 2003 NHS direct and children's A&E services: a case review. Paediatric Nursing15(5):36–39

Health for all Children 2003. The PCHR. Online. Available: http://www.healthforallchildren.co.uk/pchr.html January 2004

Health on the Net Foundation 2003 HON Code of Conduct (HONcode) for medical and health web sites. Online. Available: http://www.hon.ch

NHS Information Authority 2003 Information Governance. Online. Available: http://www.nhsia.nhs.uk/infogov/pages/default.asp January 2004

NHS Information Policy Unit 1999 Working Together With Health Information, A Partnership Strategy for Education, Training and Development. Online. Available: http://www.dh.gov.uk/ipu/develop/nip/worktoge.htm 21 April 2004

NHS Information Policy Unit 2002 Delivering 21st century support for the NHS. Online. Available: http://www.doh.gov.uk/ipu/whatnew/specs_12dexec.pdf 21 April 2004

NHS Modernisation Agency 2003 Essence of Care Programme. Online. Available: http://www.cgsupport.org/Programmes/Essence_of_Care_Programme.asp January 2004

NHS Scotland 2003 Information Management and Technology for NHS Scotland. Online. Available: http://www.show.scot.nhs.uk/imt/ January 2004

Nursing and Midwifery Council (NMC) 2002a Guidelines for records and record keeping. NMC, London

Nursing and Midwifery Council (NMC) 2002b Code of Professional Conduct. NMC, London

O'Cathain A, Webber E & Nicholl J 2003 NHS Direct: consistency of triage outcomes. Emergency Medicine Journal 20(3):289–292

Powell E & Austin A 1998 Developing a pediatric diabetes critical pathway. Pediatric Nursing 24(6):558–561

Royal College of Nursing (RCN) 2003 Clinical Governance: An RCN Resource Guide. RCN, London

Scottish Executive 2003 Scottish Executive Child health support group. Online. Available: http://www.show.scot.nhs.uk/chsg/ January 2004

Walker P & Greenfield M 2001 Tell no secrets – Tell no lies: Information Governance in the NHS. Online. Available: http://www.nhsia.nhs.uk/erdip/pages/workshops/SecurityWorkshop/ January 2004

Chapter 21

Caring for the acutely ill child at home

Sarah Neill

> **KEY ISSUES**
>
> - The majority of childhood illness takes place at home with no recourse to professional care and support.
> - Parents' ability to manage acute childhood illness at home appears to be directly related to personal control, itself related to the perceived degree of threat to the child's health.
> - When parents seek help, children with acute childhood illness at home are often cared for by healthcare professionals with no specific qualification in child healthcare.
> - Parents are reported to be often dissatisfied with care provided by General Practitioners, wanting more reassurance and information.
> - Rising demand means that alternatives to General Practitioner care are needed to support children and their families during acute childhood illness at home.
> - Future development of community services needs to provide this client group with services from appropriately qualified professionals, such as the community children's nurse, accessible to families from within the primary healthcare team.

INTRODUCTION

The majority of childhood illness is of short duration and takes place in the child's own home. However, research into community healthcare of children has focused primarily around the care of the chronically ill or highly dependent child. 'Theoretical developments regarding family process during acute illness have been limited' (Rennick 1995) to the experience of the hospitalised child. This chapter focuses on the acutely ill child at home. The literature is critically reviewed to identify what is known about the experiences of children and families and the involvement of health services in their care at these times. From this analysis the chapter considers the implications of this knowledge for both contemporary and future models of care. Examples of contemporary practice are included. Throughout the chapter, where parents are referred to, the following definition will be applied: 'the child's birth parents, his/her legal guardians or permanent parent substitute (those who usually care for him/her)' (Neill 1996).

WHAT IS MEANT BY 'ACUTE CHILDHOOD ILLNESS' FROM A COMMUNITY PERSPECTIVE?

Acute childhood illness is characterised by a rapid onset, severe symptoms and is of brief duration. Services to provide care for acutely sick children at home are not well developed in most areas (Meates 1997). This chapter is, therefore, concerned primarily with acute illness in children whose illness is not of sufficient severity to warrant hospitalisation. The term 'common childhood illness' is also often used to refer to acute childhood illness in the community. Such illness includes:

- coughs and colds
- upper respiratory tract infections
- childhood infectious diseases (mumps, measles, chickenpox)
- gastroenteritis
- acute exacerbations of chronic conditions such as asthma
- otitis media
- other febrile illness.

The terms 'acute illness', 'minor illness' and 'minor ailments' will be used interchangeably, as these terms all appear in the literature reviewed.

HEALTHCARE SERVICE USE DURING ACUTE CHILDHOOD ILLNESS AT HOME: THE STATISTICS

Children aged under 16 years comprise 20% of the UK population (Office for National Statistics 2002). Some 9% of these are from minority ethnic groups. One-third of the ethnic minority population consists of children, in contrast to 20% of the total population of the UK. In some areas with large minority ethnic populations, the childhood population is continuing to expand (Leicester City Council 2001). Children make up 17–19% of consultations with doctors in general practice and 15% of consultations with Practice Nurses (PNs) (McCormick et al 1995). The 0–4-year age group consults more often than any other group except the elderly. Acute childhood illness constitutes a high proportion of these consultations, the most common reason for consultation being diseases of the respiratory system, two thirds of consultations for the under-5-year age group and one third of consultations in the 5–15 year age group. Data suggest that between 11 and 12% of 0–9-year-olds suffered from acute illness in the 2 weeks prior to data collection in the most recent Health Survey for England to focus on children (Health Committee 1997).

Whilst no statistics are centrally available concerning the involvement of other community nursing services in the care of the acutely ill child at home, Health Visitors (HVs), School Nurses (SNs) and District Nurses (DNs) are variously involved in providing care to children in the community with minor ailments. In a few areas, where there are Hospital at Home services for children, Community Children's Nurses (CCNs) may also be involved.

IMPACT ON THE WORK OF HEALTHCARE PROFESSIONALS IN THE COMMUNITY

The statistics show that children with acute childhood illness at home constitute a significant proportion of the workload of General Practitioners (GPs) and PNs, roughly parallel to the proportion of children in the population. In areas with a higher proportion of children in the population, such as areas with large minority ethnic communities, this workload can be expected to be higher. For example, in Leicester 35% of the population belongs to minority ethnic groups (Leicester City Council 2001), in contrast to the national figure of 7.9% (Office of National Statistics 2002). These figures are even more relevant when considered in the light of evidence that minority ethnic groups also have an increased incidence of socio-economic deprivation (Webb 1996). This potentially leads to higher rates of health service use per head of the population due to the associated increased morbidity. These suggestions are supported by the findings of Carr-Hill et al (1996) who found higher consultation rates for patients from the Indian subcontinent, Clarke and Hewison (1991), who found higher consultation rates in 'Asian' groups with increased scores for severity of illness and Watson (1991) who found that Bengali children were reported to suffer more severe symptoms, coughs and colds than children from the indigenous group.

A further factor affecting the uptake of health services for the acutely ill child in the community is poverty. Consultation rates are higher in lower socio-economic groups (Carlisle & Johnstone 1998). This is not surprising as virtually all aspects of health are worse in children living in poverty than those living in affluent families (Reading 1997). These children are likely to represent a considerable proportion of healthcare professionals' workload, as approximately one third of children are living in conditions of poverty in Britain today (Office of National Statistics 2003). These children will be ill more often (Mayall 1986, Reading 1997) and more seriously than children in more affluent circumstances (Wyke et al 1990, Clarke & Hewison 1991, Watson 1991). Spencer (1984) suggests that these parents are most vulnerable to breakdown of parenting skills and will therefore fail to respond to their child's symptoms, seeking help at a later stage of the child's illness.

IMPLICATIONS OF EXISTING SERVICE PROVISION FOR THE QUALITY OF CARE

Qualifications of healthcare professionals involved in care

Few PNs hold a children's nursing qualification, yet 15% of their workload involves children (McCormick et al 1995). Many GPs, HVs, SNs and DNs hold no formal qualification relevant to the care of the sick child and it is not mandatory for them to do so. It would be unthinkable for a doctor or nurse caring for the adult community not to have a qualification in the care of adults. Clearly children are still considered to be 'little adults' or at least of lesser importance (Learning from Bristol 2001). The quality of care provided for children during acute childhood illness at home has to be less than optimal. As the Health Committee (1997) pointed out: 'as a matter of principle, sick children need and deserve no less (than adults)' (para 49). It is expected that the National Service Framework (NSF) for children will lay down some criteria for appropriate qualifications for all practitioners working with children (Department of Health 2003).

Community children's nursing services' involvement in childhood acute illness

In contrast to those currently providing most care to these children, children's nurses have access to, and are undertaking in increasing numbers, the degree course leading to the qualification of specialist practitioner in community children's nursing, equivalent to the DN and HV qualifications. It would seem that the obvious person to care for the acutely ill child at home is the CCN. However, where community children's nursing services exist, few families are likely to be able to access them for help during acute childhood illness. There are a small number of Hospital at Home schemes providing care for the acutely ill child in the community but these do not usually provide care for children who are not seriously ill enough to warrant hospitalisation, as the rationale for developing such services is usually to speed discharge or to replace hospital in-patient services (Cramp et al 2003). Most do not accept direct parent referrals meaning that families can only access such services if the GP or Paediatrician deems it to be relevant. A majority of community children's nursing services remain small, limiting their ability to address the needs of children with more minor acute illness in the community (Cramp et al 2003). Few have the ability to offer an adequately resourced 24-hour service to the children on their caseloads (see Chapter 15). This situation leaves parents of an acutely ill child who is not ill enough for hospitalisation with limited choice and access to professional support.

Historically, the early community nursing services for children were designed to care for acutely ill children at home (see Chapter 2). Their aim was to prevent hospital admissions and therefore reduce the potential for cross-infection (Gillett 1954, Smellie 1956, Shrand 1965). Aspects of this earlier pattern of care are now informing contemporary developments in some areas (see Chapter 15 p 178).

EXPERIENCES OF THE CHILD AND FAMILY WHEN A CHILD IS ACUTELY ILL AT HOME

Whose voice is being heard in this research?

Most of the research that considers the care of the sick child fails to ask children themselves, preferring to research the views of their parents (Alderson 1993, 1995). The assumption made here is that the client is the child's parent, not the child (Alderson 1993). As a result little is known about the influence of the child's characteristics on the family's needs for support during acute childhood illness at home or of the older child's development of knowledge about self-care. Wilkinson's (1988) review of the literature, and report of his own research, addresses the child's understanding of what is meant by health and illness but does not specifically address their experiences or needs during acute childhood illness.

Parental perception of the child's minor illness

Parents develop a sense of what is normal for their child as they develop in their role as parents. They learn about developmental changes with the first child and then apply this knowledge with their subsequent children (Spencer 1984, Mayall 1986, Cunningham-Burley 1990, Cunningham-Burley & Maclean 1991, Irvine & Cunningham-Burley 1991, Pearson 1995). It is from this reference point that the identification of illness is made. For example, parents attribute many symptoms of minor illness to teething (Spencer 1984, Mayall 1986, Irvine & Cunningham-Burley 1991), a process seen as a normal part of child development. It follows, then, that some illnesses are, in themselves, perceived to be normal for an individual child. Likewise, a specific illness such as chickenpox may itself be viewed as a normal childhood illness (McKenna & Hunt 1994). Children with persistent illness were also viewed as essentially healthy, the illness being attributed to an innate predisposition in that child (Mayall 1986, Irvine & Cunningham-Burley 1991). Some symptoms are particularly worrying to parents (Spencer 1984, Mayall 1986, Cornford et al 1993, Holme 1995, Hopton et al 1996, Kai 1996a):

- respiratory symptoms, particularly a persistent cough
- high temperature
- vomiting and pain, especially if the pain is severe, unrelieved and unexplained.

Altered breathing and/or coughing are the commonest reason for parents to consult a doctor about their child's health (Cunningham-Burley & Irvine 1987, Holme 1995).

Parents also fear not recognising serious illness in their children (Kai 1996a). They may even worry about common symptoms if they do not know what is wrong (Allen et al 2002). For some parents this was linked to 'past frights', when their child had been diagnosed by doctors to be much more seriously ill than they had thought before seeking medical advice (Hopton et al 1996). This 'fright' reduces the parents' confidence in their own ability to judge the state of their child's health. Houston & Pickering's (2000) more recent research found that parents whose child had been ill previously were more willing to hand over responsibility to the doctor, also suggesting a loss of confidence in their own abilities.

Parents' actions in response to illness in their child

Parents constantly monitor the state of their child's health so that they are able to make a judgement about the normality or abnormality of the child's state of health (Cunningham-Burley 1990, Kai 1996a). When parents notice that there is something wrong with their child their first action is to wait and see (Spencer 1984, Cunningham-Burley & Irvine 1987, Allen et al 2002). When symptoms persist, their treatment of the child may consist of nursing actions and/or the use of over-the-counter (OTC) remedies (Spencer 1984, Mayall 1986, Cunningham-Burley & Irvine 1987, Cunningham-Burley & Maclean 1987, Cornford et al 1993, Cantrill et al 1996). The majority of OTC remedies are already present in the home (Cantrill et al 1996). Generally children are given extra attention and time (Mayall 1986), providing the child with increased emotional support (Spencer 1984). Overall, parents make every effort to treat the child themselves and are reluctant to 'bother the doctor' (Cunningham-Burley & Maclean 1991, Houston & Pickering 2000, Kai 1996a). Difficulties in obtaining an appointment may be one reason for this reluctance (Cantrill et al 1996). Although parents in Houston & Pickering's research (2000) commented that reluctance to call the doctor was about not wanting to impose, for some it was a feeling that is was important to be seen to cope. They found this difficult to balance with doing the right thing for the child. Between 59% and 99% of all episodes of acute childhood illness at home are managed without recourse to health professionals (Holme 1995, Mayall 1986).

The role of family and friendship networks

Parents use what is described as a 'lay network' of family and friends to seek information about caring for their child (Mayall 1986, Kai 1996a, Allen et al 2002). This includes suggestions of diagnoses, advice on nursing their child, home remedies and when to refer to the doctor. Where this supportive network is smaller, an increased use of general practice services results (Mayall 1986, Houston & Pickering 2000). Social support for mothers results in better health for their children, an effect that is strongest in families living in poverty (Oakley et al 1994). The importance of a supportive network of family and friends reflects a key theme within the dominant philosophy of children's nursing: the need for children to be viewed and cared for within the context of their families (Royal College of Nursing 2003).

Factors affecting parents' use of health services

The published literature seems to indicate that the family doctor is perceived to be the main source of help available to families once their own resources have been exhausted. Allen et al's (2002) recent research mentions other healthcare professionals but with caveats for the ill child: HVs are seen as more personal than GPs and an important source of advice for young children, although they are recognised as not necessarily the best person for the sick child. PNs are perceived as for immunisations or for less serious illness; and NHS Direct is seen as useful, easy to access but slow to ring back and tending to refer to GPs. Parents' decisions to consult their doctor are based on the following:

- abnormal symptoms (Cunningham-Burley 1990, Hopton et al 1996) or symptoms associated with meningitis (Allen et al 2002)
- behavioural change (Hopton et al 1996, Kai 1996b)
- perceived increased severity of illness (Wyke et al 1990, Clarke & Hewison 1991, Cornford et al 1993)
- feelings of helplessness, lack of confidence in own management or of being unable to cope (Morrison et al 1991, Kai 1996b, Houston & Pickering 2000)
- when their own attempts to treat the child have failed (Cunningham-Burley & Irvine 1987, Hopton et al 1996, Allen et al 2002).

Parents' ability to cope with their child's illness seems to be closely related to their perceptions of the extent to which the illness is a threat to the child's life (Kai 1996a). This logically suggests that the greater the perceived threat to the child's health the more likely it is that a parent will decide to seek professional help and advice.

Parents' perceptions of healthcare services

When parents decide to seek help from health services, the most common desire is for the reassurance that they have not missed anything serious. This is followed closely by their need for information about their child's illness and care (Mayall 1986, Clarke & Hewison 1991, Irvine & Cunningham-Burley 1991, Morrison et al 1991, Cornford et al 1993, Kai 1996b, Allen et al 2002). Such information helps parents to understand their child's illness and the necessary treatment, reducing the perceived threat of the illness to the child's life and, therefore, increasing the parents' ability to continue to manage the episode of illness at home. Parents also seek information from sources other than healthcare professionals, often learning more from the media, in the form of books, parenting magazines, the internet, television dramas and publicity campaigns (Allen et al 2002, Kai 1996b). Parents wish to have their views respected and their competence as a parent recognised. Mothers, in particular, report that they are made to 'feel stupid' or 'silly' by doctors when consulting for a minor illness when all they wanted was reassurance (Cunningham-Burley & Maclean 1991). Allen et al (2002) identified a patronising attitude from healthcare professionals as a barrier to accessing healthcare.

Contrary to popular medical opinion, a minority of parents want medication for their child (Cunningham-Burley & Irvine 1987, Clarke & Hewison 1991). There is further conflict between parents and doctors here, as parents also misunderstand the reasons for the prescription of antibiotics. Parents' desire for antibiotics is based on their perception of the severity of their child's illness, rather than on an understanding of bacterial versus viral infection (Kai 1996b). There is an obvious mismatch here between the desires of parents and what GPs provide. From the doctor's perspective, their practice may be influenced by the necessity to see large numbers of patients in a short period of time, with the average GP consultation time being 9.4 minutes in the UK (Deveugele et al 2002). The extent to which the reassurance and information needs of families can be met in such a short time period must be limited.

At the end of such short consultations, parents may be no clearer about what is wrong with their child, or why they have or have not been given a prescription and their confidence in their own ability to care for their child may have been reduced. This situation may result in parents resorting to hospitalisation for their child (Meates 1997) or further GP consultations. Clearly the opposite may also occur where parent's needs are met. These parents may feel more confident in their ability to care for their child and reassured that their child is not seriously ill (Cornford et al 1993, Kai 1996a). Consequently their children may be less likely to be admitted to hospital as they feel able to care for them at home.

IMPLICATIONS OF THE EXPERIENCES OF CHILDREN AND THEIR FAMILIES DURING ACUTE CHILDHOOD ILLNESS FOR HEALTHCARE SERVICE DELIVERY

Demand for GP services to children aged one to 15 years is increasing (Health Committee 1997). In addition, general practice is facing a recruitment crisis with fewer doctors wanting to move into this field of work. GPs tried to manage the rising demand for out-of-hours services through the creation of GP cooperatives (Jessopp et al 1997). The style of each consultation is unlikely to change, creating even more demand as parents' needs continue to be unmet. Demand also appears to be rising due to the increased accessibility of these services, compared with the individual GPs doing their own on-call. Alternative options for managing the continually increasing demand need to be considered, in particular the role of other health professionals in helping parents to care for the child during acute childhood illness at home.

OPTIONS FOR THE INVOLVEMENT OF CHILDREN'S NURSES IN THE CARE OF THE ACUTELY ILL CHILD AT HOME

Integrated primary care model

This model involves CCNs based within and integrated into primary healthcare teams (PHCTs). Some of the advantages of this approach are:

- an appropriately qualified professional providing care for children and their families
- accessibility of services to children and their families at their local health centre
- ease of communication with the PHCT
- self-referrals and direct referrals from GPs, PNs, HVs, SNs and DNs to the CCN
- services can be developed in response to the specific needs of the local population, enabling the specific needs of minority ethnic groups to be met more easily.

Minimal research has been conducted which addresses this area. However, one project in Sheffield has provided valuable evidence of the feasibility of using children's nurses to care for the acutely ill child at home (Drew et al 2002, 2003). Drew's findings of the evaluation of the project demonstrate the feasibility of children's nurses working within PHCTs. In other areas of the country a few children's nurses are beginning to work with, and be based within, PHCTs. The increase in information and the accessibility of support will improve parents' personal control and therefore their ability to care for their child (Kai 1996b, Meates 1997), with an accompanying reduction in demand for GP consultations and attendance at accident and emergency (A&E) departments (Meates 1997). In addition, the reduction of parental anxiety will reduce the child's level of anxiety, potentially facilitating a faster recovery. Examples of the success of a minor-ailments clinic combined with home visits is provided in the case studies.

Hospital at Home services

Hospital at Home services are being developed to facilitate early discharge or to prevent hospital admission (Box 21.1 and Case study 21.1). Evidence suggests a small number of the generic community children's nursing teams provide care for children with acute illness. Early research comparing these services to traditional hospital care has shown that they are much preferred by families and are cost neutral to the NHS (While 1992, Sartain et al 2001, 2002, Bagust et al 2002).

Box 21.1 The Rugby Hospital at Home Service

- Established 2000
- Aims to prevent/limit admissions
- 4.6 G Grade community-based CCNs work with children and their families/carers in their homes to increase understanding of/confidence in looking after their child's illness
- Referrals from GPs/local A&E/Paediatricians at the nearest children's ward in Coventry (15 miles away)
- Referring doctors (over half of which are GPs) maintain clinical responsibility

- Team visits children with acute illness, e.g. gastroenteritis/bronchiolitis/wheezy episode/continuation of intravenous therapy
- Team available 7 days a week/08.00–22.00 hours/on-call every night for telephone advice to families on caseload
- On referral, telephone triage undertaken, followed by visit according to need, several times a day if necessary
- Care plans in partnership with the child/parents
- Discharged when both CCN/parents happy with the child's condition

Case study 21.1 Example of care provided by a Hospital at Home service

A&E referred 8-year-old Sophie following a scald injury to her chest. Sophie would normally have been visited by the Hospital at Home team after 48 hours, but was visited the next day as her dressing was not intact. Telephone advice had already been given about the use of analgesia for pain relief. Sophie was naturally apprehensive so the use of Entonox was explained to her and her mother. Sophie used it with good effect whilst her dressing was removed and her injury assessed/redressed. Written and verbal advice was given about the injury and visits continued to review/redress the injury, using Entonox for pain relief. Sophie and family were pleased that she could be cared for at home rather than have to visit A&E repeatedly for dressings. (Résumé of Hospital at Home Team and case study provided by Margaret Simmonds, Rugby Children's Hospital at Home Team 2003)

Ambulatory care

This concept has been defined as 'the non-inpatient hospital services and the provision of care to sick children at home or in their local environment' (Meates 1997). This approach includes units such as children's admission units, day case units, rapid-response outpatient clinics, children's A&E and hospital outreach children's nursing services (Glasper & Lowson 1998). Meates (1997) describes the presence of children's nurses in the A&E department as making 'a huge difference to the care of children'. In the best examples, each of these units is able to refer children to a community-based generic CCN for follow-up visits and support.

The ambulatory care approach does prevent some unnecessary admissions, but many of the services delivered under this label do involve hospital attendance (Glasper & Lowson 1998, Macleod et al 2000). Consequently, it does disrupt family life as the child has to travel to the hospital, usually at a greater distance from home than the local health centre. Although these units do minimise hospital attendance, this is not community care. Much of the care given in this way could be given at home. Concentrating these services within the hospital environment is convenient for health professionals, not for families. It also reflects the resource constraints within the current climate of the NHS.

Inevitably hospital-based services are limited by the nature of their referral system. Referrals usually come from other hospital services. As a result, the service is not accessible to families whose children are not referred to the hospital or who do not attend the A&E department. Both the Royal College of Nursing (2000) and the Royal College of Paediatrics and Child Health (RCPCH) (RCPCH 2002) provide further examples of new patterns of service provision for the ill child at home.

Further developments in primary healthcare are likely to have a significant effect on the provision of services for the acutely ill child at home. The contract for GPs, implemented from April 2004, allows GPs to contract out of providing out-of-hours care, moving services currently provided by GP cooperatives into the management of Primary Care Trusts. It poses the questions:

- Will these Trusts see the value of employing CCNs to augment out-of-hours services when GPs are becoming a scarce commodity?
- How will CCNs work within such services?
- Will they be the first point of contact for families seeking help for their children?

CONCLUSION

The majority of childhood illness takes place at home with no recourse to professional care and support. Despite this, children with acute childhood illness constitute a significant proportion of the GP's workload. Various professionals are currently involved in the care of these children in the community, most of whom do not hold a qualification in child healthcare and/or a specific community qualification. Parents are often dissatisfied with the care provided by GPs, wanting more reassurance and information. The average consultation time with their family doctor is far too short for parents' needs to be met in this way. Rising demand and the non-expansion of GP services means that alternatives to GP care are needed to support children and families during acute illness.

The strategic development of services that integrate CCNs within PHCTs and primary care groups has the potential to meet parents' needs for information and reassurance. In doing so, CCNs are enabling parents to continue to care for their child at home, thus reducing the pressure on both hospital and GP services. The continuing move towards community care and centralisation of tertiary care across the NHS make the further development of local services, which enable children and families to cope at home, an essential prerequisite for the management of rising demands for services.

REFERENCES

Alderson P 1993 Children's consent to surgery. Open University Press, Buckingham

Alderson P 1995 Listening to Children. Children, Ethics and Social Research. Barnado's, Ilford

Allen J, Dyas J & Jones M 2002 Minor illness in children: parents' views and use of health services. Journal of Community Nursing 7(9):462–468

Bagust A, Haycox A & Sartain S 2002 Economic evaluation of an acute paediatric hospital at home clinical trial. Archives of Disease in Childhood 87(6):489–492

Cantrill J A, Johannesson B, Nicolson M & Noyce P R 1996 Management of minor ailments in primary schoolchildren in rural and urban areas. Child: Care, Health and Development 22(3):167–174

Carlisle R & Johnstone S 1998 The relationship between census-driven socio-economic variables and general practice consultation rates in three town centre practices. British Journal of General Practice 48(435):1675–1678

Carr-Hill R A, Rice N & Roland M 1996 Socioeconomic determinants of rate of consultation in general practice based on fourth national morbidity survey of general practices. British Medical Journal 312(7037):1008–1012

Clarke A & Hewison J 1991 Whether or not to consult a general practitioner: decision-making by parents in a multi-ethnic inner city area. In: Wyke S & Hewison J (eds) Child Health Matters. Open University Press, Milton Keynes, ch. 7, p 74

Cornford C S, Morgan M & Ridsdale L 1993 Why do mothers consult when their children cough? Family Practice 10(2):193–196

Cramp C, Tripp S, Hughes N & Dale J 2003 Children's home nursing: results of a national survey. Paediatric Nursing 15(8):39–43

Cunningham-Burley S 1990 Mothers' beliefs about and perceptions of their children's illnesses. In: Cunningham-Burley S & McKeganey N P (eds) Readings in Medical Sociology. Tavistock/Routledge, London, ch 4, p 85

Cunningham-Burley S & Irvine S 1987 'And have you done anything so far?' An examination of lay treatment of children's symptoms. British Medical Journal 295:700–702

Cunningham-Burley S & Maclean U 1987 The role of the chemist in primary health care for children with minor complaints. Social Science and Medicine 24(4):371–377

Cunningham-Burley S & Maclean U 1991 Dealing with children's illness: mothers' dilemmas. In: Wyke S & Hewison J (eds) Child Health Matters. Open University Press, Milton Keynes, ch. 3, p 29

Department of Health 2003 Getting the right start. National Service Framework for Children. Emerging Findings. The Stationery Office, London

Deveugele M, Derese A, van den Brink-Muinen A, Bensing J & De Maeseneer J 2002 Consultation length in general practice: cross sectional study in six European countries. British Medical Journal 325(7362):472–477

Drew J, Nathan D & Hall D 2002 Role of a paediatric nurse in primary care 1: research issues. British Journal of Nursing 11(22):1352–1360

Drew J, Nathan D & Hall D 2003 Role of a paediatric nurse in primary care 2: research findings. British Journal of Nursing 12(1):34–42

Gillett J A 1954 Domiciliary treatment of sick children. The Practitioner 172:281–283

Glasper E A & Lowson S 1998 Innovations in Paediatric Ambulatory Care. A Nursing Perspective. Macmillan, Basingstoke

Health Committee 1997 House of Commons Health Select Committee. Health services for children and young people in the community: home and school. Third report. The Stationery Office, London

Holme C 1995 Incidence and prevalence of non-specific symptoms and behavioural changes in infants under the age of two years. British Journal of General Practice 45:65–69

Hopton J, Hogg R & McKee I 1996 Patients' accounts of calling the doctor out of hours: qualitative study in one general practice. British Medical Journal 313:991–994

Houston A M & Pickering A J 2000 'Do I don't I call the doctor': a qualitative study of parental perceptions of calling the GP out-of-hours. Health Expectations 3:234–242

Irvine S & Cunningham-Burley S 1991 Mothers' concept of normality, behavioural change and illness in their children. British Journal of General Practice 41:371–374

Jessopp L, Beck I, Hollins L, Shipman C, Reynolds M & Dale J 1997 Changing the pattern out of hours: a survey of general practice cooperatives. British Medical Journal 314:199–200

Kai J 1996a What worries parents when their pre-school children are acutely ill, and why: a qualitative study. British Medical Journal 313:983–986

Kai J 1996b Parents' difficulties and information needs in coping with acute illness in preschool children: a qualitative study. British Medical Journal 313:987–990

Learning from Bristol 2001 The report of the public inquiry into children's heart surgery at the Bristol Royal Infirmary 1984–1995. The Stationery Office, London

Leicester City Council 2001 City Statistics. Area Profile for the City of Leicester: Demographic and Cultural. Leicester City Council, Leicester

McCormick A, Fleming D & Charlton J 1995 Morbidity statistics from general practice 1991–2. Series MB5. No. 3. Office of Population Censuses and Surveys. HMSO, London

McKenna S P & Hunt S M 1994 A measure of family disruption for use in chickenpox and other childhood illnesses. Social Science and Medicine 38(5):725–731

Macleod C, McElroy G, O'Loan D, Kennedy F, Kerr R-M, Jenkins J & Lim J 2000 Ambulatory paediatrics; does it work. Royal College of Paediatrics and Child Health, London

Mayall B 1986 Keeping children healthy. Allen & Unwin, London

Meates M 1997 Ambulatory paediatrics – making a difference. Archives of Disease in Childhood 76:468–472

Morrison J M, Gilmour H & Sullivan F 1991 Children seen frequently out of hours in one general practice. British Medical Journal 303:1111–1114

Neill S J 1996 Parent participation. Part 1. British Journal of Nursing 5(1):34–40

Oakley A, Hickey D & Rigby A S 1994 Love or money? Social support, class inequality and the health of women and children. European Journal of Public Health 4:265–273

Office for National Statistics (ONS) 2002 Social Focus in Brief: Children. ONS, London

Office for National Statistics (ONS) 2003 Census 2001: Households Below Average Income. ONS, London

Pearson P 1995 Client views of health visiting. In: Heyman B (ed.) Researching User Perspectives on Community Health Care. Chapman & Hall, London, Ch. 6, p 106

Reading R 1997 Poverty and the health of children and adolescents. Archives of Disease in Childhood 76:463–467

Rennick J E 1995 The changing profile of acute childhood illness: a need for the development of family nursing knowledge. Journal of Advanced Nursing 22:258–266

Royal College of Nursing (RCN) 2000 Children's community nursing. Promoting effective teamworking for children and their families. RCN, London

Royal College of Nursing (RCN) 2003 Children and young people's nursing: a philosophy of care. Guidance for nursing staff. RCN, London

Royal College of Paediatrics and Child Health (RCPCH) 2002 Old Problems, New Solutions. 21st Century Children's Healthcare. RCPCH, London

Sartain S, Maxwell M & Todd P 2001 Users' views on hospital and home care for acute illness in childhood. Health and Social Care in the Community 9(2):108–115

Sartain S, Maxwell M & Todd P 2002 Randomised controlled trial comparing an acute paediatric hospital at home scheme with conventional hospital care. Archives of Disease in Childhood 87(5):371–375

Shrand H 1965 Behaviour changes in sick children nursed at home. Pediatrics 36(4):604–607

Smellie J M 1956 Domiciliary nursing service for infants and children. British Medical Journal i:256

Spencer N J 1984 Parents' recognition of the ill child. In: Macfarlane J A (ed.) Progress in Child Health, vol 1. Churchill Livingstone, Edinburgh, p 100

Watson E 1991 'Appropriate' use of child health services in East London: ethnic similarities and differences. In: Wyke S & Hewison J (eds) Child Health Matters. Open University Press, Milton Keynes, Ch 8, p 88

Webb E 1996 Meeting the needs of minority ethnic groups. Archives of Disease in Childhood 74:264–267

While A 1992 Consumer views of health care: a comparison of hospital and home care. Child: Care, Health and Development 18:107–116

Wilkinson S R 1988 The Child's World of Illness. The Development of Health and Illness Behaviour. Cambridge University Press, Cambridge

Wyke S, Hewison J & Russell I T 1990 Respiratory illness in children: what makes parents decide to consult? British Journal of General Practice 40:226–229

Chapter 22

Delivering and funding care for children with complex needs

David Widdas and Anna Sidey
with Sue Dryden

KEY ISSUES
- Incidence, prevalence and location of care.
- Sociopolitical influences.
- Continuing care framework.
- Delivering complex care within multi-agency frameworks.
- Respite care.
- The role of the key worker.

INTRODUCTION

Innovations in medical practice and technological advances have meant that children are now surviving once-fatal diseases (Birch et al 1988, Roberton 1993). Often their care is complex due to a reliance on technology (Kirk 1998). For example 'A third of parents with a severely disabled child under the age of two use more than three pieces of equipment daily to provide basic care' (DoH 2003 p 28).

These factors have implications for meeting the needs of this population. This chapter examines the issues influencing the provision of integrated and appropriate support for these children and their families in the community.

INCIDENCE, PREVALENCE AND LOCATION OF CARE

The prevalence of chronic illness in childhood more than doubled between 1972 and 1991 (Office of Population Censuses and Surveys 1991) and in 1996 it was estimated that 14% of under-16-year-olds had a chronic illness (Perkins 1996).

- The Avon Lifetime Service identified 123 children aged 0–19 years with a wide range of rare conditions within a population of 411 800, a prevalence of 1.28 per thousand. Within this number children with non-malignant life-threatening illness outnumbered children with malignant disease by two to one (Lewis 1999).

- In 1999, 141 children dependent on long-term ventilation were identified (Jardine et al 1999).

Demand and capacity for care has expanded and moved into the community for a number of reasons which include:

- Medical advances enabling long-term survival from once-fatal disorders which have preceded legal and ethical guidance (Youngblut et al 1994).
- Greater availability of medicines, therapies and portable technology to support associated care needs (Social Policy Research Unit 2003).
- Government agenda and supporting policies that have pursued a shift from secondary care to primary care alongside a philosophy of increasing consumer expectations.
- The availability and recognition of community children's nursing as a separate community resource (United Kingdom Central Council 1994).

An increasing body of knowledge on the advantages and disadvantages of these fundamental shifts acknowledges the costs and benefits of home care. These benefits are summarised by Linter et al (2000) and Whiting et al (2001). Family nursing as a framework for community children's nursing practice together with the development of emotional intelligence are described by Muir & Sidey (2003). The costs of caring include the adverse effects on siblings, social isolation, lack of privacy, financial loss and parental stress (Dobson & Middleton 1998, Warner & Wexler 1998, Murphy 2001a, 2001b).

Recent research considers the feelings of children with complex care needs living at home: 'even those with the most severe impairments are able to communicate about their feeling, about their lives and the treatment they receive ... children are not passive victims' (Joseph Rowntree Foundation 1999 p 1).

SOCIOPOLITICAL INFLUENCES

Government policies and recommendations have continued to advocate for children to be cared for in their own homes and for appropriate services to be provided (Ministry of Health 1959, DoH and Social Security 1976, DoH 1991, NHS Executive 1996, Health Committee 1997). Published as guidance rather than formal requirements they have resulted in local interpretation and a disparity in the provision of community children's nursing services. By 1997 only 50% of children in the UK had access to such services (Health Committee 1997). The first specific Government funding of community children's nursing was in 1998 in memory of Diana, Princess of Wales. The accompanying guidance formally identified, for the first time, the need for multiprofessional teams (English National Board for Nursing, Midwifery and Health Visiting & DoH 1999). In addition the DoH discussion document Partnership in Action (DoH 1998a) advocated the integration of health and social services as the most advantageous way of delivering care to individuals with complex health needs. This policy initiative has now come to the forefront with the advent of Children's Trusts (see Chapter 3).

CONTINUING CARE FRAMEWORK

In 1994 the Ombudsman's report 'Failure to provide long term NHS care for a brain damaged patient', referred to as The Leed's Case (Health Circular 1994), prompted the Government to develop the continuing care policy (DoH 1995). The aim of this policy was to provide for long-term complex healthcare once hospital treatment was no longer required, by establishing a distinction between nursing (health) care and social care, and funding continuing nursing care accordingly. Responsibility for the development of eligibility criteria for this 'continuing care' was devolved to health and local authorities. Some welcomed the ability to interpret and define the policy at a local level while others believed that this contributed to disparity of service provision across the country (Thomas 1996).

The continuing care policy primarily focused on the needs of the elderly with no reference to the specific needs of children. It excluded children by defining the age of the client group as 18 years and older (DoH 1995). Some local policies, prompted by CCNs, identified the need for further development of explicit eligibility criteria for children's services. In 1999 a crucial judgement made in the Court of Appeal (R v. North and East Devon Health Authority ex parte Coughlan) stated when it was lawful to fund nursing care, in part or in full, from Local Authority (LA) resources. This is termed Coughlan compliance and applies if required nursing services are:

- 'merely incidental or ancillary to the provision of the accommodation which the local authority is under a duty to provide
- of a nature which it could be expected that an authority, whose primary responsibility is to provide social services, could be expected to provide'.

The significance of this judgement is that care above this level would become an NHS responsibility and therefore free at the point of delivery as opposed to LA means-tested care. This is central to the formulation of Strategic Health Authority (SHA) and LA criteria for continuing care that is funded at three levels:

1. NHS-funded care (free at the point of delivery)
2. NHS/LA-funded care (a percentage means tested)
3. LA-funded care (means tested) (DoH 2001a, 2001b, Health Circular 2003).

It should be noted that the Health Circular 2003 only applies to individuals aged 18 years and older, whilst Coughlan compliance is not defined by age. Primary Care Trusts (PCTs) consequently have had to make their own decisions on applicability to children. (The publication of the Children's National Service Framework (NSF) will rectify this anomaly.)

Given the continuing existing inequalities in community children's nursing services within the UK (Health Committee 1997) this policy widened the gulf between the parity of care provision for those who have access to the service and those who do not. Where services exist, CCNs are uniquely placed to contribute to the development of eligibility criteria for their client group and to ensure that the total needs of individual children are recognised and met (NHS Executive 1998). SHAs/LAs may elect to draw up children's continuing care funding criteria based on the existing health service circulars and the Coughlan judgement although this is not widespread practice. Alternatively, individual PCTs can choose to apply existing criteria to children and to concentrate on a more child-focused assessment process. Some areas are focusing continuing care funding on a specialist commissioner model where the decisions are made by a lead commissioner based on existing SHA criteria as in Warwickshire (D Widdas & M Karn, unpublished work, 2002).

DELIVERING COMPLEX CARE

Assessment

Assessment for home care is commenced when a child and family make an informed decision that care is to be undertaken at home. 'Statutory authorities should not assume that a relative will automatically be able to put their life on hold in order to become a carer' (Warner & Wexler 1998 p 16). Four key principles underpin the assessment process:

1. Parents are the experts and primary carers.
2. Home is the centre of caring.
3. Assessment should be carried out within the context of family life and the community and culture in which they live.
4. Coordination to produce a single interdisciplinary and multi-agency assessment (Association for Children with Life-threatening or Terminal Conditions and their Families & Royal College of Paediatrics and Child Health 2003).

The document 'Framework for the Assessment of Children in Need and their Families' provides information to assist in the joint planning of continuing care needs of children in the community (DoH 2000).

Assessing and managing risk

An ongoing principle used by The Avon Lifetime Service is that if a greater than 10% chance of a risk exists an event should be actively planned for. An example may include the interruption of electric power that would render loss of oxygen flow from an oxygen concentrator and an ability to visually monitor a child's condition. Local Clinical Governance departments provide risk assessment tools that may be adapted for use by CCNs. The formulation of risk management plans that include protocols and identifiable roles and responsibilities should accompany the child at all times. In addition and where appropriate an accepted and agreed resuscitation statement should be available (Linter et al 2000).

Delivery models

Unfortunately, the void which exists as a result of the absence of a national strategy for community children's nursing (see Chapter 10) has resulted in individual service models that have evolved around isolated children with complex care needs. For example, research indicates that this results in enormous differences in the level of available support for children with central hyperventilation syndrome from between one night each week to 24-hour nursing care (Noyes et al 1999). Anecdotal evidence suggests that a substantial number of individual care packages rely on nursing agency staff. External working groups of the NSF considered the best practice available to date and it is to be expected that guidance on workforce planning will follow.

Skill mix and competencies

The growth of teams has led to a need to consider workforce planning and introduce skill mix that includes non-nursing support workers. This intensifies the need for robust competency-based training (Linter et al 2000). Given the isolated nature of the practice of some CCNs a judgement may need to be considered on the appropriateness of skill mix. Some sources consider it inappropriate for CCNs to assume responsibility for the training of non-nursing support workers as 'in so doing jeopardise their professional position' (Murphy 2001b p 26). Dimond (Chapter 12 p 140) states: 'If a health professional were to give negligent advice to a patient or to the carers and, in reliance on that advice, harm was caused, then, if the advice was given knowing that it would be relied upon, the health professional or employer could be held accountable'. The Nursing and Midwifery Council (NMC) state:

> 'You may be expected to delegate care delivery to others who are not registered nurses or midwives. Such delegation must not compromise existing care but must be directed to meeting the needs of and serving the interests of patients and clients. You remain accountable for the appropriateness of the delegation and for ensuring the person who does the work is able to do it and that adequate supervision and support is provided' (NMC 2002).

To facilitate appropriate and safe delegation of care, competency frameworks have developed. An example is based on Steinaker and Bell's model of learning (1979). These frameworks allow non-nursing support workers and registered nurses to learn new skills in a structured way. In addition, CCN assessors can demonstrate the required teaching skills and record the levels of competency achieved (D Widdas, unpublished work, 2002). The information and record of activity contained within a competency framework system should contain key elements common to all frameworks. These elements are then adapted and expanded for individual application according to individual patient, family and carer/worker (formal or informal) needs. The key elements of a competency framework are the 'principles': (1) the 'areas of concern', (2) the 'skills and knowledge' and (3) the 'levels of competency/learning' (D Widdas, unpublished work, 2002).

Principles
- For use with named child only
- For use by named worker only
- Time limited (depending on level reached)
- Child centred
- Includes psychological care
- Signed by carer/worker and CCN educator.

The actual structure of the competency has three parallel elements.

1. Areas of concern
   - Basic anatomy and physiology
   - Psychological implications
   - Demonstration of skill
   - Complications and trouble shooting
   - Safety routines
   - Record keeping (DoH 2001b)
   - Privacy and dignity (DoH 2001b).

2. Required skills and knowledge
   - Each area of concern is broken down into its component parts, grouped into sections and signed by worker and teacher/assessor when completed at each of the following competency levels.

3. Levels of competency:
   - Exposure – initial teaching
   - Participation – supervised practice
   - Identification – safe to practise
   - Internalisation – competent/confident to practice (risk of over confidence)
   - Dissemination – safe to teach/research (Steinaker & Bell 1979).

Following on from a competency frameworks system the next consideration is the application, maintenance and audit of the system. Widdas (D Widdas, unpublished work, 2003) suggests the implementation of a competency cycle based on recommendations of the Bristol Enquiry (Kennedy 2001) (Fig. 22.1).

Agreements of care

Intensive home care is invariably accompanied by an array of complex social boundary issues that may include care of siblings, domestic tasks and maintenance of the parental role. Early complex packages of care were not supported within proactively planned frameworks aimed at preventing conflict and misunderstandings between family and non-family carers

Fig. 22.1 Competency cycle based on recommendations from the Bristol Enquiry (Kennedy 2001).

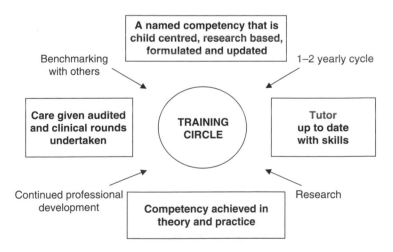

(Murphy 2001b, Beale 2002). A variety of contracts and agreements have been formulated in response to perceived and identified needs and aim to formalise and agree arrangements between families and formal care givers (Box 22.1).

Box 22.1 An example of a generic agreement of care between a family and the Community Children's Nursing Service

Agreement of Care

Patient's Name:

To be reviewed on:

The purpose of this agreement is to make clear what you can expect us to provide and what agreements we need from you to safely provide the care that *Child/Young Person* requires.

Our responsibilities:
1. We will provide a Nurse/Carer.
2. We will treat you with respect and value your opinions. You will always remain the lead people in *Child/Young Person's* care with the final say and ultimate responsibility for *Child/Young Person's* care.
3. Nurse/Carer will only discuss *Child/Young Person's* care on a need to know basis with members of the wider team.
4. We will supply, clean and maintain all equipment.
5. We will supply and maintain adequate stock levels of all supplies.
6. We will respect your home and clean up any untidiness we make.
7. We will respect your privacy and leave if asked, but you must take over all *Child/Young Person's* care for that shift.
8. In the event of a Nurse/Carer being ill we will try to find a replacement but this cannot be guaranteed.

Your responsibilities:
1. You always retain overall responsibility for *Child/Young Person's* care.
2. You need to keep us informed of any changes to the support you require; if the Nurse/Carer arrives for work and you are not there, they will be redeployed and no staff will be provided for the shift.
3. Our staff need access to a kitchen, toilet and a small cupboard to store tea, coffee and cups.
4. Will you provide milk? Yes/No (please delete).
5. Our staff are employed to look after *Child/Young Person*. Please do not ask them to do domestic tasks.
6. Nurse/Carer will need to hand over to you 15 minutes before they leave.
7. It is NHS Policy that care will be withdrawn if staff are verbally or physically assaulted.
8. Family are invited to add their own responsibilities.

(D Widdas, unpublished work, 2001)

Joint working

The DoH (1998b) has acknowledged that 'health and social care are often one and the same' (para. 2.29). The need to break down existing barriers and pursue integrated health and social care provision has also been recognised within the NSF's Emerging Findings document (DoH 2003). The Partnership in Action discussion document (DoH 1998a, p 6) stated that (see Chapter 15):

'Joint working is needed at three levels:
1. *Strategic planning: agencies need to plan jointly for the medium term, sharing information about how they intend to use their resources toward the achievement of common goals.*
2. *Service commissioning: when securing services for their local populations, agencies need to have a common understanding of the needs they are jointly meeting and the kind of provision likely to be most effective.*
3. *Service provision: regardless of how services are purchased or funded, the key objective is that the user receives a coherent integrated package of care and that they, and their families, do not face the anxiety of having to navigate a labyrinthine bureaucracy.'*

Most joint services are achieved by Health, Social Services and Education undertaking their own specific tasks within whole packages of care (DoH 2003). In order to encourage agencies towards more coordinated thinking the Government developed the concept of Children's Trusts (DoH 2002). These Trusts are viewed as a way of supporting joined up working in a more formalised way by enabling the development of services based on local needs. In addition the first Trusts are involving local and national voluntary services. It is anticipated that the NSF for children will help facilitate joint assessments, planning and commissioning (see Chapter 3).

RESPITE CARE

'The more disabled a child is – the less likely their family is to get a short break service'

(Shared Care Network 2003 p 2).

Parents remain the principal carers often required to learn complex nursing skills and assume 24-hour responsibility in order to achieve home care (While et al 1996, Townsley & Robinson 1999, Boosfeld & O'Toole 2000, Glendinning & Kirk 2000, Murphy 2001a, 2001b, Muir & Sidey 2003). Alongside the emotional burdens associated with this clinical care families can be socially isolated and virtually housebound (Patterson et al 1994, Kirk 1998). The consequences of this may be increased parental stress, deterioration of the family structure and marital problems (Andrews & Nielson 1988, Jennings 1990, Leonard et al 1993, Teague et al 1993, Hall 1996). In 2000 the Carers and Disabled Children's Act identified the caring aspects of the parental role (Kirk 2001). Under this Act parents now have the right to an assessment of their own needs as a carer. Identified services can be provided under section 17 of the Children Act (DoH 1989).

There is a shortfall in appropriate respite care provision particularly where highly specialised care is required (Hall 1996, While et al 1996, NHS

Executive 1998, Townsley & Robinson 1999, MENCAP 2003). To meet this increasing need health and social service provision is supplemented by voluntary or independent organisations and non-parent carers. To date there is no national guidance from the DoH for the training of such carers, despite being a recommendation of the 1997 Health Committee report. In order to overcome this, voluntary organisations have led the way in developing both guidance and protocols. For example 'Promoting Partnership' and 'Towards a Healthy Future' describe key policies and practices required to enable non-parent carers to care for children with complex care needs (Servian et al 1998, Rhodes et al 1999).

Respite care is most effective when it meets the expressed needs of children and their families (NHS Executive 1998, Glendinning & Kirk 2000) and is:

- accessed as and when necessary
- flexible in terms of location
- negotiable in time and length.

THE KEY WORKER

The overwhelming and sustained nature of caring for a child with complex needs is exacerbated by additional factors:

- confusion around the roles and responsibilities of the different professionals involved
- the number of visits from and to various professionals
- the need to clarify and coordinate services and equipment
- the need to act as advocate for their child (Joseph Rowntree Foundation 1999, Muir & Sidey 2003).

The varied expectations of the role of the key worker have emerged from a succession of documents. The role may be viewed on a continuum from being the responsibility of a single under-resourced nominated professional to that of a dedicated and funded key worker service (NHS Executive 1998, English National Board for Nursing, Midwifery and Health Visiting & Department of Health 1999, DoH 2003). The widely accepted definition of the role emerged in 1997 (Association for Children with Life-threatening or Terminal Conditions and their Families & Royal College of Paediatrics and Child Health 2003) (see Chapter 23 p 265). Families describe the distinguishing features of an effective key worker as:

- proactive in contact
- supportive
- open relationship
- holistic family-centred approach
- cross-agency working
- approach based on family strengths and ways of coping
- working for the family as opposed to the agency (Joseph Rowntree Foundation 1999).

Research findings quoted by the Joseph Rowntree Foundation (1999 p 2) define the role of the key worker as: 'A named person whom the parent approaches for advice about any problem related to the disabled child. The key worker has responsibility for collaborating with professionals from their own and other services. Workers performing this role may come from a number of different agencies, depending on the particular needs of the child'. The concept of the key worker has finally reached the top of the policy agenda with the launch of the NSF. The challenge remains in ensuring appropriate resources and support for the professionals undertaking this essential role.

CONCLUSION

A growing body of evidence and experience is emerging to support the provision of complex packages of care. The need for supporting complex care within community settings is established and acknowledged within Emerging Findings (DoH 2003). The reactive and ad hoc growth and development of community children's nursing has resulted in a restricting absence of a corporate identity and national strategy. To date, a tendency to similarly respond to the needs of children with complex care needs is evident. The opportunity exists to harness current legislation in order to identify need and appropriately resource and structure services for this expanding group of children and their families.

REFERENCES

Andrews M M & Nielson D W 1988 Technology dependent children in the home. Pediatric Nursing 12(2):111–114

Association for Children with Life-threatening or Terminal Conditions and their Families (ACT) & Royal College of Paediatrics and Child Health 2003a A guide to the development of children's palliative care services. 2nd edn. ACT, Bristol

Association for Children with Life-threatening or Terminal Conditions and their Families (ACT) 2003b Assessment of children with life-limiting conditions and their families. A guide to effective care planning. ACT, Bristol

Beale H 2002 Respite care for technology-dependent children and their families. Paediatric Nursing 14(7):18–19

Birch J M, Marsden H B, Morris Jones P H, Pearson D & Blair V 1988 Improvements in survival in childhood cancer: results of a population-based study over 30 years. British Medical Journal 296:1372–1376

Boosfeld B & O'Toole M 2000 Technology-dependent children: Transition from hospital to home. Paediatric Nursing 12(6):20–22

Department of Health 1989 The Children Act. HMSO, London

Department of Health 1991 The welfare of children and young people in hospital. HMSO, London

Department of Health 1995 NHS responsibilities for meeting continuing health care needs. HSG(95)8 LAC(95)5. HMSO, London

Department of Health 1998a Partnership in action. A discussion document. The Stationery Office, London

Department of Health 1998b Our healthier nation. The Stationery Office, London

Department of Health 2000 Framework for the Assessment of Children in Need and their Families. The Stationery Office, London

Department of Health 2001a Continuing Care: NHS and Local Councils' Responsibilities. The Stationery Office, London

Department of Health 2001b Health Service Circular 015. The Stationery Office, London

Department of Health 2002 Children's Trusts. The Stationery Office, London

Department of Health 2003 Getting the right start: The National Service Framework for Children, Young People and Maternity Services. Emerging Findings. The Stationery Office, London

Department of Health and Social Security 1976 Fit for the future. Report of the Committee on Child Health Services. HMSO, London

Dobson B & Middleton S 1998 The cost of childhood disability. Joseph Rowntree Foundation, York

English National Board for Nursing, Midwifery and Health Visiting & Department of Health 1999 Sharing the care. Resource pack to support Diana, Princess of Wales Community Children's Nursing Teams. English National Board, London

Glendinning C & Kirk S 2000 High-tech care: high-skilled parents. Paediatric Nursing 6(12):25–27

Hall S 1996 An exploration of parental perception of the nature and level of support needed to care for their child with special needs. Journal of Advanced Nursing 24:512–521

Health Circular 1994 'Failure to provide long term NHS care for a brain damaged patient' (The Leed's Case). Health Circular 157. HMSO, London

Health Circular 2003 The Health Service Ombudsman. NHS funding for long term care. 2nd Report. The Stationery Office, London

Health Committee 1997 House of Commons Select Committee. Health services for children and young people in the community: home and school. Third report. The Stationery Office, London

Jardine E, O'Toole M, Paton J & Wallis C 1999 Current status of long term ventilation of children in the UK; questionnaire survey. British Medical Journal 318:295–299

Jennings P 1990 Caring for a child with a tracheostomy. Nursing Standard 4(30):24–26 & 4(32):38–40

Joseph Rowntree Foundation 1999 Implementing key worker services: a case study of promoting evidence-based practice. Joseph Rowntree Foundation, York

Kennedy I 2001 The Report of the Public Enquiry into Children's Heart Surgery at the Bristol Royal Infirmary 1984–1995. Learning from Bristol. The Stationery Office, London

Kirk S 1998 Families' experiences of caring at home for a technology-dependent child: a review of the literature. Child: Care, Health and Development 24(2):101–114

Kirk S 2001 Negotiating lay and professional roles in the care of children with complex health care needs. Journal of Advanced Nursing 34(5):593–602

Leonard B J, Dwyer Brust J & Nelson R P 1993 Parental distress: caring for medically fragile children at home. Journal of Pediatric Nursing 8(1):22–30

Lewis M 1999 The Lifetime Service: a model for children with life threatening illness and their families. Paediatric Nursing 11(7):21–23

Linter S, Perry M & Cherry D 2000 Continuing care: an integrated approach. Paediatric Nursing 12(8):17–18

MENCAP 2003 Breaking Point. MENCAP, London

Ministry of Health 1959 The welfare of children in hospital. Report of the committee (chairman Sir Harry Platt). HMSO, London

Muir J & Sidey A 2003 Community Children's Nursing. In: Watkins D, Edwards J & Gastrell P (eds) Community Health Nursing Frameworks For Practice 2nd edn. Baillière Tindall, Edinburgh, pp 271–280

Murphy G 2001a The technology-dependent child at home Part 1 – In whose best interest? Paediatric Nursing 13(7):14–18

Murphy G 2001b The technology-dependent child at home Part 2 – The need for respite. Paediatric Nursing 13(8):24–27

National Health Service Executive 1996 A patient's charter: services for children and young people. HMSO, London

National Health Service Executive 1998 Evaluation of the pilot project programme for children with life threatening illnesses. The Stationery Office, London

Noyes J, Hartmann H, Samuels M & Southall D 1999 The experiences and views of parents who care for ventilator dependant children. Journal of Clinical Nursing 8:440–450

Nursing and Midwifery Council (NMC) 2002 Code of Professional Conduct. NMC, London

Office of Population Censuses and Surveys 1991 OPCS surveys of disability in Great Britain. HMSO, London

Patterson J M, Jernell J, Leonard B J & Titus J C 1994 Caring for medically fragile children at home: the parent–professional relationship. Journal of Pediatric Nursing 9(2):98–106

Perkins E 1996 Community children's nursing: generalist or specialist? NHS Executive, Leeds

Rhodes A, Lenehan C & Morrison J 1999 Promoting Partnership. Supporting disabled children who need invasive clinical procedures: A Barnardo's guide to good practice for family support services. Barnardo's, Ilford

Roberton N R C 1993 Should we look after babies less than 800g? Archives of Disease in Childhood 65:1076–1081

Servian R, Jones V, Lenehan C & Spires S for Shared Care Network 1998 Towards a healthy future. Multiagency working in the management of invasive and life-saving procedures for children in family-based services. Shared Care Network, Bristol

Shared Care Network 2003 Too Disabled for Care. Press release 13th September. Shared Care Network, Bristol

Social Policy Research Unit (SPRU) 2003 The community equipment needs of disabled children and their families. Research findings from SPRU, University of York

Steinaker N W & Bell M R 1979 The Experiential Taxonomy. A New Approach to Teaching and Learning. Academic Press, New York

Teague B R, Fleming J W, Castle A, Lobo M L, Riggs & Wolfe J G 1993 'High-tech' home care for children with chronic health conditions: a pilot study. Journal of Pediatric Nursing 8(4):226–232

Thomas B 1996 Continuing care needs for the elderly mentally ill. British Journal of Nursing 5(10):622–624

Townsley R & Robinson C 1999 What rights for disabled children? Home enteral tube feeding in the community. Children and Society 13:48–60

UK Central Council UKCC 1994 The future of professional practice – the Council's standards for education and practice following registration. UKCC, London

Warner L & Wexler S 1998 Eight Hours a Day and Taken for Granted? You just get on with it don't you? Princess Royal Trust for Carers, London

While A, Citrone C & Cornish J 1996 A study of the needs and provisions for families caring for children with life-limiting incurable disorders. King's College, London

Whiting M, Greene A & Walker A 2001 Community Children's Nursing – Delivering the Quality Agenda.

In: Sines D, Appelby F & Raymond E (eds) Community Health Care Nursing. 2nd edn. Blackwell Science, Oxford, pp 164–183

Youngblut L M, Brennan P F & Swegart L A 1994 Families with medically fragile children: a study. Pediatric Nursing 20:463–468

Legal case

R v. North and East Devon Health Authority ex parte Coughlan July 1999

Chapter 23

Meeting the palliative care needs of children in the community

Anna Sidey and Dorothy Bean

KEY ISSUES

- Defining palliative care.
- Who needs palliative care?
- Innovations and current developments in children's palliative care.
- Clinical responsibility for the child receiving palliative care.
- Other agencies in the delivery of children's palliative care.
- Respite care and support services.
- Emotional and bereavement support.
- Facing the death of a child and death at home.

INTRODUCTION

At the beginning of the twentieth century infant and child mortality were common in the UK. Davies (2000) suggests that infant mortality between 1900 and 1910 was 138 per 1000 births. Illness trajectories from diagnosis to death were often short with infections being the most frequently cited cause of death. However, a very different picture now presents principally due to developments in medical science and public health. The disappearance of infectious diseases such as scarlet fever and diphtheria has significantly reduced mortality and morbidity in childhood. In addition some childhood disorders that may have once been considered to be fatal, such as diabetes and cystic fibrosis, are treated as chronic conditions extending into adulthood and longer and fuller lives (Muir & Sidey 2003). However, there remain groups of children who continue to face death in childhood and the grinding uncertainties that this brings with it for them and their families (Gravelle 1997). They frequently face years of medical interventions, many of which are painful and frightening. Regular hospital visits, some requiring admission and supportive care will be maintained by a variety of domiciliary services complementing the care undertaken by the family and child. This commitment to care, and the duration of the interventions, has significant consequences upon the quality of life for the child and their family (Association for Children with Life threatening and Terminal Conditions and their Families & Royal College of Paediatrics and Child Health 2003). Palliative care seeks to positively contribute to quality of life and the trajectory of an illness for both the child and extended family. This chapter aims to provide an overview of the professional issues relating to the delivery of palliative care to children and their families.

DEFINING PALLIATIVE CARE

Misconceptions can occur when the term palliative care is used. It can conjure images of a child in the last days or hours of their life. However, the Association for Children with Life-threatening or Terminal Conditions and their Families (ACT) and the Royal College of Paediatrics and Child Health (RCPCH) (2003 p 6) provide the following definition:

> *'Palliative care for children and young people with life-limiting conditions is an active and total approach to care, embracing physical, emotional, social and spiritual elements. It focuses on enhancement of quality of life for the child and support for the family and includes the management of distressing symptoms, provision of respite and care through death and bereavement.'*

Similarly, Sutherland et al (1993) offer the following definition: 'care which is provided when curative treatment is not possible or not appropriate, and which personalises the care of the whole child and family, focusing on the relief of physical, emotional, social and spiritual distress and aiming for the best possible quality of life'.

The term 'palliative care' is used to describe a shared vision and approach to care that promotes the potential of each individual with a life-limiting condition until death.

Definitions of palliative care support a philosophy that promotes both physical and psychosocial wellbeing and involves (Addington-Hall & Higginson 2002, ACT & RCPCH 2003):

- a focus on quality of life including good symptom control
- a whole-person approach to care
- care for the person with the life-threatening illness and those who matter to them
- respect for patient autonomy and choice
- an emphasis on sensitive communication.

The terms life limiting and life threatening identify a distinction that centres upon the degree of potential for death in childhood. The term life limiting refers to conditions 'for which there is no reasonable hope of cure and from which children will die.' The term life threatening refers to illness where a cure, leading to full recovery, may be possible, albeit possibly with long-term consequences of treatment (ACT & RCPCH 2003 p 9). Although different, these two terms are often used synonymously.

WHO NEEDS PALLIATIVE CARE?

The number of children with life-limiting illness who may require palliative care is relatively small (Box 23.1). Conditions from which they suffer are often rare and the length of time a child requires palliative care may vary from days to years. ACT and RCPCH (2003), in the second edition of their Guide to the Development of Children's Palliative Care Services, estimated that in a Health District of 250 000 people, with a child population of 50 000, eight children are likely to die each year from a life-limiting condition (three from cancer, two from heart disease and three from non-malignant disease). In addition, approximately 50 children will actively require palliative care in any one year.

> **Box 23.1** Groups of children who may require palliative care (ACT & RCPCH 2003)
>
> 1. Where a cure may be possible but treatment may fail (e.g. cancer/organ failure)
> 2. Where there may be intensive treatment to prolong/improve quality of life but premature death is probable (e.g. cystic fibrosis/human immuno-deficiency virus infection)
> 3. Where the condition is progressive/degenerative and care is required for a number of years (e.g. Batten's disease)
> 4. Where severe neurological damage causes disability that will impact on health and may cause rapid deterioration (e.g. severe cerebral palsy)

INNOVATIONS AND DEVELOPMENTS IN THE PROVISION OF PALLIATIVE CARE FOR CHILDREN

Statistics demonstrating the numbers of children requiring palliative care are incomplete and, in parallel with many community children's nursing services, development of services may be considered to be ad hoc. Formalised palliative care is not available in some areas of the UK (ACT & RCPCH 2003). It is recognised that children with cancer or leukaemia have access to charitable funds and relatively well-established services provided by outreach care from tertiary and local hospitals. However, services to children with non-malignant disease are under-developed (Liben 1998). Community Children's Nurses (CCNs) are frequently involved in caring for children with life-limiting illnesses. A child may only be visited on one occasion or care and support for the child and family may span many years. The CCN is able to optimise and personalise the package of care received by each family (Health Committee 1997).

The lack of equitable provision and resourcing for palliative care has been a key driver to the introduction of Diana, Princess of Wales Community Children's Nursing Services and palliative care nursing posts supported by the New Opportunities Fund (NOF) (NOF 2002). The NOF posts seek to develop services that will:

- support the development of new or existing home-based palliative care services for children
- support the development of dedicated bereavement teams for families who have or will experience the death of a child resulting from a life-threatening illness

- sustain and support the development of existing good-quality provision of children's hospices.

Additional guidance from the National Service Framework (NSF) for Children is also expected to contribute positively to the development of future services (DoH 2003). Provision of transitional care and support are areas of emerging consideration and practice as more young people with life-limiting conditions live to adulthood (National Council for Hospice and Specialist Palliative Care Services 1995, ACT & RCPCH 2003) (see Chapter 32). The NSF will specify transitional arrangements for this group in health, social care, education and employment.

CLINICAL RESPONSIBILITY FOR THE CHILD RECEIVING PALLIATIVE CARE

The stage at which palliative care commences may be dependent on the type of disease, treatment options, and choices made by the family, the child and multiprofessional team. There may be a slow transition from curative treatment to palliative care or palliative care may start suddenly when it is realised that a cure is not possible (ACT & RCPCH 2003). The decision about which medical practitioner assumes clinical responsibility, and at which stage of the illness, can be complex and confusing. Parents may be unsure who is clinically responsible and professionals often do not make this explicit between themselves (While et al 1996, Read 1998).

During active, curative treatment, at a regional centre, professionals and families often assume that clinical responsibility is maintained by the paediatrician. General Practitioners (GPs) may see very few children with life-limiting conditions throughout their time in practice. This lack of experience may contribute to the family and members of the primary healthcare team losing contact with each other during acute illness and long periods of hospitalisation. However the GP may be the most appropriate physician to provide clinical responsibility during palliative or terminal care when care is transferred to the community (Goldman 1998). It is essential, therefore, that contact is maintained and positively encouraged throughout the trajectory of the illness. Appropriate primary healthcare involvement can reduce or prevent the need for a child to return to hospital. The GP and Health Visitor may be among the few professionals to have known the family before a child's illness. This can be comforting to the parents, it helps them relate to the care team as individuals in their own right as well as the parents of a sick child. A CCN may be able to facilitate the ongoing involvement of the GP by coordinating effective liaison between members of the care team at all stages of the child's illness.

AGENCIES INVOLVED IN THE DELIVERY OF PALLIATIVE CARE

In addition to CCNs other community agencies will be involved in the provision of palliative care for a child and family. These include a key worker, a named Social Worker, Diana Community Children's Nurses and hospice outreach nurses.

Key worker

ACT and RCPCH (2003) recommend that every family should have a named key worker who is responsible for the coordination of health and social care (Box 23.2). The family and the community children's nursing team may have developed a trusting relationship that began at the onset of the child's illness or, in some congenital conditions, at the child's birth. Because of this the role of key worker is most frequently designated to the CCN. However the identification of a key worker should be made in collaboration with the child and the family who need to identify the person with whom they feel able to trust and communicate (NHS Executive 1998, English National Board for Nursing, Midwifery and Health Visiting & Department of Health 1999). Children with life-limiting conditions frequently have complex medical, nursing and social needs and are the recipients of numerous services' and professionals' attention. The number of professionals and services involved can be overwhelming and leave families feeling isolated and unsupported (Stein & Woolley 1990). Many childhood conditions are extremely rare and this can increase a sense of isolation. Without the support and coordination of a key worker, input and care can be disorganised and inappropriate (Goldman 1998) (see Chapter 22 p 257).

Box 23.2 Responsibilities of the key worker (ACT & RCPCH 2003)

Key aspects of the role:

- Liaise between agencies
- Coordinate service provision
- Act as a single point of reference for communication
- Act as an advocate for the child and family
- A source of comprehensive information

To ensure that:

- Services do not overlap
- Gaps in service provision do not exist
- Communication between agencies is accurate and speedy
- Equipment is available
- The care plan is followed
- The package of care is appropriate and meets the needs of the child and family

To provide:

- Emotional support
- Access to a range of required resources

To act:

- As a link and an advocate ensuring that total care is available

---

Diana Princess of Wales Community Children's Nursing teams

The aim of Diana teams is to 'focus on enhancing the quality of life for the child and support for the family within the community by offering flexible and negotiated care which is responsive to their needs' (English National Board for Nursing, Midwifery and Health Visiting &

Department of Health 1999). This is achieved by providing community nursing and home-based respite care. The models of care by which teams may work differs. One model allocates palliative care patients to all nursing staff and thereby facilitates a balanced caseload comprising very sick and less sick children. Some teams work predominantly with terminally ill children. The strength of this model is that it allows for the development of specialist palliative care skills. The teams are multidisciplinary and comprise, for example, CCNs, psychologists, social workers (SWs), support workers and nursery nurses. Care may include packages of care for terminally ill children over 24 hours per day, 7 days a week (Diana Community Nursing Team 2003).

Named social workers

Families benefit from the support of a 'named SW' (ACT & RCPCH 2003). Named SWs, allocated specifically to a child and family, may be:

- generic SWs from local social services
- based within local authority Children's or Disability Social Work Teams
- part of a multidisciplinary team, i.e. a Diana team
- within a hospital social work department
- Sergeant Cancer Care social workers based within hospital social work teams/within children's oncology units.

Their support can include:

- liaison between social services/health
- multiprofessional assessments
- social work advice to team members
- individual work with children and families to offer support or to advocate for their needs
- facilitation of parents' groups
- bereavement support
- facilitating respite
- psychosocial care
- creating family support services
- emotional/social/financial impact of illness
- help for families to deal with practical problems
- childcare
- travel and accommodation
- advice about employment obligations/financial concerns and impact of illness/benefits/financial assistance to meet child's needs.

Anecdotal evidence suggests that a shortage of social workers, to work collaboratively with CCNs and families, may create additional and inappropriate demands on the role of the CCN (A Sidey, unpublished work, 2001). The nature of social work practice is dictated by the responsibilities of the employing organisation. Assessment is central to the social worker role and driven by the 'Framework for the Assessment of Children in Need and their Families' (DoH & Department of Education and Employment 2000).

The children's hospice outreach services

'Children's hospices support children and young people who are expected to die before or shortly after reaching adulthood ... through offering a range of services' (Association of Children's Hospices 2003). Children's hospices are predominantly voluntary-run organisations with very different histories behind their individual development. They aim to provide palliative, terminal and respite care in response to regional unmet need and consequently service provision differs between hospices. Increasingly they have developed home outreach services. Anecdotal evidence suggests that the roles of hospice outreach nurses (HONs) vary and that aspects of the development of the role may be similar to that of the ad hoc earlier development of the role of the CCN (A Sidey, unpublished work, 2001). These include a lack of both a corporate identity surrounding the development of the HON and a national philosophy underpinning the role (see Chapters 2 and 10). Furthermore, it may be unclear who securely provides professional leadership and supervision for the community practice of HONs. CCNs benefit from the opportunities provided by the recognition that community children's nursing is supported by a discrete and recordable specialist practitioner qualification. CCNs are frequently managed by children's nurses who have little or no experience of community practice or community nurses who are not children's nurses. The same would appear to be occurring with some of the developing roles of the HON who, in turn, may not have the benefit of a specialist community qualification.

RESPITE CARE AND SUPPORT SERVICES

The strain of caring for a sick child in the home is immense. Parents may suffer physical, psychological and emotional exhaustion and become isolated. Respite care aims to support parents and offer enjoyable play and social experiences to children. No one model of respite care exists for children within the UK (ACT & RCPCH 2003). Few families have access to adequate or suitable respite care facilities (Hall 1996, While et al 1996, NHS Executive 1998, ACT & RCPCH 2003) and provision varies greatly. It may be facilitated by a variety of service providers (Box 23.3).

Box 23.3 Examples of providers of respite care

- Health-service-funded nursing teams
- Diana Community Children's Nursing teams
- NOF teams
- Continuing care funding
- Charitably funded teams
- Hospices
- Hospice outreach services
- Social services homecare
- Social services residential care
- Learning disabilities residential and outreach care
- Short-term fostering (Family Link)
- Family and friends

The CCN is able to explore with the family which of the available respite providers may meet their needs. Introductions to a provider at an early stage of palliative care will avoid the possible need for unknown carers to be introduced to the child and family at a time of crisis. Respite care provision must be flexible to meet the changing needs of the child and family, and the parent should not be forced to relinquish the care of their child however tired or desperate they appear to be (Baum et al 1990, Farrell & Sutherland 1998, Miller 2002). Having suitable respite care enables families to cope through what may be many years of their child's illness and can allow them to decide where they would like to be at the time of their child's death (see Chapter 22 p 257).

EMOTIONAL SUPPORT

Grieving begins from the time a family is told their child will die (Goldman 1998); their lives are in turmoil and the whole family is disrupted. Many children still have their grandparents living and this may be the first loss that the parents have had to face. Most families are incredibly resilient and continue to function; however, the CCN needs to be able to recognise the factors that may indicate the family is finding it difficult to cope. Looking towards the death of their child is immeasurably painful (James & Johnson 1997). Few studies have assessed the impact of the child facing their own death (Blue Bond Langer 1978, Judd 1989).

Families require emotional support from the time of diagnosis. The CCN may not have been introduced to the family at this point but from their first meeting this type of support is an important part of the relationship between nurse and family. Research suggests that parental reactions to the diagnosis of a child's life-threatening or life-limiting illness may create psychological and social crises (Hendricks-Ferguson 2000, Ching Yiu & Twinn 2001). Families require a range of support strategies and networks from the time of diagnosis, at times of crisis and beyond (Olsen & Maslin Prothero 2001). Support networks include family, friends, and health and social care professionals. Coping strategies include social activities, active and purposeful problem solving and being central to decision making (Meijer et al 2002). Sick children, siblings and parents may benefit from the support of a psychologist, counsellor or from sharing experiences with other families who have experienced similar situations (Goldman 1998).

FACING THE DEATH OF A CHILD

Providing palliative care can be challenging and distressing for all professionals involved and it is recognised that staff require support (NHS Executive 1998, ACT & RCPCH 2003). Nurses are required to develop a range of different coping strategies and support systems (Davies et al 1996). Understanding the process of bereavement, which is an integral part of palliative care (ACT & RCPCH 2003), can assist in the overall care and support nurses provide. Over the last century theories, concepts and models of bereavement have been developed (Stroebe 1992, Klass et al 1996). Clinical supervision when working with bereaved families helps nurses to balance and maintain professional boundaries (Bishop 1998).

After the death parents recount how helpful it was to have planned what they would do when their child died. The CCN can help parents explore a range of options. For example it can be a relief to families to know they can keep their dead child at home for as long as practically possible (Liben 1998). The CCN will often continue to visit the family for many months after the child's death. Every family's grief is unique and bereavement support will be led by the needs and wishes of the family. They can be offered choices concerning support in their bereavement and whom they wish to be involved in the support (Goldman 1998).

The issues surrounding a 'do not resuscitate' decision are complex and become even more so in the home environment. The topic is widely discussed within the context of acute care but the following issues need to be considered within home care:

- Who decides and reviews the decision?
- Have the wishes of the dying child been sought?
- Where is the decision most appropriately documented?
- Who assumes responsibility for the decision?
- Format and location of information about the decision
- Which service providers are covered by the decision, e.g. GP, CCN, school staff, paramedics, parents, siblings, hospice staff, ward staff?
- Are there criteria for e.g. treatment, ventilation, resuscitation, use of antibiotics?

If disagreements should occur between the assessed rights of a child and the wishes of the child's parents or the healthcare team (that may be judged not to be in the child's best interest) legal opinion should be sought sooner rather than later, e.g. conflicts over requesting or accepting treatment that may be considered futile or experimental (British Medical Association, The Resuscitation Council & Royal College of Nursing 2001). Further advice may be found on www.resus.org.uk April 2004.

CONCLUSION

Demand for palliative care is unpredictable and therefore service provision needs to be flexible (NHS Executive 1998). The ACT & RCPCH (2003) reinforced earlier recommendations for the provision of palliative care. One of the main recommendations was that 'community children's nursing teams are essential for the management of children with palliative care needs' and that commissioners should facilitate their establishment or development to provide for the needs of this group of children and their families. In addition the report recognises that children and their families who need palliative care require access to 24-hour nursing support. The Diana Community Children's Nursing teams meet the needs of this distinct group (English National Board for Nursing, Midwifery and Health Visiting & Department of Health 1999). This chapter has explored some of the key issues in children's palliative care and the associated role of the CCN. The recommendations of the ACT & RCPCH report (2003) provide comprehensive guidance to enable the CCN to ensure that families receive appropriate care and support.

REFERENCES

Addington-Hall J M & Higginson I J 2002 Palliative Care for Non-Cancer Patients. Oxford University Press, Oxford

Association for Children with Life-threatening or Terminal Conditions and their Families (ACT) & Royal College of Paediatrics and Child Health (RCPCH) 2003 A Guide to the Development of Children's Palliative Care Services. ACT, Bristol

Association of Children's Hospices (ACH) 2003. Online. Available: www.childhospice.org.uk 27 April 2004

Baum J D, Dominica F & Woodward R (eds) 1990 Listen. My Child Has a Lot of Living to Do. Oxford University Press, Oxford

Bishop V 1998 Clinical Supervision in Practice. Macmillan, Hampshire

Blue Bond Langer 1978 The Private Worlds of a Dying Child. Princeton University Press, Surrey

British Medical Association (BMA), The Resuscitation Council & Royal College of Nursing (RCN) 2001 Decisions Relating to Cardiopulmonary Resuscitation. A Joint Statement. BMA, London

Ching Yiu M & Twinn 2001 Determining the needs of Chinese parents during the hospitalisation of their child diagnosed with cancer: an exploratory study. Cancer Nursing 24(6):483–489

Davies B, Clarke D, Connaughty S, Cook K, Mackensie B, McCormick J, O'Loane M & Stutzer C 1996 Caring for dying children: Nurses' experiences. Pediatric Nursing 22(6):500–507

Davies R 2000 Acheivements in child health over the first half of the 20th century. British Journal of Nursing 9(1):28–32

Department of Health and Department for Education and Employment 2000 Framework for the Assessment of Children in Need and their Families. The Stationery Office, London

Department of Health 2003 Getting the right start: National Service Framework for Children. The Stationery Office, London

Diana Community Nursing Team 2003 Online. Available: www.warwickshire.gov.uk/web/corporate 14 September 2004

English National Board for Nursing, Midwifery and Health Visiting (ENB) & Department of Health 1999 Sharing the Care. Resource pack to support Diana, Princess of Wales community children's nursing teams. ENB, London

Farrell M & Sutherland P 1998 Providing paediatric palliative care: collaboration in practice. British Journal of Nursing 7(12):712–716

Goldman A 1998 Palliative care for children. In: Fauld C, Carter Y & Woof R (eds) Handbook of Palliative Care. Blackwell Science, London

Gravelle A M 1997 Caring for a child with a progressive illness during the chronic phase: parents' experience of facing adversity. Journal of Advanced Nursing 25:738–745

Hall S 1996 An exploration of parental perception of the nature and level of support needed to care for their child with special needs. Journal of Advanced Nursing 24:512–521

Health Committee 1997 House of Commons Select Committee. Health services for children and young people in the community: home and school. Third report. The Stationery Office, London

Hendricks-Ferguson 2000 Crisis intervention strategies when caring for families of children with cancer. Journal of Pediatric Oncology Nursing 17(1):3–11

James L & Johnson B 1997 The needs of parents of pediatric oncology patients during the palliative care phase. Journal of Pediatric Oncology Nursing 14(2):83–95

Judd D 1989 Give Sorrow Words: Working with a Dying Child. Free Association Books, London

Klass D, Silvermann P R & Nickman F 1996 Continuing Bonds: New Understandings of Grief. Taylor and Francis, Washington

Liben S 1998 Home care for children with life threatening illness. Journal of Palliative Care 14(3):33–38

Meijer S A, Gerben S, Bijistra J O, Mellenburgh G J & Wolters W H G 2002 Coping styles and locus of control as predictors for psychological adjustment of adolescents with a chronic illness. Social Science and Medicine 54:1453–1461

Miller S 2002 Respite care for children who have complex special healthcare needs. Paediatric Nursing 14(5):33–37

Muir J & Sidey A 2003 Community Children's Nursing. In: Watkins D, Edwards J & Gastrell P (eds) Community Health Nursing. Baillière Tindall, Edinburgh, pp 271–280

National Council for Hospice and Specialist Palliative Care Services (NCHSPCS) 1995 Specialist Palliative Care Services Occasional Paper 8. NCHSPCS, London

NHS Executive 1998 Evaluation of the pilot project programme for children with life threatening illness. The Stationery Office, London

New Opportunities Fund 2002 Palliative Care for Children Programme: Guidance Notes. Online. Available: www.nof.org.uk 22 April 2004

Olsen R & Maslin-Prothero P 2001 Dilemmas in the provision of own-home care respite support for parents of young children with complex medical health care needs: evidence from an evaluation. Journal of Advanced Nursing 34(5):603–610

Read S 1998 The palliative care of people with learning disabilities. International Journal of Palliative Nursing 4(5):246–251

Stein A & Woolley H 1990 An evaluation of hospice care for children. In: Baum J D, Dominica F & Woodward R (eds) Listen. My Child Has a Lot of Living to Do. Oxford University Press, Oxford, p 67

Stroebe M 1992 Coping with bereavement: a review of the grief work hypothesis. Omega 26(1):19–42

Sutherland R, Hearn J, Baum J D & Elston S 1993 Definitions in paediatric palliative care. Health Trends 25(4):148–150

While A, Citrone C & Cornish J 1996 A Study of the Needs and Provision for Families Caring for Children with Life-limiting Incurable Disorders. King's College, London

Chapter 24

Meeting the mental health needs of children and young people

Kath Williamson

KEY ISSUES

- The provision of child and adolescent mental health services.
- The role of a specialist nurse in meeting mental health needs in practice.
- The use of a family systems approach.

INTRODUCTION

The mental health of children and young people is everyone's business (Mental Health Foundation 1999). An assessment of the emotional well-being of children should be a part of every health and social care intervention. All people, agencies and services are involved in this process. Their ability to contribute effectively depends on the level of training and support they receive, for example from specialist child and adolescent mental health services (CAMHS) (DoH 2003a). This chapter examines the contribution a 'specialist nurse in children's mental health' (SNCMH) can make in meeting the needs of children and young people receiving care in acute and community settings (NHS Health Advisory Service 1995). It considers how this role can facilitate communication between:

- hospital children's services
- community children's nursing services
- child and adolescent mental health services
- social services
- education services
- voluntary agencies.

The SNCMH may be a member of a community children's nursing team or a CAMHS.

INCIDENCE OF MENTAL HEALTH PROBLEMS AND DISORDERS

Kurtz (1992 p 6) defines mental health problems in children and young people as:

'abnormalities of emotions, behaviour or social relationships sufficiently marked or prolonged to cause

- *suffering or risk to optimal development in the child*
- *distress or disturbance in the family or community.'*

It is calculated that at any one time 20% of children and adolescents experience psychological problems (Mental Health Foundation 1999) whilst the prevalence of problems which meet the criteria for diagnosable mental disorder amongst children and young people aged between 5 and 15 years is estimated at 10% (Office for National Statistics 2000). There is an increased rate of mental health and adjustment problems in children with chronic health problems. Children with a chronic medical condition and associated disability that limits usual childhood activities are at a more than threefold risk of developing mental health disorders compared with their healthy peers (Wallace et al 1997). Approximately one in six children with a life-threatening condition are reported to experience a mental disorder (Office for National Statistics 2000). Furthermore, Taylor and Eminson (1994) assert that research measures commonly employed to identify increased rates of disorder in children often fail to reveal generally increased levels of distress and dysfunction within these families.

A national review of services for the mental health of children and young people in England (Kurtz et al 1994) estimated that 5–15% of children were referred to children's departments primarily because of emotional and behavioural problems. Some 70% of children's departments said they needed more support and training for staff in responding to these types of problems (Kurtz et al 1994).

PROVISION OF CHILD AND ADOLESCENT MENTAL HEALTH SERVICES

The National Service Framework for Children will address the mental health and psychological wellbeing of children and young people with a commitment to the access of high-quality services delivered in appropriate settings (DoH 2003a). Whilst there are current discrepancies in provision across the country (DoH 2003b) there is a target in England to provide a comprehensive service, including mental health promotion and early intervention, by 2006 (DoH 2003a).

Community children's nurses (CCNs) assess and highlight the needs of children and young people in their care and develop collaborative arrangements for professional support and the joint care of children with SNCMH and CAMHS. The provision of CAMHS is encapsulated in a four-tier model of service (NHS Health Advisory Service 1995) (Box 24.1).

The SNCMHs have an important role to play in strengthening the interface between child health services and professionals at Tiers 1, 2 and 3. They can facilitate partnership and joint working to meet the mental health needs of children being treated in both acute and community children's services.

Box 24.1 Four-tier model for provision of child and adolescent mental health services

Tier 1 (serving population of about 250 000)

Primary or direct contact services, including interventions by:

- General Practitioners
- Voluntary workers
- School nurses
- Health visitors
- Teachers
- Social workers

who are in a position to:

- Identify mental health problems early in their development
- offer general advice and in certain cases treatment for less severe mental health problems
- pursue opportunities for the promotion of mental health and the prevention of mental health problems

Tier 2 (serving a population of about 250 000)

Interventions offered by individual specialist CAMHS professionals including:

- Clinical child psychologists
- Educational psychologists
- Psychotherapists
- Child psychiatrists
- Community child psychiatric nurses
- Occupational therapists

offering:

- training/consultation to other professionals (who may be within Tier 1)
- consultation for professionals and families
- assessment that may trigger treatment at a different tier

Tier 3 (serving a population of about 250 000)

Intervention offered by teams of staff from specialist CAMHS including:

- Specialist assessment teams
- Individual and art psychotherapy
- Substance misuse teams
- Family therapy teams
- Day unit services

A specialist service for the more severe, complex and persistent disorders, usually a multidisciplinary team or service working in a community child mental health clinic or child psychiatry outpatient service, offering:

- assessment and treatment of child mental health disorders
- assessment for referrals to Tier 4
- contributions to the services, consultation and training at Tiers 1 and 2
- participation in research and development projects

box continues

> **Tier 4 (serving a population of about 750 000)**
> Very specialised intervention and care, using highly specialised teams, including:
>
> - patient services for young people with very complex and/or refractory problems
> - inpatient child and adolescent mental health services
> - special units for sensorily impaired young people
> - specialised neuropsychiatric services
>
> This tier comprises infrequently used but essential tertiary level services such as day units, highly specialised outpatient teams and inpatient units for older children and adolescents who are severely mentally ill or at suicidal risk. These services serve a population of about 750 000 and may need to be provided on a supra-district level.

Traditionally, psychiatric liaison and consultation services in children's services have been provided by child psychiatrists and psychologists (Lask 1994). Reference to children in the literature on liaison mental health nursing is limited and often describes the provision of services by mental health nurses to children's units (Tunmore 1997a). However, children's nurses have developed expertise in this area and the roles of specialist nurses have been developed to meet local need.

ROLE OF THE SPECIALIST NURSE IN CHILDREN'S MENTAL HEALTH

As community children's nursing services developed it became apparent that some children with chronic medical conditions were spending time in hospital as a result of family problems or emotional and behavioural difficulties. It was considered that a children's nurse, educated in child and adolescent psychiatric nursing (the SNCMH), and working with a child psychiatrist, could address some of these issues. Within the context of the four-tier model the role of the SNCMH is located within Tier 2. The role can achieve the objectives of a Tier 2 service. The objectives of Tier 2 services are shown in Box 24.2.

> **Box 24.2** Objectives of the Tier 2 services (NHS Health Advisory Service 1995 para 449 p 141)
>
> - To enable families to function in a less distressed manner
> - To enable children/families to overcome their mental health problems
> - To diagnose/treat disorders of mental health
> - To increase the skill level of all those working with children/young people/families
> - To enable children/young people/their families to benefit from their home/community/education
> - To enable children/young people/their families to cope more effectively with their life experience

The role of the SNCMH can achieve the objectives of a Tier 2 service (Box 24.3).

Box 24.3 Role of the specialist nurse in children's mental health

1. Provides consultation and support to professionals in Tier 1
2. Accepts referrals to assess/undertake direct work with children/young people and families as part of a holistic approach
3. Maintains strong links with the child and adolescent mental health services, achieved through: (a) consultation/clinical supervision with a child and adolescent mental health team (b) joint working
4. Liaises with other services involved in family's care
5. Involved in development work/research/training

Fundamental to the role of the SNCMH is a systemic approach that goes beyond seeing the child in the context of the family to viewing the family as the unit of care. This model of family nursing (Wright & Leahey 1994, Whyte 1997), acknowledges the potential for the nurse to intervene at a systems level or at individual and interpersonal levels. Consideration of the environment, ethnicity, culture, and wider social systems within which the family is operating is an integral part of this approach. The availability of the SNCMH within the children's service facilitates the identification of concerns about children and adolescents at an early stage. This is important for intervention to make a difference (Eiser 1993). In addition, if following an assessment it is agreed that the problems can be better addressed at another tier, the SNCMH acts as a bridge between services. Initial contact with and assessment by the nurse can overcome the reluctance of some families to seek help from the CAMHS and enable them to go on to receive appropriate intervention.

CONSULTATION

The term consultation is used to describe a form of collaborative work where one person helps another with a particular problem 'without taking on responsibility for the solution' (Tunmore 1997a p 207). The SNCMH provides consultation for other professionals within the children's service. For example:

- A colleague in the community team might discuss their concerns about a young person with a chronic illness who is not adhering to treatment.
- Members of the ward team may seek support in managing the difficult behaviour of a child or young person on the ward.

Professionals who already know the family are often the most appropriate people to undertake the work with them. They can be enabled to do this by having the opportunity to reflect on the problem and explore different possible interventions. The SNCMH is accessible to colleagues and can offer continuing support by being based in the children's service and attending ward and team meetings.

LINKS WITH THE CHILD AND ADOLESCENT MENTAL HEALTH SERVICE

Formal channels for liaison with the CAMHS are essential to the framework of the role of the SNCMH. They include individual consultation, group supervision and a monthly joint consultation meeting with professionals from the children's team and child and adolescent mental health service. Joint work is undertaken with workers from this service when their expertise is required, or when they believe they can benefit from the specialist experience of working with children with physical illness.

WORK WITH CHILDREN, YOUNG PEOPLE AND FAMILIES

Referrals to the SNCMH are accepted from all members of the multi-professional team. However, it is important that the referral is discussed and agreed within the team to ensure that the referral is appropriate. This prevents duplication of the work that could have adverse effects on the family. The specialist nurse is not involved in the assessment of children and young people who deliberately self-harm as this service is provided by the CAMHS. Reasons for referral of children and young people are shown in Box 24.4.

Box 24.4 Examples of reasons for referral to the specialist nurse in children's mental health

Emotional and behavioural problems in addition to a physical problem, for example:

- Pre-school child who has asthma and a sleep problem
- School-age child who has recently been diagnosed as having Type 1 diabetes and become anxious about attending school
- Young person with a chronic illness who has become withdrawn following a deterioration in their condition

Emotional and behavioural problems as the primary reason for referral to the children's service, for example:

- Child with behavioural difficulties that might be diet-related psychosomatic problems
- Recurrent abdominal pain when an organic cause has been excluded

Difficulties associated with adapting to and coping with chronic and life-threatening illness/treatments/procedures

- Bereavement work with carers and siblings

ASSESSMENT, INTERVENTION AND EVALUATION

A systematic approach to assessment is used which includes gathering information about the family and extended structure, history and beliefs. These are considered within the context of the family's culture. Drawing a genogram can be useful as part of this process (Wright & Leahey 2000). Information about the child's development, education, medical history, current treatment and interaction with systems providing health, education and social care is gathered. How the child and family perceive the problem and what issues they feel they need help with may differ from the opinions of the referrer. The assessment process can be therapeutic in itself, enabling families to explore their perception of the difficulties and reflect on their experience. This can enable them to identify their own problems and mobilise their own coping resources (Whyte 1997). Alongside stories of sickness and suffering, stories of strength and tenacity can emerge (Wright & Leahey 2000). A care plan is then formulated with the family.

The role of the SNCMH requires the ability to offer a variety of approaches according to the needs of the child and family (Sharman 1997). Interventions may involve working with the family together, or individually with a child or parent. A plan for a child who has difficulties with constipation and soiling may include a combination of behavioural and family work. In this work, self-awareness and the ability to reflect upon and recognise the limitations of one's practice is essential. In some cases it is more appropriate to refer to another service, for example CAMHS, child psychology or social services. This may lead to the nurse working jointly with another professional.

Evaluation is undertaken with the family and considers the impact of actions undertaken or changes within the family. It can provide an opportunity to emphasise further the family's strengths and highlight small changes that have taken place over a period of time. Key issues where further work is needed can be clarified or it may be decided that it is appropriate for the intervention to end (Whyte 1997).

It is important that professionals undertaking psychological work with children who have physical illness have some knowledge and understanding of that illness, its current treatment and the impact it can have on children, siblings, parents and other carers. This understanding is particularly helpful when initially engaging the family in the therapeutic process and when exploring the family and child's perception and understanding of the illness. Equally important is the ability to listen to children and find ways to communicate effectively with them. This requires creativity, imagination (Sharman 1997) and a range of techniques the worker must be able to adapt according to the needs of the child or young person. Some of these skills are demonstrated in Case study 24.1.

EDUCATION FOR CHILDREN'S NURSES IN CHILD AND ADOLESCENT MENTAL HEALTH

Education for nurses in child and adolescent mental health is not comprehensive. Hooton (1999) found that those involved in mental health and children's nurse education each believed the other was responsible for teaching in this area. In practice nurses often lack the training and confidence to manage mental health problems amongst children and young people. Access to education and ongoing support from specialist staff is essential if a comprehensive CAMHS is to be realised (DoH 2003a). The knowledge, skills and experience of children's nurses provide a firm foundation for further training in working with children and young people with mental health problems. Whyte et al (1997 p 80), argue that 'a fuller understanding of family transitions and interaction, and the development of therapeutic skills in working with families, is a logical expansion of the role of paediatric nurses'. This would provide CCNs with an opportunity to expand their holistic approach to family-centred care.

Case study 24.1

Eight-year-old David has cystic fibrosis (CF) diagnosed aged 6 weeks. He lives with his parents and brother, aged 10. David's treatment includes physiotherapy/nebulisers/vitamins/enzymes/dietary supplements/frequent courses of antibiotics. He was referred during an admission to hospital for his first course of intravenous (IV) antibiotics and overnight nasogastric feeding.

Practitioners working within the CF team were concerned at David's reluctance to communicate. He was described as not cooperating fully with treatment and as clinically depressed. Initially, the SNCMH discussed with the team how far David's behaviour was a reaction to the deterioration in his condition and his admission to hospital and what intervention, if any, was appropriate to help him adjust to his changed circumstances. As a result it was decided that he did not meet the diagnostic criteria for clinical depression.

The SNCMH undertook an initial assessment with David and his mother in hospital. Throughout this assessment David was willing to play table football but reluctant to talk about his illness. He simply expressed a strong desire to go home. His mother thought that David saw himself as 'no different to anyone else' and he considered his admission to hospital to be an imposition that prevented him getting on with his life.

Anger and resentment about his illness were perhaps part of the origin of David's difficult behaviour in hospital. His parents were not as anxious about his mental health as the hospital staff. They did not feel they experienced the same difficulties with treatment at home and reported that he was doing well at school and socialised with his peers. They addressed questions about CF as David raised them, but they had not talked about it recently. They agreed that it might be appropriate to address the issues raised by the deterioration in David's condition and the need for more treatment. The SNCMH arranged to visit at home to continue to build a relationship with David and engage him in thinking about his condition.

The SNCMH liaised closely with the CCN and physiotherapist and visited the family at home. When still unable to engage David in talking about anything other than football, football was used as a metaphor for talking about CF and as a way of externalising aspects of his illness (White 1990). It was suggested that David drew his own football team of all the players who were helping him to beat CF and he immediately responded to this. He chose his team and supporters and drew intricate cartoon figures of the people he saw as being on his side. This included friends, family, teachers and health professionals. There was shared humour here as David portrayed the individual characteristics of the people he selected. It was decided to stick the drawings to a football pitch poster and this formed a literary/pictorial record of the work (White & Epston 1990). David called the team CF Football Club (CFFC). As the pictures were stuck to the pitch, David was able to talk about how these individuals were helping him and the different tactics he and the team could use. This provided information about how David perceived his condition and understood his treatment. It revealed gaps in his knowledge/ understanding which were discussed with him and with his permission, passed on to other members of the CF team to enable them to provide him with more information. At the end of the session David shared the work with his mother.

In the next session David thought about the opposing team which he chose to call 'Illness Football Club' (IFC). He chose a black marker and wrote directly on the pitch personifying some of the aspects of his illness including coughs/feeling tired/aches/sputum/ enzyme deficiency as football players. The influence of his Christian beliefs could be seen in the inclusion of the devil on this team. He was able to express some of his anger and said he felt this team was winning. This was acknowledged and he was encouraged to think about some of the reasons why he might feel like that at that time.

With the SNCMH he then went on to think about some of the tactics and strategies that were successful and how CFFC might use these to get back in the lead. These included ways in which aspects of his treatment might help him to score against the other team. It was important to do this without giving David a message that his negative feelings were unacceptable or had been dismissed.

A few weeks later David required admission to hospital for a further course of IV antibiotics. This was a short admission as the treatment was to be completed at home. He took his football poster with him and put it up on the wall of his cubicle. He shared aspects of it with some of the ward team and recruited a network of supporters (White & Epston 1990). The hospital staff reported that David appeared more relaxed, communicative and inclined to participate in his treatment. David had a new strategy and his CFFC team was winning. When asked how they were winning he gave a broad grin and said he had his Dad on his side and they were 'going to rip the legs off' the opposing team. It appeared that he had been able to channel some of his anger in a more positive way.

CONCLUSION

It has been suggested that nurses practising at the traditional boundaries of different clinical services, or on clinical problems at the interface of mind and body, have the potential to identify new and evolving specialisms and shape the future delivery of nursing care (Tunmore 1997b). Specialist nurses in child and adolescent mental health have a valuable role within children's services working with children, young people and families, and offering consultation and support to colleagues in the multiprofessional, multi-agency team. They can assess and treat mental health difficulties at an early stage, prevent the development or consolidation of mental health problems and facilitate appropriate referrals to other agencies.

REFERENCES

Department of Health 2003a Getting the right start. National Service Framework – Emerging Findings. The Stationery Office, London

Department of Health 2003b National Child and Adolescent Mental Health Service Mapping Exercise. The Stationery Office, London

Eiser C 1993 Growing up with a chronic disease: the impact on children and families. Jessica Kingsley, London

Hooton S 1999 Results of a survey undertaken to establish the degree to which pre-registration programmes address child and adolescent mental health. English National Board for Nursing Midwifery and Health Visiting, London

Kurtz Z 1992 With health in mind. Action for Sick Children. In association with South West Thames Regional Health Authority, London

Kurtz Z, Thornes R & Wolkind S for South West Thames Regional Health Authority 1994 Services for the mental health of children and young people in England: a national review. Report to the Department of Health. HMSO, London

Lask B 1994 Paediatric liaison work. In: Rutter M, Taylor E & Hersov L (eds) Child and adolescent psychiatry: modern approaches, 3rd edn. Blackwell, Oxford, Ch. 58, p 996

Mental Health Foundation 1999 Bright Futures: Promoting Children and Young People's Mental Health. Mental Health Foundation, London

NHS Health Advisory Service 1995 Together we stand: the commissioning role and management of child and adolescent mental health services. HMSO, London

Office for National Statistics 2000 The mental health of children and adolescents in Great Britain: the report of a survey carried out in 1999 by Social Survey Division of the Office for National Statistics on behalf of the Department of Health, the Scottish Health Executive and the National Assembly for Wales. The Stationery Office, London

Sharman W 1997 Children and Adolescents with Mental Health Problems. Baillière Tindall, London

Taylor D C & Eminson D M 1994 Psychological aspects of chronic physical sickness. In: Rutter M, Taylor E & Hersov L (eds) Child and Adolescent Psychiatry: Modern Approaches, 3rd edn. Blackwell, Oxford, Ch. 42, p 737

Tunmore R 1997a Liaison mental health nursing and mental health consultation. In: Thomas B, Hardy S & Cutting P (eds) Mental Health Nursing: Principles and Practice. Mosby, London, Ch.15, p 207

Tunmore R 1997b Mental health liaison and consultation. Nursing Standard 11(50):46–53

Wallace S A, Crown L M, Cox A D & Burger M 1997 Child and Adolescent Mental Health: Health Care Needs Assessed. Radcliffe Medical Press, Oxford

White M 1990 Stories: knowledge and power. In: White M & Epston D 1990 Narrative Means to Therapeutic Ends. Dulwich Centre, Adelaide

White M & Epston D 1990 Narrative Means to Therapeutic Ends. Dulwich Centre, Adelaide

Whyte D A 1997 Explorations in Family Nursing. Routledge, London

Whyte D A, Baggaley S E & Rutter C 1997 Chronic illness in childhood. In: Whyte D A (ed.) Explorations in Family Nursing. Routledge, London, Ch. 4, p 54

Wright L M & Leahey M 1994 Nurses and Families: A Guide to Family Assessment and Intervention, 2nd edn. F A Davis, Philadelphia

Wright L M & Leahey M 2000 Nurses and Families: A Guide to Family Assessment and Intervention, 3rd edn. F A Davis, Philadelphia

Chapter 25

Meeting the needs of children with learning disabilities

Melanie Coombes and Jo Holder

KEY ISSUES

- Historical context.
- What is a learning disability?
- Children with profound learning disabilities and associated healthcare needs in the community.
- The needs of the child and family and the associated stressors.
- Integration of services to meet the needs of children and their families.
- Who is the appropriate nurse?
- The transition from child to adult services.

INTRODUCTION

This chapter focuses on the issues surrounding the care of children with profound learning disabilities and their families and their associated healthcare needs in the community. After briefly setting the historical context, sources of stress for the prime caregivers will be considered. The chapter concludes by considering the transition process from child to adult services.

HISTORICAL CONTEXT

The disciplines concerned with nursing children have experienced dramatic changes during the past 50 years. A profound revolution has occurred in the field of learning disability nursing. In the 1960s social conscience and an analysis of human values preceded and informed the theory and implementation of normalisation (Hughson & Brown 1992). Implementing the concepts of normalisation in practice led to the de-institutionalisation movement and eventually to community care (Department of Health and Social Security 1976, 1981, Brown 1992). Political reform also initiated the term 'learning disability' as less socially stigmatising than 'mental handicap' (Ayer & Alaszewski 1984). These changes in ethos have led to increased numbers of children with learning difficulties being cared for by parents at home (Elfer & Gatiss 1990, Orr et al 1991).

Recent advances in medical knowledge together with technological interventions appear to have preceded detailed legal or ethical guidance as to the 'reasonable effort' involved in preserving life (Youngblut et al 1994). Consequently, more children are surviving birth with increasingly complex needs and medical dependence (Teague et al 1993, Fradd 1994). This has coincided with the emphasis on home care (While 1991, Heaman 1995). The white paper 'Valuing People – a New Strategy for Learning Disability for the 21st Century' (DoH 2001) took this one stage further and looked at quality care within the community and positive strategies for giving young people with learning disabilities rights as valued individuals in society. The document supports the roles of community nurses in improving the services provided to children with learning disabilities.

WHAT IS A LEARNING DISABILITY?

The most recent definition from the Department of Health (DoH) (used to plan and deliver services) states that a learning disability includes the presence of:

- a significantly reduced ability to understand new or complex information or to learn new skills (impaired intelligence)
- a reduced ability to cope independently (impaired social functioning) which started before adulthood with a lasting effect on development.

Low intelligence quota (below 70) alone is not an indicator of learning disabilities; in addition, social functioning and communication skills are key areas for assessment. On this same basis not all those broadly termed as having 'learning difficulty' in education legislation will have learning disabilities from a health perspective. It is estimated that there are approximately 210 000 people with severe and profound learning disabilities of which 65 000 are children and young adults (DoH 2001). Evidence suggests that this number may increase by 1% per annum for the next 15 years as a result of a number of factors (DoH 1999). These include:

- increased life expectancy
- increases in technological advances, resulting in children with complex and multiple disabilities surviving longer
- increased awareness of disabilities that are now being diagnosed (Gordon et al 2000).

THE NEEDS OF THE CHILD AND FAMILY

When planning care for a child with a learning disability it can be too easy to become enveloped by the family's needs and forget that this child is a child first and has a learning disability second. The child may not be able to communicate their wishes and their need for independence, and families can engulf them with well-intentioned protectiveness (DoH 1998). 'Disabled children and young people' in Valuing People (DoH 2001) includes messages voiced by consulted disabled children. They mirror previous work in this area (Russell 1998):

- treat us more like our brothers and sisters
- we want to do things other children do, not always 'something special'
- give us a chance to be independent, get a job and have a home.

A family that has a child with learning disabilities as a member will be subjected to increased stressors when compared to an 'average' family (Beresford 1994, Keeley et al 1995). A family and each family member will develop different coping strategies to overcome these stressors. These stressors include:

- diagnosis
- developmental milestones
- daily burden of care
- future concerns, particularly transition from child to adult services.

The nurse can aid the child and family through these difficult times.

Diagnosis

There will always be a proportion of children without a clearly defined diagnosis and for these families the 'unknown' can itself be more distressing than the 'known' (Waisbren 1980, Maxwell 1993). Families require, where possible and within a context of honesty, clear information about their child's disability that initially focuses on the positives and what their child may achieve as opposed to the negatives and what their child may not achieve. Where a genetic link can be made the family will require genetic counselling. The process itself can be distressing as apportioning blame can create a negative feeling towards both the child as well as the carrier of an abnormality. There is an increased chance that the family may reject the child and initial support can help the whole family to overcome their feelings and fears (Richards & Reed 1991).

Developmental milestones

The first sign of a previously undiagnosed learning disability may be the child's failure to meet developmental milestones and these significantly broaden as the child becomes older (Cullen et al 1991, Keeley et al 1995). It is helpful for the nurse to break a child's development down into small, achievable and retainable targets and celebrate each achievement as a step forward no matter how small it may seem.

Daily burden of care

Fatigue is commonly reported among family members when they are looking after a child with learning disabilities (Taanila et al 1996). Simple daily tasks take on an increased complexity, require more energy and take longer for families undertaking the same daily regimes for a young adult as they would expect to with a child, i.e. feeding, washing, dressing, etc. The Government have recognised this burden of daily care and earmarked £60 million to increase home-based help for families. The introduction of direct payments allows more flexibility for parents and young adults aged 16/17 to say how services are delivered to them (DoH 2001). However, parents have reported how intrusive it can be when they have carers working in their homes and providers of services need to ensure that families do not feel deskilled and devalued (Ward 2001).

Future concerns

The availability of funding and resources are frequently major factors when planning for the future. Coupled with the families' fear of letting go, this can be one of the most stressful times for any parent, in particular a parent of a disabled child whose physical condition may not be stable (Morris 1999). Many parents describe this period as the 'great unknown' and 'falling off a cliff into a great chasm'. They feel they have not been adequately prepared for transition and the change can come as a profound shock (Ward 2001). A child with a learning disability will not 'get better' in terms of their learning disability but can strive to become more independent.

The Community Children's Nurse (CCN) may play a key role in the future planning or transition stage of an older child with learning disabilities (see Chapter 32).

WHO IS THE APPROPRIATE NURSE?

'Valuing People' (DoH 2001) sets out the Government's objective as:

'To promote holistic services for people with learning disabilities through effective partnership working between all relevant local agencies in the commissioning and delivery of services' and 'people with learning disabilities have the same right of access to mainstream health services as the rest of the population.'

Not all children with learning disabilities will have healthcare problems directly attributable to their learning disability.

Children and their families have the right to receive healthcare from appropriately skilled and available professionals and have their care coordinated by a key worker. 'Lack of key workers leads to poorly co-ordinated inter-agency support' (Ward 2001). The need for a key worker to coordinate services is the top of the wish list for parents with a disabled child (DoH 1998, 2001, Ward 2001). Following initial assessment a child's healthcare needs should be prioritised in terms of the most prevalent need for the family and child. These should then be matched to the individual specialist skills of the multidisciplinary team. This individual could then become the key worker for the child and family (see Chapter 23 p 265).

Case study 25.1

Emma has learning disabilities and associated complex medical needs that render her technology dependent. The family receives care and support from a Learning Disability Nurse (LDN) and CCN. The predominant amount of care has been provided by the LDN as for many years the needs associated with Emma's learning disabilities have outweighed those requiring nursing care. The CCN has been available for advice and support and the teaching, assessment and evaluation of the additional nursing care provided by the LDN and family as required or requested. Emma's condition is deteriorating and, in addition, she requires palliative care. A decision needs to be taken as to which nurse assumes responsibility for (i) her care at this stage of her life and (ii) the role of the key worker (KW) as recommended by ACT & RCPCH (2003). The LDN has undertaken the role of KW throughout Emma's care. The identification of a KW was made some years ago (shortly following initial referral to the LDN) in collaboration with the child and family, who identified the person they felt able to trust and communicate with freely (NHS Executive 1998, ENB & DoH 1999). The LDN/KW and CCN have worked collaboratively and within their individual role boundaries. As Emma's needs become more complex the children's palliative care team are also involved. However the KW remains the LDN as he can most effectively fulfil this role for Emma and her family even when, as she nears the end of her life, her nursing needs outweigh the needs associated with her learning disabilities.

TRANSITION FROM CHILD TO ADULT SERVICES

The change from childhood to adulthood takes place through dimensions of many different experiences, for example biological, legal, social, cultural, emotional and attitudinal. However, the concepts 'childhood' and 'adulthood' are ambiguous and hard to define (Jones & Wallace 1992). Transition to adult services can be a difficult time for young people with a learning disability and their families. Transition is not a process that has neat beginnings and ends. In 'Hurtling in to the void' Morris (1999) highlights problems faced in transition by young people with 'complex health and support needs' (see Chapter 32).

The Education Act 1993 and the associated code of practice for the identification and assessment of special needs students, outlines the duties and regulations that local authorities should follow for young people with statements of special educational need approaching adulthood. 'Valuing People' (DoH 2001) sets out the Government's strategy on how transition should be implemented. This includes the new service 'Connexions', for 13–19-year-olds, that offers support, guidance and advice for each person using personal advisers. Advisers identify all young people who have a learning disability and attend school reviews from year nine onwards. The service works with the school and other relevant professionals and agencies to draw up a transitional plan. It has responsibility for arranging a review for the young person with a learning disability, in their nineteenth year, with local learning and skills councils and employment services. Learning Disability partnership boards are charged with ensuring continuity in health care and since 2003 all young people moving between children and adult services have a person-centred plan (DoH 2001). Social Services under the Social Care Quality Framework, are expected to ensure that good links are in place between child and adult services.

There is no singular definition of successful transitional outcomes though there are many overlapping dimensions. These may be summarised as being any desired outcome in residence, education or social environment: i.e. social support, personal satisfaction, friendships (Halpern 1994, McGrew et al 1994, Tisdall 1994, Chadsey-Rusch & Heal 1995).

SUPPORT IN THE DECISION–MAKING PROCESS

A carefully planned transition programme should meet all needs by including the following elements:

- offering the young person a well-structured careers education and guidance programme
- the opportunity to visit a range of post-school taster days
- availability of link courses
- a process of career guidance and action planning commencing in year nine
- opportunity to assess the options against their own skills
- parents/carers engaged in the process with (i) accessible information about options, (ii) clear information about transition planning, (iii) guidance on how the process of assessing options fits in to the process, (iv) explanation of professionals' roles, (v) identification of a key link person and (vi) the availability of an advocate
- schools and supporting professionals sharing understanding of transitional planning and the assessment process, clear agreed time scales and a structure for cooperative working
- professionals benefiting from a clear understanding of each other's roles with agreement about information sharing, facilitation and shared assessments.

Case study 25.2 Mandy and her transition plan

Mandy, now aged 15, had achieved normal developmental milestones until her third birthday, when she was involved in a road traffic accident. She sustained severe damage to her spinal column together with a cerebral insult and bleed that resulted in brain damage. Mandy lost her verbal communication skills, social skills, mobility, required ventilation at night and had severe, uncontrolled epilepsy. She attends a special school and receives a package of care and support that includes a CCN, respite care, a Social Worker and LDN.

Transition plan

- Initial information (school year 8–9, approximate age 13–14 years)
- Preparation for transition review (school year 9, approximate age 14 years)

Transition review

- Transition plan
- Review of transition plan (school year 10–11, approximate age 15–19 years)
- Leaving school (school year 11, approximate age 16–19 years)
- Post-school plan

Age 18+

- Adult services aged 18–25

CONCLUSION

There is evidence that many young people with learning disabilities and their families experience a failure by health and social services to meet their needs. Structured programmes ensure that needs and aspirations are met (DoH 2001). 'Connexions' is part of this process. Children with profound learning disabilities may have multiple needs and LDNs and CCNs have an essential role to play as members of a multiprofessional team in providing for assessed need. This group and their families challenge traditional nursing boundaries and collaboration and commitment are required to ensure each child is seen as an individual and that the interactions with both them and their families is appropriate. It is important to recognise professional limitations and ensure open and effective communication with other practitioners to ensure high standards of care.

REFERENCES

Association for Children with Life-threatening or Terminal Conditions and their Families (ACT) & Royal College of Paediatrics and Child Health 2003 A guide to the development of children's palliative care services. ACT, Bristol

Ayer S & Alaszewski A 1984 Community Care and the Mentally Handicapped. Croom Helm, Beckenham

Beresford B A 1994 Resources and strategies: how parents cope with the care of a disabled child. Journal of Child Psychology & Psychiatry 35(1):171–209

Brown J 1992 The residential setting in mental handicap: An overview of selected policy initiatives 1971–1989. In: Thompson T & Mathias P (eds) Standards and mental handicap: keys to competence. Baillière Tindall, London

Chadsey-Rusch J & Heal L W 1995 Building consensus from transition experts on social integration outcomes and interventions. Exceptional Children 62:165–187

Cullen J C, Macleod J A, Williams P D & Williams A R 1991 Coping, satisfaction and the life cycle in families with mentally retarded persons. Issues in Comprehensive Pediatric Nursing 14:193–207

Department of Health 1998 Disabled Children. Directions for their future care. The Stationery Office, London

Department of Health 1999 Facing the Facts: Services for People with Learning Disabilities: Policy impact study of Social Care and Health Services. The Stationery Office, London

Department of Health 2001 Valuing People: a new strategy for learning disability for the 21st century. The Stationery Office, London

Department of Health and Social Security 1976 The Court Report. Fit for the future: the report of the committee in child health services. HMSO, London

Department of Health and Social Security 1981 Care in the community: a consultative document on moving resources for care. HMSO, London

Elfer P & Gatiss S 1990 Charting child health services. National Children's Bureau, London

English National Board for Nursing, Midwifery and Health Visiting (ENB) & Department of Health 1999 Sharing the care. Resource pack to support Diana, Princess of Wales community nursing teams. ENB, London

Fradd E 1994 Whose responsibility? Nursing Times 90(6):34–36

Gordon D, Parker R & Loughran F 2000 Disabled Children in Britain, a re-analysis of the Office of Population Censuses and Surveys Disability Surveys. The Stationery Office, London

Halpern A 1994 Quality of life for students with disabilities in transition from school to adulthood. Social Indicators Research 33:193–236

Heaman D J 1995 Perceived stressors and coping strategies of parents who have children with developmental disabilities. Journal of Pediatric Nursing 10(5):311–319

Hughson E A & Brown R I 1992 Learning difficulties in the context of social change: a challenge for professional action. In: Thompson T & Mathias P (eds) Standards and Mental Handicap: Keys to Competence. Baillière Tindall, London

Jones G & Wallace G 1992 Youth, family and citizenship. Open University Press, Buckingham

Keeley D, Dennis J & Hart C 1995 The parents of a severely dependent child. The Practitioner 239:505–512

McGrew K S, Johnson D R & Bruininks R H 1994 Factors analysis of community adjustment outcome measures for young adults with mild to severe disabilities. Journal of Psychoeducational Assessment 12:55–66

Maxwell V 1993 Look through the parents' eyes, helping parents of children with a learning disability. Professional Nurse December:200–202

Morris J 1999 Hurtling into the Void. Pavilion Publishing, London

National Health Service Executive 1998 Evaluation of the pilot project programme for children with life threatening illness. The Stationery Office, London

Orr R, Cameron S J & Day D M 1991 Coping with stress in families with children who have mental retardation: an evaluation of the double ABCX model. American Journal on Mental Retardation 95(4):444–450

Richards C & Reed J 1991 Your baby has Down's Syndrome. Nursing Times 87(46):60–61

Russell P 1998 Council for Disabled Children. Having A Say? Partnership in decision-making with disabled children. National Children's Bureau, London

Taanila A, Kokkonen J & Jarvelin M 1996 The long-term effects of children's early-onset disability on marital relationships. Developmental Medicine and Clinical Neurology 38:567–577

Teague B R, Fleming J W, Castle A, Kiernen B A, Lobo M L & Riggs S 1993 'High tech' home care for children with chronic health conditions. Journal of Pediatric Nursing 8:226–232

The Education Act 1993. HMSO, London

Tisdall E K M 1994 Why not consider citizenship? A critique of post school transitional models for young disabled people. Disability & Society 9:3–17

Waisbren S E 1980 Parents' reactions after the birth of a developmentally disabled child. American Journal of Mental Deficiency 84:345–351

Ward C 2001 Family Matters. Counting families in. A report from the family carers working group. The Stationery Office, London

While A 1991 An evaluation of a paediatric home care scheme. Journal of Advanced Nursing 16:1413–1421

Youngblut J M, Brennan P F & Swegart L A 1994 Families with medically fragile children: a study. Pediatric Nursing 20:463–468

Chapter 26

Young carers and community children's nursing

Lorly McClure

KEY ISSUES

- Self-identified experiences and needs of young carers.
- The rights of children.
- Community children's nurses and families.
- Multi-agency partnerships.
- Conflicts and dilemmas.

INTRODUCTION

The success of modern medicine in the Western world has generated a growing need and demand for long-term care of chronically sick and disabled people of all ages. This, together with the philosophy of family-centred care can result in the close involvement of all family members in the care of their sick or disabled child or sibling. Children with complex healthcare needs are increasingly being cared for at home, often with inadequate community children's nursing and respite care provision (Health Committee 1997). The assumption is that adult members of the family, normally the mother, will provide the care. However, there is increasing evidence that siblings from a very early age can be socialised into becoming caregivers, a role which can affect their health and development (Frank et al 1999). The Office of National Statistics estimated in 2001 that the number of young carers in Britain was 175 000, a figure considered by the Children's Society to be 'the tip of the iceberg' (Frank 2002). Community nurses and Health Visitors have direct contact with caregivers of all ages. Community Children's Nurses (CCNs) work closely with families, encountering parents as carers, and in some cases younger members of the family. This chapter will explore the experiences and needs of young carers, consider the rights of children and the role that CCNs might have in supporting them. The opportunities for multiprofessional working will be examined and some conflicts and dilemmas discussed.

FAMILY CARERS AND YOUNG CARERS

The vulnerability and support needs of carers of all ages has been recognised by the Government in 'Caring about Carers, A National Strategy for Carers' (DoH 1999). This report complements the focus on multi-agency working and collaborative approaches to community care as outlined in the white paper 'Modernising health and social services' (DoH 1998). The most significant and consistent care 'by the community' continues, as it always has, to be provided by family members. Indeed government initiatives in supporting carers are astute. Estimates indicate that the work carers undertake saves the taxpayer £57 billion a year (Holzhausen 2002).

Public awareness of the experiences of young carers has been informed over the past decade by a number of research studies. In the 1980s collaborative research was undertaken by local authority social services departments in conjunction with the education department and the Carers National Association (CNA) (O'Neill 1988). Further work, funded by the DoH, built on the previous research and recognised the complexity of the issues faced by such children (Meredith 1990, 1991, 1992). These studies were mainly descriptive and quantitative, whilst later work attempted to expose the life experiences of young carers through qualitative studies by profiling those who care and those who are cared for (Aldridge & Becker 1993, Becker et al 1995, Frank et al 1999).

DEFINITIONS, EXPERIENCES AND NEEDS OF YOUNG CARERS

Several official definitions of young carers have been developed over the last decade to direct the guidance and legislation that has informed practice at national and local government level. In 1995 the DoH defined a young carer as 'A child or young person who is carrying out significant caring tasks on a regular basis and assuming a level of responsibility for another person which would usually be taken by an adult' (DoH 1995).

Also in 1995, the CNA, now known as Carers UK, indicated that young carers were 'Children and young people under the age of 18 years whose lives are in some way restricted because of the need to take responsibility for the care of a person who is ill, has a disability, is experiencing mental distress or is affected by substance misuse or HIV/AIDS' (CNA 1995). More recently the Advisory Group on Young Carers 1999 stated that a young carer is 'Any child or young person under 18 years whose life is restricted by the emotional or physical dependence or care of another family member/s' (Advisory Group on Young Carers 1999).

Because of their age, and the nature of their situation, there is a problem with young carers being able to identify and define themselves. Family life is complex, embracing reciprocal responsibilities and strong emotional ties (Newman 2002). When considering school nurses' perceptions of school-age carers it was found that most children appeared to have enduring love for and loyalty to their families. 'They had an old fashioned attitude that families should manage, and would do anything for their parents' (McClure 2001).

Baker (2002) points out that identifying young people with caring responsibilities for a relative at home is difficult. They may not have the language, confidence or self-awareness to relay the physical and/or emotional impact of living with a relative who requires care, or identify themselves as having caring responsibilities. Maya Angelou suggests that 'children's talent to endure stems from their ignorance of alternatives' (Small 1992 p 10). However, through research and the work undertaken by voluntary and statutory agencies since 1995, the voices of some young carers expressing their experiences and needs are starting to be heard. Young carers can be involved in the care of family members of all ages and, depending on their family situation, be involved in a wide range of activities (Box 26.1).

Box 26.1 Some facts about young carers (Dearden & Becker 1998)

- Children aged 2–18 years act as young carers with an average age of 12 years
- 54% of young carers live in a lone-parent family
- 58% of young carers care for their mother
- 17% of young carers care for a sibling
- 63% of young carers cared for a relative with physical health problems
- 29% of illnesses and conditions relate to mental health issues
- One in three young carers of compulsory school age experience educational difficulties
- 57% were girls, 43% boys
- One in ten young carers care for more than one person
- 60% are involved in general care, assisting with mobility and giving medication
- One in five provide intimate care
- One in four had no external support

Research has also indicated that the experiences of these children and young people can differ along a continuum from a well-adjusted child who has the support and recognition of their family, to an overburdened child who is struggling with inappropriate roles and responsibilities (Lamorey 1999). It would appear that the nature, experiences and therefore needs of these children and young people will differ from one another, to the same extent that the nature, experiences and needs of each family will differ (Box 26.2).

Box 26.2 Types of caring (Frank 2002)

A young carer may undertake some or all of the following:

- Practical tasks such as cooking/housework/shopping
- Managing the family budget/collecting benefits/prescriptions
- Physical care such as lifting
- Personal care such as dressing/washing/helping with toilet needs
- Giving medication/helping with physiotherapy
- Ensuring safety

---

box continues

- Looking after/parenting younger siblings
- Giving emotional support or worrying
- Interpreting (either because of sensory impairment or of English not being the first language of the family)

YOUNG CARERS AND THEIR SIBLINGS

Those young carers who are involved in the care of a disabled or chronically sick sibling are more likely to be encountered by CCNs. Living with a sibling who has a disability can have both positive and negative consequences for a young carer. Maturity and consideration, as well as worry and stress can be demonstrated (Banks et al 2001) and significantly less time can be spent at school (Boyce et al 1991). Young carers of all ages are involved in undertaking a range of tasks for their parents and siblings. Tasks can be measured in hours but the emotional support they provide and the ensuing consequences can be difficult to calculate. These are identified in a study of adults who had been young carers. The findings revealed a 'conspiracy of silence' with concealed consequences such as influences of family dynamics, personal health and wellbeing and life chances (including education and future opportunities), finally leading to social exclusion and isolation (Frank et al 1999). One young carer states:

'At times being a carer is soul destroying. I battle against an invisible disease in my brother that means his health deteriorates ... I am the only one who can give him emotional support when he is feeling down. It is me who's left to make him smile. However much hard work it is to achieve this it's always worthwhile for the smiles and looks he gives me'

(Bibby & Becker 2000 p 69).

Experiences of young carers can be found in a wide range of literature and websites, for example from the award winning 'Bubblycrew' of the Hammersmith and Fulham Young Carers. Some of their stories are echoed in Case study 26.1.

Case study 26.1

Thomas's story

As the elder child and only son Thomas, aged 11 years, feels very protective of his three sisters, especially Emma aged 7 with autism. She has social and behavioural difficulties and often becomes noisy and destructive. Emma requires constant supervision. Sophie aged 10 and Sally aged 9 are great friends and help to look after each other as both parents are fully occupied either caring for Emma or working. On return from school Thomas helps with household chores, goes to the shops and watches over Emma to give his mother a break. His mother is receiving treatment for depression and his father for hypertension. Thomas loves his sister Emma. He feels guilty when her behaviour is beyond his control and she has to return to the protective environment of her specially adapted, padded playroom. He rarely invites school friends home. On occasion, Thomas feeds Emma, changes her incontinence pads and administers her medicines. He does not really understand what autism is and wonders about her future.

CCNs themselves could possibly identify scenarios similar to Thomas's story from their caseloads. The stories found in the literature all testify, in varying degrees, to children who assume a role that can be found difficult to sustain by most adults, often with very little support from health professionals (Frank 2002).

THE NEEDS OF YOUNG CARERS

Thomas's needs could be said to include assessment, counselling and peer support, information relevant to his cognitive level, and the freedom to be a child and brother to Emma. These are assumed needs and if he could be asked they might be very different. Recently, through the work of Carers UK and the Children's Society, attempts have been made to identify what it is that young carers think that they need (Box 26.3). A series of three Young Carers Festivals organised by the Children's Society and the Young Men's Christian Association have, to some degree, given them a voice.

> **Box 26.3** Summary of needs expressed by young carers (Frank 2002)
>
> - Better understanding towards disability and carers. It hurts our feelings when someone says something about our families
> - (People) to find out more about young carers so that teachers understand and are more aware of our situation at home
> - Attention and caring
> - Our voices heard, not next week or tomorrow but now!
> - More flexible responses from health and social services
> - Prompt assessment of families' needs
> - Care packages flexible enough to respond to illnesses episodic in nature
> - Assessments that take crisis provision into account

In 2002, four young carers presented a summary of the 2001 Young Carers Festival to the House of Lords 'All Parliamentary Group for Children' (Frank 2002):

- Agencies need to recognise that it is vital to consult with young carers and their families because they know their situation best.
- Young carers want schools to respect and understand the issues they have to deal with at home and to promote more awareness and tolerance of disability and illness.
- Young carers want health services to communicate with them about the medical care of parents and siblings in a clear and simple way, e.g. what to expect in the way of illness and behaviour and what to do in case of an emergency.
- Young carers want social workers to understand that all families are different and that it is important to consider the family members and their needs, not just one member. They want social workers to provide a flexible service because circumstances can change, affecting the level of support young carers need.

Overall young carers say that they wish to be listened to, understood and believed. They also wish to be valued, consulted and respected

(Frank 2002). Before any of these needs are met it is necessary that young carers are recognised by the health and social care professionals they encounter, all of whom will be fully aware of the policies and legislation related to the rights of children.

THE RIGHTS OF CHILDREN

Children are autonomous members of our society as acknowledged by the Children Act (DoH 1989) and the United Nations Declaration of Children's Rights (United Nations General Assembly 1959). They have the right to be respected, express their own wishes and be able to maximise their health and developmental potential. Frank et al (1999) identify a lack of a culture in the UK that listens to children who, as a consequence, have difficulty in making their needs known.

In relation to children as carers, ethical issues begin to emerge that involve the concepts of free will, choice and advocacy. Do children and young people act as carers of their own free will and are they given a choice as to whether they undertake such duties or not? Aldridge and Becker (1993) suggest that they have little choice in commencing the role and are in fact socialised into the caring act. They recognise that care receivers, similarly, have little choice.

There are, however, concerns being expressed in relation to the focus on the rights of young carers. The wide range of research and literature related to young carers that has emerged over the past decade has led to a debate between the disability rights movements and advocates of young carers rights (Keith & Morris 1995, Olsen 1996, Newman 2002). Despite having raised the profiles of families affected by illness and disability, it has been expressed that:

- the preoccupation with the rights of young carers has diverted attention, and possibly resources, from the needs of families
- the notion that family illness and disability poses a threat to young carers could have a distressing and detrimental effect on disabled and ill parents and siblings (Newman 2002).

The response to these concerns is to encourage agencies to refocus on the needs of the whole family rather than regarding either care recipient or carer as patient or client (Bibby & Becker 2000, Aldridge & Becker 2003). This debate appears to be stimulating a healthy tension which could help to enhance research and thereby raise to the surface critical issues related to chronic illness and disability which have for too long been submerged.

THE ROLE OF THE COMMUNITY CHILDREN'S NURSES IN HELPING TO MEET YOUNG CARERS' NEEDS

CCNs in their daily work may encounter a range of 'young carers' providing support to their parents and siblings as part of their normal family life. These activities could enhance their development, promoting responsibility, maturity and self-esteem or they could be overburdened, exhausted and made anxious by them. CCNs will have the opportunity to recognise young carers, identify their needs and where appropriate offer help and support. Family-centred assessment and care includes the whole family (While 1997). CCNs' communication skills will enhance their ability to recognise young carers and their needs. In partnership with parents they will be in a position to offer age-appropriate information about the condition and prognosis of the child receiving care. However, their workload may not allow them the resources to meet all the needs of young carers. Knowledge of their community and the range of services available can enable them to be both resource and advocate. They can advise young carers which websites to access, where they can go for help and support or refer them to other professionals such as the school nursing service, social services or appropriate voluntary agencies. They can also ensure that the young carer and family are aware of and understand their rights to assessment within the Carers Act (DoH 1995) and the Children Act (DoH 1989).

MULTI-AGENCY WORK

The profile of young carers has been raised by many local and national initiatives. As a result a significant number of young carers' projects and websites have been developed both nationally and locally. Young carers and their families have been supported in a number of ways, including the provision of information, opportunities to network and counselling and leisure activities. Collaborative projects with schools have also encouraged a multi-agency approach to the issues that frequently occur for young carers. Bullying and teasing by peers, attrition or aggressive behaviour, insensitive reaction by peers and adults to disability and the consequences of being a carer are frequently reported (Aldridge & Becker 1993). An example of a supporting project is in Surrey where caring and disability issues have been incorporated into the personal, social and health education curriculum (Arnot 1998). Lesson plans and a resource pack, available nationally, have been developed which contain case studies and background information.

The needs of young carers may fall between organisational divisions and agency boundaries. They are often recognised as a priority only when a family crisis point is reached. It is essential, therefore, that a multi-agency approach is used to assess the needs of young carers and implement support and advice. Strategies could then be developed within communities that take into account local and national policies, existing resources and current service provision. The expertise, enthusiasm and commitment of CCNs can ensure that the needs and rights of young carers are constantly on the agenda.

CONFLICTS AND DILEMMAS

CCNs can frequently have difficulty in helping young carers when their carer role is covert and concealed. They may be reluctant to draw attention to themselves and their families because of not wanting 'interference' from schools and social services (Banks et al 2002). Furthermore, dilemmas related to confidentiality may arise. A CCN may be aware of a young carer in need of help but could be unwilling to risk a trusting relationship with the family by making a referral to other agencies. If the young carer could be classified as a 'child in need' (DoH 1989) support will be required from colleagues and through clinical supervision. An ethical dilemma occurs if a young person requests teaching in nursing techniques such as lifting or undertaking technical or invasive procedures. How safe is it to teach these skills? How safe is it for the young carer to covertly undertake these tasks without instruction?

It can be seen that where siblings are acting as carers, embracing the concept of the family as client (Muir & Sidey 2003) could challenge the beliefs and values of some CCNs. A consequence could be confusion and conflict to those who might see their role exclusively as advocate for the sick or disabled child. Conversely, it could be argued that CCNs have a commitment, not only to the family as client, but to the development of stronger networks within the community and a public health role. These conflicts and dilemmas need to be debated in the light of a changing society and Government policies.

CONCLUSION

While there are families, illness, disability and handicap there will be young carers. Accidents and disease can strike children at any time, leading to their siblings finding themselves providing varying degrees of support and care. Young carers will live within poor or affluent families, capable or dysfunctional families and represent all social classes, ethnic groups and cultures. CCNs can make a difference by assessing the whole family and identifying the needs of young carers. Their intervention and referral could help to prevent future debilitating consequences for individuals and families and help to influence allocation of resources to children and families in need.

REFERENCES

Advisory Group on Young Carers 1999 Report on Young Carers in Oxfordshire: Where are we? What is needed? A Way Forward. Children's Strategy Group, Oxford

Aldridge J & Becker S 1993 Children Who Care – Inside the World of Young Carers. Loughborough University, Leicester

Aldridge J & Becker S 2003 Caring roles. Journal of Family Therapy 21(3):303–320

Arnot J 1998 Information Pack for Teachers. Surrey Education Service, Kingston-on-Thames

Baker G 2002 Unseen and Unheard: The Invisible Young Carers. Carers Lewisham, Princess Royal Trust for Carers, London

Banks P, Coggan N, Deley S, Hill M, Riddell S & Tisdall K 2001 Seeing the invisible children and young people affected by disability. Disability and Society 16(6):794–814

Banks P, Cogan N, Riddell S, Deeley S, Hill M & Tisdall K 2002 Does the covert nature of caring prohibit the development of effective services for young carers? British Journal of Guidance and Counselling 30(3):229–246

Becker S, Aldridge J, Brittain D, Clasen J, Dietz B & Gould A (eds) 1995 Young Carers in Europe: An Exploratory Cross-national Study in Britain, France,

Sweden and Germany. Loughborough University, Leicester

Bibby A & Becker S (eds) 2000 Young Carers in Their Own Words. Calouste Gulbenkian Foundation, London

Boyce G C, Barnett S & Miller B C 1991 Time use and attitudes among siblings: A comparison in families of children with and without Down's syndrome. Poster presented at the biennial meeting of the Society for Research in Child Development, April

Carers National Association 1995 Debate on definition of young carers. Unpublished communication. Carers National Association, London

Dearden C & Becker S 1998 Young Carers in the UK: A Profile. Carers National Association, London

Department of Health 1989 The Children Act. HMSO, London

Department of Health 1995 Chief Inspector letter C1(95)12

Department of Health 1998 Modernising health and social services: national priorities guidance. The Stationery Office, London

Department of Health 1999 Caring about carers: a national strategy for carers. The Stationery Office, London

Frank J 2002 Making it Work: Good Practice with Young Carers and their Families. The Princess Royal Trust for Carers and the Children's Society, London

Frank J, Tatum C & Tucker S 1999 On Small Shoulders. The Children's Society, London

Health Committee 1997 House of Commons Select Committee. Health services for children and young people in the community: home and school. Third report. The Stationery Office, London

Holzhausen E 2002 Without Us ... ?: Calculating the Value of Carers' Support. Carers UK, London

Keith L & Morris J 1995 Easy targets: a disability rights perspective on the 'children as carers' debate. Critical Social Policy 44/45 Autumn:36–57

Lamorey S 1999 Parentification of siblings of children with disability. In: Chase N (ed) Burdened Children, Theory, Research and Treatment of Parentification. Sage Publications, London

McClure L 2001 School-age caregivers: Perceptions of school nurses working in central England. The Journal of School Nursing 17(2):76–82

Meredith H 1990 A new awareness. Community Care. February 22:viii

Meredith H 1991 Young carers. Contact Summer 4:14–15

Meredith H 1992 Supporting the young carer. Community Outlook May 2(5):15–18

Muir J & Sidey A 2003 Community children's nursing. In: Watkins D, Edwards J & Gastrell P (eds) Community Health Nursing. Baillière Tindall, Edinburgh, pp 271–280

Newman T 2002 'Young carers' and disabled parents: time for a change of direction. Disability and Society 17(6):613–625

Olsen R 1996 Young carers: challenging their facts and politics of research into children and caring. Disability and Society 11:41–54

O'Neill A 1988 Young Carers: The Tameside Research. Tameside Metropolitan Borough Council, Tameside

Small E 1992 Growing up fast. Social Work Today 23(34):10

United Nations General Assembly 1959 Declaration of the Rights of the Child. UNICEF, Geneva

While A 1997 Explorations in Family Nursing. Routledge, London

Chapter 27

Play therapy within community children's nursing

Debbie Mills

KEY ISSUES

- The developing role of the community play specialist within community children's nursing.
- The role of the play specialist in a Diana Community Children's Nursing team.
- Parameters of the role.
- A consideration of the types of therapeutic play.

INTRODUCTION

The benefits of play have been recognised as fundamental in helping a child cope during an illness (Save the Children Fund 1989). The report recommends that a child's emotional and psychological needs should be supported through play. 'Play Specialists do far more than occupy children. They can reduce uncertainty by providing play that is familiar, a welcome relief after all the strange sights, sounds and bodily discomfort' (Lansdown & Goldman 1988 p 557). Play aims to provide the child with a medium in which to deal with the often threatening and unfamiliar experience of hospitalisation. Peterson (1989) suggests that play can be used as an indirect factor in removing the formality of the medical experience. McMahon (1992 p 55) states 'It is recognised that the stress of a hospital stay can be further reduced and a child's recovery hastened by the provision of play'. Brimblecombe (cited in Weller & Oliver 1980) called attention to the value of professional hospital play specialists.

Traditionally the role of the play specialist has been limited to the hospital setting. 'It has been recommended that all children staying in hospital have access to a play specialist' (DoH 2003). Increasing numbers of children with complex health needs are cared for at home and therefore a more focused and specialised play therapy role that extends beyond the acute setting is required. Community play specialists are employed in a range of settings and frequently within Diana Community Children's Nursing Teams (DCCNTs). Their roles vary according to the needs and criteria of the employing service. Play specialists, both in acute and primary sectors, may be confused with play therapists. Their methods may be similar but the training is different and therapists tend to use more structured models of practice relating to psychological issues.

> 'There is no single professional preparation for play therapy in Britain. Play therapists arrive at their own knowledge by a variety of idiosyncratic routes. Hospital Play Specialists and child development centre workers use play in their work with sick, disabled and developmentally delayed children, occasionally psychiatrists and clinical psychologists will use play methods in work with children and families' (McMahon 1992 p 57)

This chapter outlines the role of a community play specialist (CPS). It uses examples from practice, considers the role of a CPS within a DCCNT and describes some of the types of play employed to support children and families.

DEVELOPMENT OF A COMMUNITY PLAY SPECIALIST ROLE

The DCCNT within Leicestershire and Rutland provides a multiprofessional service supporting children, young people and their families where there are acute, critical care, continuing care or palliative care needs. The focus of the CPS role is to provide therapeutic play for individual children and their families in the safe environment of their own home. The role complements that of the Community Children's Nurses (CCNs) and aims to encourage the integration of the knowledge and skills of different disciplines within the multidisciplinary team in order to provide the most effective care for the child and their family (Knott 1999) (Box 27.1).

Box 27.1 Components of a community play specialist's role

- Preparation for children and their families
- Developmental play
- Play therapy and chronic illness
- Play therapy in adolescence
- Distraction therapy
- Play therapy and phobias
- Play therapy in bereavement

The play service within the DCCNT was established in 2001 and there are 1.5 play specialists. Referral criteria, documentation, toy libraries and research into resources were established prior to developing a caseload and undertaking home visits.

REFERRALS

As a member of the DCCNT the CPS is accountable to the team leader, with whom referrals are discussed. Referrers are restricted to members of the DCCNT team. Following referral, the CPS undertakes an initial assessment either before discharge from hospital or in the child's home. Time taken with the family, to identify both actual and potential problems, enables individual and effective play programmes to be developed. These highlight and focus on the needs of the siblings as well as those of the sick child. At this stage, issues in relation to the parameters of the service are discussed and mutually negotiated (Box 27.2).

Box 27.2 Parameters of the service

- Acknowledgement of boundaries/length of each session/number of visits
- Confidentiality issues
- Identification of objectives and evaluation mechanisms
- Recognition of ending the relationship
- Future open access to the service if required

After this initial assessment joint visits with associated healthcare professionals are undertaken as appropriate. A large proportion of referrals are patients and families receiving palliative care and involve massage and relaxation, emotional play and pre- and post-bereavement support.

PREPARATION

The safe and familiar environment of home provides ideal surroundings to implement play therapy in preparation for planned treatment and care. Taylor (1991) suggests that the presence of the parents is important during preparation as they know their child intimately. Over time the CPS is able to develop a relationship with the child and family, and therefore be aware of the most appropriate methods of preparation in individual cases. This is captured in Case study 27.1.

Case study 27.1

Three-year-old Christie was due to receive a course of radiotherapy. A play programme was designed to prepare her for the experience that involved Christie lying on a large sheet of paper on which her outline was drawn. The purpose of this was to explain the importance of lying still during the radiotherapy session. To emphasise this, a water spray was used to show that when she moved it was difficult to spray the correct part of her body. A family game of sleeping lions was also used to reinforce the concept. Christie's mother was taught a visualisation exercise which she audio-taped and used during the radiotherapy, allowing Christie to hear her mother's voice whilst focusing on a favourite image. Her mother became involved with the treatment and both acquired a sense of control.

Whitting (1993) comments that simply telling a child a story about their procedure is no indication that the child has understood what is involved, and this may result in misconceptions. As children are used to accepting information through their play, the preparation, as described above, can be a positive experience for all involved (Reid 1988). Enabling the child to play out the experience provides the professional with a window into the child's thoughts.

DISTRACTION THERAPY

The importance of distraction therapy following preparation provides an effective combination of play therapy techniques to ensure a child's confidence in the nursing or medical experience remains intact (Box 27.3). Distraction focuses the attention away from what is happening. The professional or parent can be actively involved in the distraction whilst the child remains passive; this can be important when a child is required to lie still. Conversely, the child may be actively involved in the distraction.

Box 27.3 Distraction techniques

- Bubbles: Breathing techniques give the child a sense of control over a situation
- Counting: Using number games to count up, down, backwards and forwards
- Imagery: Using imagery to guide a child through a previously agreed subject
- Music relaxation: Music may develop a sense of repose
- Puppets and dolls: Allow a child and the carer to talk through a third person

---

DEVELOPMENTAL PLAY

Children with developmental delay are encouraged to reach their maximum potential through the provision of different types of play. Honeyman (1994) showed that careful planning and knowledge of a child's capabilities are essential to ensure that the type of play offered is not only challenging to the child but also gives pleasure (Case study 27.2). The CPS aims to empower the parents to have fun with their children and treat the child as normally as possible. Close liaison with relevant professionals ensures that a collaborative outcome is achieved.

Case study 27.2

Fourteen-month-old Lottie was chronically ill with a progressive muscular disorder. She was referred because of difficulties in manipulating and playing with objects. A play programme was designed with the dietician and physiotherapist. This included the introduction of messy play using food, such as jelly, pasta and yoghurt, which helped Lottie to have a greater awareness of her hands whilst developing skills in feeding herself. Her parents were actively involved in promoting her development in this playful way.

SUPPORT FOR ADOLESCENTS

Adolescents with ill health may experience reduced self-confidence and self-esteem alongside developmental regression at an already turbulent time of life. Respecting their needs and taking time to listen can provide opportunities for emotional space and personal growth. Referral to the CPS may give the adolescent permission to play games or be involved in activities that may normally be associated with a younger child. This provides opportunities for an undemanding escape. Alternatively, others feel the need to be more creative through artwork or constructive activities.

> *'Play specialists have an important role in providing an appropriate environment for adolescents. They can ensure that the relevant information is available and that other staff are aware of the adolescents' needs for privacy and independence. They should encourage group activities and encourage patients to meet each other and share experiences, anxieties and their own methods of coping with hospital life'*

> (National Association for the Welfare of Children in Hospital 1990 p 12)

MASSAGE AND RELAXATION

Within the DCCNT the CPS offers massage to children and teaches parents/carers massage strokes. Massage encourages tactile development, improves sleep patterns and increases the production of endorphins, giving improved pain relief (Porter 1996, Buckle 1997, 1999, Kemper 2001). Teaching parents to massage their children could be seen as a way of empowering them to regain control in one area (Darbyshire & Morrison 1995). This enables them to carry out the massage at times best suited to them and their child (Case study 27.3).

Case study 27.3

Sixteen-year-old Sally had profound cerebral palsy. Her joints were stiff and she received regular physiotherapy. She considered this to be a 'procedure' not a form of relaxation. The CPS shared several sessions with the parents teaching them massage strokes with closed curtains, dimmed lights and soft music. Sally therefore differentiated between this and her physiotherapy. Although she had limited vocal communication Sally was skilled at expressing her needs and feelings through facial expressions and hand movements. She chose her own massage music, which tended to be the same classical CD, and always gave her permission prior to the massage. The movements enabled her to relax her muscles and her mother observed her arms relax in a way she had not seen for several years. Sally rarely refused a massage, it was always followed by a relaxing sleep. Both parents used this techniques to help Sally and spend quality one-to-one time with her in a relaxing manner.

PLAY THERAPY AND PHOBIAS

Children, for example those requiring growth hormone replacement therapy, often experience needle phobias. This may be associated with the fact that they are not physically ill and find it difficult to understand why they need treatment. A collaborative approach by the CCN and CPS can provide age-appropriate information alongside a play programme to help the child comprehend the nature of their disorder and necessary treatment. The use of real equipment for play purposes can help familiarise children with the planned treatment. Play can be in the form of syringe painting or involve injecting water into oranges.

BEREAVEMENT SUPPORT

A CPS is able to offer a range of different play techniques using sand therapy, puppetry and expressive play to enable the ill child/young person and their siblings to express and verbalise their feelings and emotions in a safe and familiar manner (Box 27.4). Thomas and Charmers (2001) describe how children need honest information about death from someone they know and trust and that this should take into account age, life experience, maturity, and the family's cultural and spiritual beliefs.

Box 27.4 Pre- and post-bereavement play activities

- Story-telling using puppets
- Therapeutic sand play
- Stained glass memory windows
- Treasure/memory boxes
- Hand and foot prints
- Sealed letters/pictures (to place in coffin)
- Feelings collages/masks
- Feelings trees
- Salt sculptures

CLINICAL SUPERVISION

Clinical supervision should be an integral part of professional practice under the clinical governance agenda (Royal College of Nursing 1998). The aim is to sustain and develop practice through a formal process with a chosen colleague. Jones (1988) states that supervision is designed to explore issues related to the effectiveness of professional practice. However, in order ultimately to ensure the delivery of safe and effective care, respect and trust must be gained by all involved. The roles described in this chapter may be viewed as an extension of the hospital play therapist's role, which at times involves delicate and distressing situations on a long-term basis. Clinical supervision for the CPS in the DCCNT takes place monthly and is facilitated by a child psychotherapist. This provides the opportunity to reflect upon the therapeutic programme of care for each child.

CONCLUSION

The CPS is in a unique position to draw upon the knowledge and skills of the multiprofessional team in supporting children and families who require their specialist intervention. The availability of a CPS within a community children's nursing service adds to the therapeutic repertoire of skills available.

REFERENCES

Buckle J 1997 Clinical Aromatherapy in Nursing. Arrowsmith Limited, Bristol

Buckle J 1999 The use of complementary therapy for chronic pain. Alternative Therapies Health Medicine 5(5):42–51

Darbyshire P & Morrison H 1995 Empowering parents of children with special needs. Nursing Times 91(32):26–28

Department of Health 2003 Standard for Hospital Services. The Stationery Office, London

Honeyman L 1994 Play for children with special needs. Paediatric Nursing 6(3):18–19

Jones A 1988 Building professional relationships. Nursing Times Learning Curve 2(4):12–13

Kemper K 2001 Complementary and alternative medicine for children does it work? Archives of Disease in Childhood 84(1):69

Knott M 1999 Integrated nursing teams: developments in general practice. Community Practitioner 72(2):23–24

Lansdown R & Goldman A 1988 The psychological care of children with malignant disease. Journal of Child Psychology and Psychiatry 29(5):555–567

McMahon L 1992 The Handbook of Play Therapy. Routledge, London

National Association for the Welfare of Children in Hospital (NAWCH) 1990 Setting standards for adolescents in hospital. NAWCH, London

Peterson G 1989 Let the children play. Nursing 3(41):22–25

Porter S 1996 The use of massage in neonates requiring special care. Complementary Therapies in Nursing and Midwifery 2:93–96

Reid J 1988 Playing away the pain. Nursery World 7 April:10–11

Royal College of Nursing (RCN) 1998 Guidance for Nurses on Clinical Governance. RCN, London

Save the Children Fund 1989 The Case for Hospital Play Schemes. Save the Children Fund, London

Taylor D 1991 Prepare for the best. Nursing Times 87(31):64–66

Thomas J & Charmers A 2001 Responding to children bereaved by sudden death. The Child Bereavement Trust, High Wycombe

Weller B & Oliver G 1980 Helping Sick Children Play. Baillière Tindall, London

Whitting M 1993 Play and surgical patients. Paediatric Nursing 5(6):11–13

SECTION 4

Advancing Community Children's Nursing Practice

SECTION CONTENTS

Community children's nursing is evolving at an astounding rate. The need to support and inform this evolution through creative thought and research-based evidence is essential. This final section provides stimulating accounts of 'new' practice and the potential and very real opportunities that lie ahead. Contributions offer different perspectives on the advancement of community children's nursing practice including an expanded and rewritten chapter on complementary therapies.

Chapter 28

Complementary therapies in community children's nursing

Julia Fearon

KEY ISSUES

- Increasing numbers of families are using complementary therapies.
- Community Children's Nurses are well placed to discuss, advise and support families who wish to explore the potential of complementary therapies for their child.
- Integrating complementary therapies into nursing practice requires careful consideration, appropriate training and education and should not compromise or fragment existing care.

INTRODUCTION

Complementary therapy (CT) is difficult to define, embracing as it does, well over 100 different therapies (British Medical Association 1993). It is also important to consider that some therapists may see their therapy as alternative rather than complementary and would not expect individuals utilising the therapy to avail themselves of mainstream medicine at the same time. The term 'complementary and alternative medicine' (CAM) is frequently used, but it is suggested that Community Children's Nurses (CCNs) utilise the term complementary therapies (CTs) which implies they are an adjunct to mainstream care rather than CAM which could imply 'instead of' mainstream care. The Royal College of Nursing (RCN) (1995) define CTs as 'A range of interventions which may be of therapeutic benefit and support when used in addition to any other treatments and procedures offered to the patient in the orthodox healthcare setting'.

The popularity of CTs continues to increase amongst the UK population (Botting & Cook 2000, Ernst & White 2000, Harris & Rees 2000). There is limited research relating to the use of CTs by children in the UK with the majority of the literature from other countries. However, this demonstrates increasing use of CT by children and CCNs need to be aware of the issues surrounding its use. Amongst children, CTs are most commonly used by those suffering from chronic conditions, especially where mainstream medicine has limited success in offering sustained relief such as musculoskeletal disorders, oncological, skin and respiratory diseases (Spigelblatt et al 1994, Grootenhuis et al 1998, Sikand & Laken 1998, Armishaw & Grant 1999, Ernst 1999, Simpson & Roman 2001, Davis & Darden 2003). CTs can also play a role in providing psychological support for children and families (Kemper 2001, Buckle 2003, Fearon 2003) and teach children coping strategies (Burgess 2001, Kemper 2001, Brue & Oakland 2002). The increasing popularity of CTs is accompanied by a trend towards greater integration of CTs into mainstream care. This is supported by The Prince of Wales Foundation for Integrated Health (Prince of Wales FIH), formally the Foundation for Integrated Medicine (Prince of Wales FIM) (Prince of Wales FIM 1998, Prince of Wales FIH 2003).

A House of Lords scientific and technology select committee published a report on complementary and alternative medicine (House of Lords 2000) in which several recommendations were made and subsequently endorsed by the DoH (2001). Among the recommendations, the report called for stronger regulation of the CT disciplines (currently only osteopathy and chiropractic are regulated by law), better training for therapists, more research, higher-quality information and more integration with mainstream care. Work towards self-regulation is currently advanced among homeopaths, ongoing amongst the aromatherapy professional bodies and reflexology is also taking steps in this direction. The quality of training and education for therapists is an important issue for nurses wishing to actually practice a complementary therapy. The RCN has recently issued guidance on the integration of complementary therapies into nursing and midwifery practice and this document contains information about accessing appropriate education (Avis 2003). The Prince of Wales FIH has also issued a document to guide individuals considering training in CT (Williams 2003).

The role of the CCN in relation to CTs for children is likely to be focused on providing families with advice, support and perhaps the integration of selected CT techniques into their nursing practice rather than the actual provision of a complementary therapy (Richardson 2001). This is primarily because the CCN's role is a nursing role and not a complementary therapy role. If the child is to receive a CT then that therapy is best provided by a complementary practitioner. However, there may be CT techniques that can legitimately be incorporated into the CCN's nursing care.

Box 28.1 Complementary therapy techniques to incorporate into nursing practice

- Foot massage
- Head massage (during hair wash)
- Guided imagery
- Aromatherapy bubble baths
- Diffusion of essential oils
- Reflexology

Careful thought must be given as to how therapies and techniques can be integrated into practice. Nurses integrating therapies must be sure of the safety and relevance of therapies to be used and therapies should not compromise or fragment existing areas of practice and care (Avis 2003). This is especially important in the background of limited, quality research in the field of complementary therapy. It is vital too, that the nurse providing the therapy has the knowledge and skills to perform the technique and is aware of personal accountability and responsibility in line with the Nursing and Midwifery Council (NMC) Code of Professional Conduct (NMC 2002). The CCN must also ensure adherence to local Trust policies and procedures when incorporating CTs into practice. If such local policy does not exist then, from a clinical governance perspective, it would not be appropriate to continue with the integration until such time as local policy on the issue has been developed.

More importantly than actually providing a therapy is the ability of the CCN to knowledgeably, openly and honestly discuss issues surrounding CT provision for children with families in their care. The research highlights that many families are reluctant to disclose use of CTs for their child (Grootenhuis et al 1998, Ernst 1999, Scrace 2003), fearing that their disappointment in conventional care will be revealed, that the topic will not be well received or that their orthodox carers will be cynical and have little or no knowledge of the therapies (Scrace 2003). CCNs should encourage open and honest discussion about CT with families. This will demonstrate understanding and empathy, promote better support for the child and family, foster a good relationship with the family and help the family to make informed choices about using CTs for their child. CCNs should not underestimate the role that therapies can play in providing psychological support for families especially where parents themselves choose to provide the therapy. This can be very important in empowering parents at a time when they feel they have little control over what is happening to their child and enables them to take an active part in being able to do something positive for their child (Fearon 2003, Scrace 2003). When encouraged to discuss CTs, parents may well look to their CCN to provide them with information about how to access CTs, training for CTs and for recommendations about CT practitioners. Ethically it is not appropriate for individual nurses to make such recommendations, but it is acceptable for a nurse to tell parents the sort of questions they should be asking a complementary therapist in order to determine their suitability to provide therapies for their child. CCNs should also be aware that an independent CT practitioner may not have been subject to an enhanced criminal record bureau check and that a therapist should expect to be chaperoned.

Box 28.2 Questions to ask a complementary therapist

- How long have you been practising?
- Where did you train, i.e College of Further Education/University, night school, private establishment?
- How long was your training course, i.e. a few days, a few weeks, a few months, more than a year?

box continues

- Was your training accredited by a professional body?
- Did it include theoretical and practical tuition and assessment?
- Are you registered with a professional body?
- Do you have (professional indemnity) insurance to practice?
- Do you have a specialised client group/specialise in one particular area, e.g. children, stress, palliative care?

Accessing CTs can be expensive and the CCN will need to be aware of the local charges. It is most likely that families will have to pay for CT for their child, but there may be local options for charity provision, for example, through parent support organisations and occasionally a General Practitioner's (GP) practice will provide access to a therapist but even this may have a cost attached. In a very few areas, therapies can be accessed via the NHS. It is helpful if nurses are cognisant of what is available locally.

If CCNs incorporate therapies into their practice, a mechanism for assessment, evaluation, supervision and support for practitioners with specialists in the field of complementary medicine should be established (Nicoll 1995). Within that process, a range of issues that arises from practice can be explored, such as consent (Stone & Matthews 1996) and clinical effectiveness.

ACUPUNCTURE/ ACUPRESSURE

Acupuncture/acupressure involves stimulation of specific points on the body, usually by the insertion of fine needles (acupuncture) for therapeutic and/or preventative effects (Zollman & Vickers 2000, Tavares 2003). The involvement of needles would at first make it seem an unlikely therapy to be used for children, but there is some evidence to suggest that children tolerate the therapy remarkably well, especially where it is effective in providing symptom relief, and that acupressure can be equally effective (Broide et al 2001, Kemper & Wornham 2001). It is important to recognise that acupuncture is only one part of a complete system of Traditional Chinese Medicine (TCM) that seeks to diagnose, treat, cure and prevent disease. In TCM, the workings of the human body are believed to be controlled by a life force known as 'Qi' and based upon the Daoist concepts of Yin and Yang and the Five Elements (fire, earth, metal, wood, and water). There exists a dynamic relationship between yin and yang; if there is an excess of one, there will be a deficiency of the other. TCM including diet, herbs, massage and exercise as well as acupuncture aims to maintain a dynamic balance of energy within the body. The Qi circulates along 12 meridians corresponding to major functions of the body. Inserting needles/applying pressure to points along the meridians enables the flow of Qi to be realigned or redirected. Prior to treatment the initial consultation by a traditional acupuncturist is likely to take some considerable time, as every aspect of the child and their life is explored, in order to make a diagnosis of problems that may need to be addressed. Acupuncture is currently in the consultation process to become a statutory regulated profession.

AROMATHERAPY

Aromatherapy is the use of concentrated plant extracts (essential oils) for their therapeutic properties. Essential oils are aromatic material extracted from a wide variety of plants, for example trees, flowers, herbs and fruit, using techniques such as expression and steam distillation. Aromatherapy does not seek to treat and diagnose illness, rather to promote relaxation and a sense of wellbeing. The oils can be applied in a variety of ways including through massage, inhalation, compresses, creams, lotions and in baths. It is complex to analyse exactly how it exerts its effects because a treatment has many component parts. For example, the therapist/child/family relationship, the effects of massage (if used), the sense of smell and the psychological effects of aromas and the relaxation induced will all play a part in how the child reacts to the treatment.

Research has demonstrated how applying oils through massage can result in a marked reduction in anxiety (Acolet et al 1993, Field et al 1998) but even the inhalation of the aroma of a couple of drops of essential oil applied to a child's pillow can have a marked effect. Care must be exercised when choosing blends. Aroma, by virtue of its action on the limbic system, may evoke memories or emotional reactions, or put in place future memories, either positive or negative, which can then be associated with the smell of the oils used.

For skin application, because essential oils are very concentrated they are first diluted in an inert carrier oil (vegetable oil) such as sweet almond oil (*Prunus amygdalis* var. *dulcis*) or grape seed oil (*Vitis vinifera*). Where nut allergies are suspected, grape seed oil may be used as a substitute for nut oils (Price 1999). For an adult it is usual to blend up to four essential oils together in the carrier oil in up to 3% dilution (that is, approximately nine drops in 10 millilitres of base oil (different manufacturers have different sized drop dispensers) (Olleveant et al 1999)). With children caution must be exercised. They have different rates of absorption and excretory pathways, immature physiological systems and there is the possibility of adverse reactions to some of the constituents of particular oils. Safe application must be ensured (Fowler & Wall 1997). Essential oil choice is more limited (Worwood 2001) and blends must be much more dilute than for adults. For example, Price and Price Parr (1996) recommend dilutions as in Table 28.1. Even greater care must be taken if using oil for neonates and pre-term infants who have fewer layers of epidermis

Table 28.1 Suggested dilutions for essential oil and carrier oils (Price & Price Parr 1996)

Weight of child	Number of drops of essential oil in 50 ml carrier oil
Up to 12 kg	5
12–25 kg	8
25–38 kg	8
38–50 kg	8
>50 kg	Up to 15

(Tisserand & Balacs 1995) and in order not to interfere in the mother and baby bonding process, which is, in part, related to the infant's sense of smell and recognition of the mother by smell.

The quality of oils is important. Good-quality essential oils should always be labelled with the country of origin and the Latin name as a minimum. Essential oils do not last indefinitely once opened, deteriorating with exposure to light and air. They should be stored in a cool, dark place with great care. They are highly flammable liquids, some are extremely toxic if ingested and it is unusual to find oils supplied with tamper-proof caps.

Box 28.3 Conditions that may benefit from aromatherapy

- Stress-related conditions
- Pain
- Constipation (Mantle 1996, Ernst 2001)
- Skin problems
- Migraines
- Infections
- Anxiety
- Sleeping problems
- Children with special needs
- Mucositis (Gravett 2000)

Aromatherapy offers the opportunity to develop a different and more positive relationship between child and parents/carers who often choose to learn massage. It can also enhance the relationship between child and nurse. Inducing a relaxation response and encouraging enjoyment and fun may promote stimulation of the child's immune responses (Pert 1998) and hence healing.

Case study 28.1

Ann's 7-year-old son had never slept through the night. Physically he was fit and well. When he came in from school he would run wildly for an hour at a time. They had both survived a traumatic attack some 5 years earlier and were receiving counselling. Ann was taught a basic back massage technique and blended 1% equal quantities of Roman Camomile (*Anthemis nobilis*) and Sweet Marjoram (*Origanum majorana*) in a grape-seed carrier oil. That evening, after his bath and before bedtime, she lay him on the settee and massaged his back. He was happy to lie still and receive the massage and after 20 minutes he told his mother he was tired and wanted to go to bed. He slept through the night for the first time. He has had sleep-disturbed nights since, but Ann continues to massage him two to three times a week, sometimes with an essential oil blend, sometimes with plain oil, and his sleep patterns have continued to improve.

HERBALISM

Herbalism is the medicinal use of preparations that contain exclusively plant material (Ernst 2001). CCNs need to be aware that many parents will seek such remedies for their children (Kemper 2001, Simpson & Roman 2001, Sawni-Sikand et al 2002). There have been examples of herbal medicines reacting with orthodox drugs and toxicity of herbal preparations. Kemper (2001) and Ernst (2001) highlight that the risk of adverse effects is probably greater than with most other CTs. This again emphasises the need for CCNs to be able to encourage open and honest discussion with families about herbal medicines they may be using. It is also important that CCNs know where to go for advice and information about possible interactions between herbal and orthodox treatments, for example the local poisons unit or local hospital pharmacy. It might be appropriate to identify a local herbalist who may be able to advise or a local GP who is qualified in herbal medicine.

HOMEOPATHY

Homeopathic preparations are made by diluting substances from natural sources many, many times in a water and alcohol base with each successive dilution being shaken very vigorously, a process known as succussion (Atherton 2001). Orthodox scientists claim that the resulting liquid is nothing more than water, but homeopaths believe the energetic imprint or 'memory' of the original source remains in the substance. The homeopath works on the assumption that you treat like with like. Hence a symptom of vomiting will be treated with this extreme dilution of an emetic. Homeopathy is thought to be very safe which is probably why it is one of the more commonly used CTs in children (Ernst 1999, Lee & Kemper 2000, Simpson & Roman 2001). However, CCNs should be aware that in around 20% of cases treated with homeopathy an aggravation of symptoms will be seen and that some homeopaths will advocate rejection of orthodox treatments such as immunisation (Ernst 2001, Lee & Kemper 2000).

REFLEXOLOGY AND REFLEX ZONE THERAPY

In reflexology, gentle, manual pressure is applied to specific areas or zones of the feet (and sometimes hands and ears) that are believed to correspond with different parts of the body (Ernst 2001). It is suggested that reflex zones run in specific lines through the body and are reflected on the surface of the hands and feet. Stimulating and manipulating these reflexes effects change in other parts of the body and promotes wellbeing and relaxation (Griffiths 2001). Reflexology can be used to reduce anxiety and lower blood pressure (Griffiths 2001), and relieve chronic constipation and encopresis (Bishop 2003). Children cannot tolerate the same length or depth of treatment as an adult (Bayly 1982) and the practitioner must be conversant with contraindications.

THERAPEUTIC MASSAGE

Massage offers a means of communicating through caring touch, which is very different to the 'clinical' touch associated with much of nursing (Estabrooks 1992). It can be used to bring about changes in soft tissues and the circulation and to promote a range of physiological and psychological effects such as reduction in anxiety (Field et al 1992), relief from problems such as constipation, relief of muscle tension and pain relief (Fritz 1995, Holey & Cook 2003).

The beneficial effects of massage are well researched and recognised (Holey & Cook 2003). Cullen and Barlow (2002a, 2002b) have had extremely promising results from teaching a 'touch therapy programme' (simple massage techniques) to parents of children with learning disabilities and autism. Parents reported improvements in their child's muscle tone, joint mobility, sleeping patters and bowel movements. When implementing massage for children in the community, children should always be approached with respect and openness and with an understanding of verbal and non-verbal cues to ensure that the contact is appropriate and respectful. It is also important that a parent or carer is present during the massage, unless the child is able to give consent to therapy in their own right and would be embarrassed at having a parent or carer present. In the main, children enjoy physical contact, but Horgan et al (1996) stress the importance of careful assessment of need, their body language and the relevant history. Children cannot usually tolerate long sessions and so a massage treatment, as with most other therapies, should be given over a short time, such as 30 minutes.

Case study 28.2

A boy aged 13 months, with profound global developmental delay as a result of a genetic abnormality, was offered massage. His mother gave permission and stayed close by as contact was made with him. As the massage proceeded, the child started to make very specific eye contact and demonstrated non-verbally his pleasure and seeming contentment with the contact (Harrison 1995). Particular attention was paid to his hands to encourage stretching of tight muscles. The mother was shown how to carry out the massage, which she performed several times a week. She was asked for her assessment of her son's responses to the massage. He had responded very well and she found it therapeutic and relaxing for both of them. Her son's hands relaxed sufficiently to allow him to pick up and grip toys which benefited his overall development.

VISUALISATION AND GUIDED IMAGERY

Creative visualisation is the technique of using thought processes for the purpose of improving a situation or resolving a problem in life (Payne 2000). A form of relaxed, focused concentration, visualisation can be used as a means of distraction such as before an intervention (Payne 2000). Guided imagery has been described as 'engaging the child's imagination and concentrating on a specific event to modify a particular response' (Doody et al 1991). Visualisation and guided imagery can be used to teach the child and parents relaxation techniques and can be useful coping strategies for children who have to undergo repeated invasive procedures (Turner et al 2002). These techniques can enable the child to cooperate with treatment, for example immunisations, venepuncture, bone marrow aspirations, biopsies and radiotherapy (Decker & Cline-Elsen 1992). Visualisation can easily be learned and used as an adjunct to the care of toddlers and pre-school children, as well as older children who are experiencing anxiety and pain, both acute and chronic (Bullock & Shaddy 1993, Oberlander 2001, Ott 1996). Self-esteem may be improved by enabling a child to see how they have coped positively with a difficult situation. Visualisation should not be used for those who are experiencing emotional instability. It can be harmful to those who are freely disassociating or acutely psychotic (Ott 1996, Payne 2000).

The therapist must prepare for visualisation in order to be relaxed, 'centred' and focused on the child and their needs. Parents should be informed of goals and permission for the visualisation obtained. The therapist should have an open and honest relationship with the child about the visualisation, listen to any expressed concerns and then help the child to re-focus anxiety to the goals and images.

CONCLUSION

CCNs can use complementary therapy techniques to encourage trust and coping behaviours in children and their carer(s), as identified by Pederson (1994). To apply complementary therapies effectively, sound education and skills acquisition through accredited organisations are required, together with access to supervision by experienced practitioners. For CCNs greater awareness of CTs can enhance children's health and well-being, empower parents and provide a wider range of care choices.

REFERENCES

Acolet D, Modi N, Giannakoulopoulos X, Bond C, Weg W, Clow A & Glover V 1993 Changes in plasma cortisol and catecholamine concentrations in response to massage in preterm infants. Archives of Disease in Childhood 68(suppl 1):29–31

Armishaw J & Grant C C 1999 Use of complementary treatment by those hospitalised with acute illness. Archives of Disease in Childhood 81(2):133–137

Atherton K 2001 In: Rankin-Box D (ed) The Nurses' Handbook of Complementary Therapies, 2nd edn. Churchill Livingstone, Edinburgh

Avis A 2003 Complementary Therapies in Nursing, Midwifery and Health Visiting Practice: RCN Guidance on Integrating Complementary Therapies into Clinical Care. Royal College of Nursing, London

Bayly D 1982 Reflexology Today – The Stimulation of the Body's Healing Forces Through Foot Massage. Thorsons, Wellingborough

Bishop E 2003 Reflexology in the management of encopresis and chronic constipation. Paediatric Nursing 15(3):20–21

Botting D A & Cook R 2000 Complementary medicine: knowledge and attitudes of doctors. Complementary Therapies in Nursing and Midwifery 6(1):41–47

British Medical Association (BMA) 1993 Complementary Medicine – New Approaches to Good Practice. BMA, London

Broide E, Pintov S, Portnoy S & Barg J 2001 Effectiveness of acupuncture for treatment of childhood constipation. Digestive Diseases and Sciences 46(6):1270

Brue A W & Oakland T D 2002 Alternative treatments for attention deficit disorder/hyperactivity: does evidence support their use? Alternative Therapies in Health and Medicine 8(1):68–74

Buckle S 2003 Aromatherapy and massage: the evidence. Paediatric Nursing 15(6):24–27

Bullock E A & Shaddy R E 1993 Relaxation and imagery techniques without sedation during right ventricular endomyocardial biopsy in pediatric heart transplant patients. Journal of Heart and Lung Transplantation 39:215–217

Burgess C 2001 Complementary therapies: guided imagery and infant massage. Paediatric Nursing 13(6):37–41

Cullen L & Barlow J 2002a Increasing touch between parents and children with disabilities. Journal of Family Health Care 12(1):7–9

Cullen L & Barlow J 2002b 'Kiss, cuddle, squeeze': the experiences and meaning of touch among parents of children with autism attending a touch therapy programme. Journal of Child Health Care 6(3):171–181

Davis M & Darden P M 2003 Use of complementary and alternative medicine by children in the United States. Archives of Pediatric and Adolescent Medicine 157(4):393–397

Decker T W & Cline-Elsen J 1992 Relaxation therapy as an adjunct in radiation oncology. Journal of Clinical Psychology 48:388–393

Department of Health 2001 Government response to the House of Lords Select Committee on Science and Technology's report on complementary and alternative medicine. CM5124. The Stationery Office, London

Doody S B, Smith C & Webb J 1991 Non-pharmacological intervention for pain management. Critical Care Nursing Clinics of North America 3(1):69–75

Ernst E 1999 Prevalence of complementary/alternative medicine for children: a systematic review. European Journal of Pediatrics 158(1):7–11

Ernst E 2001 Complementary and Alternative Medicine: an Evidence-based Approach. Mosby, Edinburgh

Ernst E & White A 2000 The BBC survey of complementary medicine use in the UK. Complementary Therapies in Medicine 8(1):32–36

Estabrooks C A 1992 Toward a theory of touch: the touching process and acquiring a touching style. Journal of Advanced Nursing 17:448–456

Fearon J 2003 Complementary therapies: knowledge and attitudes of health professionals. Paediatric Nursing 15(6):31–35

Field T, Morrow C, Valdeon C, Larson C, Kuhn S & Schanberg S 1992 Massage reduces anxiety in child and adolescent psychiatric patients. Journal of the American Academy of Child & Adolescent Psychiatry 31(1):125–131

Field T, Henteleff T, Hernandez-Reif M, Martinez E, Mavunda K, Kuhn C & Schanberg S 1998 Children with asthma have improved pulmonary function after massage. Journal of Pediatrics 132(5):854–858

Fowler P & Wall M 1997 COSHH and CHIPS: ensuring the safety of aromatherapy. Complementary Therapies in Medicine 5:112–115

Fritz S 1995 Fundamentals of Therapeutic Massage. Mosby Lifeline, New York

Gravett P 2000 Aromatherapy treatment of severe oral mucositis. The International Journal of Aromatherapy 10(1):52–53

Griffiths P 2001 Reflexology. In: Rankin-Box D (ed) The Nurses' Handbook of Complementary Therapies, 2nd edn. Churchill Livingstone, Edinburgh

Grootenhuis M A, Last B F, de Graaf-Nijerk J H & der Wel M 1998 Use of alternative treatment in paediatric oncology. Cancer Nurse 21(4):282–288

Harris P & Rees R 2000 The prevalence of complementary and alternative medicine use among the general population: a systematic review of the literature. Complementary Therapies in Medicine 8(2):88–96

Harrison J 1995 An introduction to aromatherapy for people with learning disabilities. British Journal of Learning Disabilities 23:37–40

Holey E & Cook E 2003 Evidence-based Therapeutic Massage, 2nd edn. Churchill Livingstone, Edinburgh

Horgan M, Choonara I, Al-Waidh M, Sambrooks J & Ashby D 1996 Measuring pain in neonates: an objective score. Paediatric Nursing 8(10):24–27

House of Lords 2000 Complementary and Alternative Medicine. Select Committee, Science and Technology. 6th report. The Stationery Office, London

Kemper K 2001 Complementary and alternative medicine for children: does it work? Archives of Disease in Childhood 84(1):6–10

Kemper K J & Wornham W L 2001 Consultations for holistic pediatric services for inpatients and outpatient oncology patients at the children's hospital. Archives of Pediatrics and Adolescent Medicine 155(4):449–454

Lee A C & Kemper K 2000 Homeopathy and naturopathy: practice characteristics and pediatric care. Archives of Pediatrics and Adolescent Medicine 154(1):75–80

Mantle F 1996 Eliminate the problem. Nursing Times 92(32):50–51

Nicoll L 1995 Complementary therapies and nurse education – the need for specialist teachers. Complementary Therapies in Nursing and Midwifery 1(3):60–72

Nursing and Midwifery Council (NMC) 2002 Code of Professional Conduct. NMC, London

Oberlander T F 2001 Pain assessment and management in infants and young children with developmental disabilities. Infants and Young Children 14(2):33–47

Olleveant N A, Humphris G & Roe B 1999 How big is a drop? A volumetric assay of essential oils. Journal of Clinical Nursing 8(1–3):299–304

Ott M J 1996 Imagine the possibilities! Guided imagery with toddlers and pre-schoolers. Paediatric Nursing 22(1):34–38

Payne R 2000 Relaxation Techniques, 2nd edn. Churchill Livingstone, Edinburgh

Pederson C 1994 Ways to feel comfortable: teaching aids to promote children's comfort. Issues in Comprehensive Pediatric Nursing 17:37–46

Pert C 1998 Molecules of Emotion. Simon & Schuster, London

Price L 1999 Carrier Oils for Aromatherapy and Massage, 3rd edn. Riverhead, Stratford-upon-Avon

Price S & Price Parr P 1996 Aromatherapy for Babies and Children. Thorsons, London

Prince of Wales Foundation for Integrated Health 2003 Setting the Agenda for the Future. The Prince of Wales Foundation for Integrated Health, London

Prince of Wales Foundation for Integrated Medicine 1998 Integrated Healthcare: a way forward for the next five years. Prince of Wales Foundation for Integrated Medicine, London

Richardson J 2001 Integrating complementary therapies into health care education: a cautious approach. Journal of Clinical Nursing 10(6):793–798

Royal College of Nursing (RCN) 1995 Complementary Therapies, Issues Series. Document 24. RCN, London

Sawni-Sikand A, Schubiner H & Thomas R L 2002 Use of complementary/alternative therapies among children in primary care pediatrics. Ambulatory Pediatrics 2(2):99–103

Scrace J 2003 Complementary therapies in palliative care: a literature review. Paediatric nursing 15(3):36–39

Sikand A & Laken M 1998 Pediatricians' experience with and attitudes toward complementary/alternative medicine. Archives of Pediatric and Adolescent Medicine 152(11):1059–1064

Simpson N & Roman K 2001 Complementary medicine use in children: extent and reasons. A population-based study. British Journal of General Practice. 51(472):914–916

Spigelblatt L, Laine-Ammara G, Pless B I & Guyver A 1994 The use of alternative medicine by children. Pediatrics 94(6):811–814

Stone J & Matthews J 1996 Complementary Medicine and the Law. Oxford University Press, Oxford

Tavares M 2003 National guidelines for the use of complementary therapies in supportive and palliative care. The Prince of Wales Foundation for Integrated Health, London

Tisserand R & Balacs T 1995 Essential Oil Safety – A Guide for Health Care Professionals. Churchill Livingstone, London

Turner M A, Unsworth V & David T J 2002 Intravenous long-lines in children with cystic fibrosis: a multi-disciplinary approach. Journal of the Royal Society of Medicine 95:11–22

Williams L 2003 Choosing a course in complementary healthcare: a student guide. Prince of Wales Foundation for Integrated Health, London

Worwood V A 2001 Aromatherapy for your Child. Thorsons, London

Zollman C & Vickers A 2000 ABC of Complementary Medicine. BMJ Books, London

Chapter 29

Nurse prescribing: an opportunity for community children's nursing

Mark Jones

KEY ISSUES

- Overview of the 20-year quest for nurse prescribing rights.
- Summary analysis of the Crown I and Crown II reports.
- Extended and Supplementary prescribing.
- Challenges facing community children's nurses should they wish to prescribe.

INTRODUCTION

Over 20 years ago the quest toward achieving prescribing rights began when a group of district nurses put their case to the Royal College of Nursing (RCN) (RCN 1978). The case was a logical and reasonable one, in that the nurses believed they had the knowledge base required to make prescribing decisions for a range of wound care products they used, and that time would be saved for both patients and the General Practitioners they had to harangue into signing off prescriptions for items that they did not really understand too well.

These basic tenets of knowledge base and competency, time saving and improved patient care have been at the centre of the nurse prescribing debate. A range of 'official' reports has supported the original stance that nurses who are competent should be able to prescribe from a specific formulary to meet their patients' care needs. The Cumberlege report (Department of Health and Social Security 1987) notably recommended to ministers that community nurses with a district nursing or health visiting qualification should be able to prescribe from a limited formulary. This was followed by the report of a Government review group specifically charged with the task of determining whether prescribing by nurses was a viable concept. The 'Crown report' (DoH 1989) once more endorsed the concept of prescribing by competent nurses with health visiting and district nursing qualifications. Crown suggested that these nurses should be able to 'prescribe' in three ways (Box 29.1).

Box 29.1 Proposals on nurse prescribing in the Crown report

■ Nurses could prescribe from a limited formulary as a medical practitioner would.
■ Nurses could alter the timing and dosage of administration of a medicine that had already been prescribed.
■ Nurses would be able to use a protocol to select medicines for administration from a list agreed with a medical practitioner prescriber.

Encouraged by these reports and ongoing examples of how nurses might benefit from prescribing, the RCN lobbied the Government to introduce legislation to allow nurses to prescribe. In a climate of Government reticence resulting from a burgeoning NHS drugs bill, the RCN used its political influence to encourage a Member of Parliament (MP), Roger Sims, to put forward a Private Member's Bill to facilitate nurse prescribing when he was given the opportunity to do so by Parliament (Gardener & Sims 1999). Before Sims presented his Bill, the RCN had primed MPs through an opinion poll and distribution of information supporting the nurse prescribing argument. Together with covert Government support, this lobby activity ensured the Sims Bill passed through Parliament, receiving Royal assent and entering the statute books as the Prescription of Medicinal Products by Nurses Etc. Act 1992.

PILOT SITES AND NATIONAL ROLL OUT

Even though the law had now been changed to allow nurses to prescribe it was not until Baroness Julia Cumberlege, a champion of nurse prescribing, became Junior Minister for Health that a series of pilot or 'demonstration' projects was set up. These pilots evaluated well and proved that nurses, with appropriate education and training, could prescribe effectively for their patients without increasing the drugs budget. The next move, therefore, was to have the Government extend the pilot projects to all eligible health visitors and district nurses.

Using the Government's own analysis of the pilot sites, the RCN argued that the ability of health visitors and district nurses to prescribe from their formulary without problem warranted extension of the scheme. Consequently, just before the Secretary of State for Health was to make a keynote address to the 1998 RCN congress, his office telephoned the author to ask how much this would cost and how many health visitors and district nurses would be involved. Time was pressing and a 'back of an envelope' calculation led to an insertion into the speech agreeing a budget of £14 million to extend the current model of prescribing.

WHY JUST DISTRICT NURSES AND HEALTH VISITORS?

The original case had been made by district nurses and a key factor was the time wasted having to hassle GPs into signing prescriptions. The general feeling was that community nurses would be best advantaged if allowed to prescribe given that they did not have the same access to medical colleagues as nurses working in acute-care environments. The Cumberlege report, with a remit only for community nursing, picked up on this theme (Department of Health and Social Security 1987). When Crown's team reported in 1989, they too considered prescribing only for community-based practitioners (DoH 1989). Both Cumberlege and Crown believed that prescribing should be reserved for nurses with post basic qualifications. At the time their work was carried out the only such qualifications existing in community practice were those of health visiting and district nursing. This is now recognised as being anachronistic, especially as there are now a range of specialist recordable qualifications in community practice, such as community children's nursing and practice nursing, in addition to those for health visiting and district nursing.

The area of 'hot debate' is, of course, whether nurses should be able to prescribe in their own right, without the sanction of another healthcare professional (i.e. medical practitioner). The second Crown review team considered this issue in some detail, and agreed with the evidence presented to it by the RCN (1997) that there was a case for competent nurses to be able to prescribe products to meet their patients' nursing care needs (DoH 1999).

EXTENDED PRESCRIBING

Bolstered by the success in achieving at least limited prescribing rights for those nurses having district nursing and health visiting qualifications, the nursing profession continued to lobby for these rights to be extended to other nurses. This culminated in the Medicines Control Agency (MCA) consultation on the possibility of extended prescribing rights to nurses working in areas of health promotion, palliative care, minor injuries and treating minor ailments (MCA 2001: MLX 273). These areas of practice were selected as, in the Government's opinion, they would gain most from prescribing nurses. The proposals also advocated adding: (i) in excess of 100 prescription-only medicines (POMs), (ii) pharmacy only (P) medicines and (iii) general sales list (GSL) medicines (relevant to the fields of practice above) to the nurse formulary. Despite some ardent lobbying against the inclusion of a handful of common antibiotics (with restricted use) in the proposed formulary, the consultation had a positive result.

However, it was not simply to be the case that existing nurse prescribers would get access to the new drugs and products. Rather, a new 25-day classroom-based course with 12 days learning in practice was devised for would-be 'extended nurse prescribers'. This course was open to all registered nurses including children's nurses, working in one of the above areas of practice, who could demonstrate a positive benefit for their patients should they become prescribers. The Government set a target of some 10 000 new extended prescribers to be trained by 2004.

SUPPLEMENTARY PRESCRIBING

Whilst the extension of prescribing rights to a wider range of nurses utilising a broader formulary was to be welcomed, the nursing profession still pointed out that much more could be done with an even wider formulary (e.g. RCN 2001). The Crown II review team had also proposed the second category of nurse prescriber, the dependent prescriber. Following further lobbying, the DoH was won over (DoH 2002) and the MCA consulted on the possibility of introducing this model of prescribing (MCA 2002: MLX 284). In the eyes of Government, this type of prescribing was to be seen as an adjunct to that of the medical practitioner and as such the Crown term 'dependent prescribing' was altered to 'supplementary prescribing'. Again the consultation responses were positive, and in the spring of 2003 it became legal for nurses to become supplementary prescribers. The educational requirement was to follow the same course as independent prescribers with an additional supplementary prescribing module. In effect this brought about the adoption of a generic 26-day theoretical course, including a 12-day practice-based programme, for all would-be nurse prescribers.

Supplementary prescribing is the model to which children's nurses should be turning to maximise their potential to improve healthcare for their patients. Unlike the independent prescribing model there are no real restrictions to the formulary for the supplementary model. At the time of going to press, controlled drugs were exempt along with unlicensed medicines. At the core of the supplementary prescribing model is a Clinical Management Plan (CMP) agreed between the supplementary nurse prescriber and independent prescribing doctor. It is the doctor's role to check that the diagnosis is correct (they do not necessarily have to make the diagnosis) and agree the nurse may take up the role of supplementary prescriber for the patient concerned. The CMP is drafted to indicate the category or class of medication that may be utilised with reference to local or national guidelines concerning the condition and care needs being addressed. Once the CMP is drafted and agreed the nurse is free to choose the appropriate medication, including dose, formulation, route of application, etc.

It should be clear that supplementary prescribing is only going to be of real benefit in chronic or enduring conditions. The effort involved in drafting the CMP makes this model inappropriate for acute care or 'one off' presentation episodes. The nurse who completes the nurse prescribing course today will:

- engage in mixed modality prescribing using independent prescriber competencies (when the formulary permits) to address immediate care needs
- use supplementary prescribing (once a CMP has been agreed) to deal with longer-term needs.

Although not prescribing per se, Patient Group Directions (PGDs) can still be used to supply and administer medication when the intricacy of a CMP is not required, although as more nurses train to be prescribers this model should be used less.

HOW DOES THIS APPLY TO THE COMMUNITY CHILDREN'S NURSE?

The challenge for all nurses wishing to prescribe will be to demonstrate the competencies required to justify either independent or supplementary prescribing rights. Aside from the need to be equipped with prescribing skills per se (pharmacological knowledge, ethics and accountability in prescribing, legal aspects of prescribing, etc.), CCNs will need to identify the attributes their particular speciality of nursing has to underpin their prescribing practice. Only those nurses who can demonstrate diagnostic and assessment ability will be considered for independent status. No doubt some CCNs fall into this category, but not all. Perhaps many more will qualify as supplementary prescribers as they find themselves in situations where they are sufficiently au fait with the drugs used to treat children in their care on a regular basis. In addition, they need to demonstrate the ability to alter dosages or prescribe medicines within the confines of a CMP agreed with an independent medical prescriber. Identifying the criteria by which some nurses (i) are independent prescribers, (ii) are supplementary prescribers, and (iii) have no prescribing rights at all, is a significant challenge for community healthcare nurses. It is essential that this process is completed in a coordinated way, leading to a high degree of consensus. If nurses cannot agree amongst themselves there will be little chance of convincing those who will determine their prescribing rights in the future.

A MOVING TARGET

Having dragged itself into existence over a two decade period despite interprofessional, intraprofessional and Government intransigence, developments in nurse prescribing are 'hotting up' and represent a fast-moving target. At the time of writing, the body which replaced the MCA in 2003, the Medicines and Healthcare Products Regulatory Agency (MHRA) was consulting, once again, on the extension of the independent nurse prescribers formulary (MHRA 2003: MLX 293). This consultation concerns proposals to add more drugs to the formulary in addition to widening the scope of prescribing practice. The drugs involved are not particularly relevant to paediatric practice but the proposal to allow nurses to prescribe 'off label' will set a useful precedent for children's nurses for the time when the formulary does include a more significant range of products associated with childhood conditions and illness.

CONCLUSION

Nurse prescribing is moving on apace. The extended nurse prescribers formulary is certainly more radical in content than that which is accessible to district nurses and health visitors who trained under the old model derived from the Crown recommendations. Supplementary prescribing no doubt reinforces the prejudice that specialist nurses still need to have the oversight of a medical practitioner, but it is certainly possible for children's nurses to maximise the potential of this model as they take up a more comprehensive role in the medicine management of their patients. With increased prescribing powers comes increased accountability for this significant new role. As the range of skills available to nurses is expanded so the expectations of the consumer will increase.

The securing of full independent prescribing rights for all CCNs cannot be guaranteed but at last there is an opportunity to pursue this expanded role, which should enhance the overall quality of care to children and their families. However, there are questions that still remain to be considered and answered (Box 29.2).

Box 29.2 Questions for consideration

- How will CCNs demonstrate the competencies required for independent or supplementary prescribing practice?
- What additional products should be included in the independent prescriber's formulary?
- Will patients and their carers accept prescribing by CCNs?
- What challenges might face the 'would be' prescriber?

REFERENCES

Department of Health 1989 Report of the advisory group on nurse prescribing (Crown report). Department of Health, London

Department of Health 1999 Review of prescribing, supply and administration of medicines. Final report (Chair Dr June Crown). Department of Health, London

Department of Health (DoH) 2002 Groundbreaking new consultation aims to extend prescribing powers for pharmacists and nurses. Press release: 2002/0189. DoH, London

Department of Health and Social Security 1987 Neighbourhood nursing – a focus for care (Cumberlege report). HMSO, London

Gardener E & Sims R 1999 Nurse prescribing – the lawmakers. In: Jones M (ed.) Nurse Prescribing – Politics to Practice. Baillière Tindall, London, p 67

Medicines Control Agency (MCA) 2001 Extended prescribing of prescription only medicines by independent nurse prescribers: Amendment to the Prescription Only Medicines (human use) Order 1997. MLX 273. MCA: London

Medicines Control Agency (MCA) 2002 Proposals for supplementary prescribing by nurses and pharmacists and proposed amendments to the Prescription Only Medicines (human use) Order 1997. MLX 284. MCA, London

Medicines and Healthcare Products Regulatory Agency (MHRA) 2003 Nurse prescribers extended formulary: proposals to extend range of prescription only medicines. Nurse prescribers extended formulary: proposals to amend requirements as to use, route of administration, or pharmaceutical form of prescription only medicines. Proposal to amend article 12 of the prescription only medicines (human use) order 1997 to include independent nurse prescribers and supplementary prescribers and consequential amendment to the medicines (pharmacy and general sale – exemption) order 1980. MHRA, London

Royal College of Nursing (RCN) 1978 District nurses dressings. Report to the Community Nursing Association. RCN, London

Royal College of Nursing (RCN) 1997 Review of prescribing, supply and administration of medicines. Update on the evidence submitted by the Royal College of Nursing. Unpublished evidence to the Crown II review. RCN, London

Royal College of Nursing (RCN) 2001 Extension of prescribing rights for nurses: Comments to the Department of Health from the RCN of the UK. RCN, London

Chapter 30

The Advanced Children's Nurse Practitioner within General Practice

Tracey Malkin

KEY ISSUES
- Development of advanced children's nursing roles in primary care.
- Characteristics of the Advanced Children's Nurse Practitioner role.
- Implications for nurse-led services in the community.
- Opportunities for community children's nursing.

INTRODUCTION

Nurse-led services within primary care are well established (Fulton & Philips 1998) and endorsed by the Chief Nursing Officer's ten key roles for nursing (DoH 2002). However, developing such initiatives within community children's nursing is a new phenomenon. This chapter describes the development of a nurse-led service for the child population of a general practice. The Advanced Children's Nurse Practitioner (ACNP), with enhanced nursing skills in health assessment and physical examination, provides an accessible and holistic primary health care service for the 0–16-year-old population and their families. Whilst the drive for this initiative was based on local health need it reflected the modernisation agenda of the NHS (DoH 1997).

DEVELOPMENT OF NURSE-LED SERVICES IN THE UK

The growth of nurse-led services in the UK has been informed by a number of political, professional and educational influences (Muir & Burnett 2000).

Political

Healthcare reforms of the 1990s contributed to the position of General Practitioners (GPs) as gatekeepers of health provision with incentives to consider more effective and efficient means of delivering healthcare to their clients (DoH 1989a, 1992). Reducing doctor's hours provided similar opportunities in ambulatory and acute care settings (Calman 1993). More recently, the drive for developing nurse-led initiatives is endorsed by the current Government's agenda to strengthen the contribution of nurses to healthcare delivery (DoH 1999a).

Professional

The UK Central Council (UKCC 1992) in the publication of 'The Scope of Professional Practice' positively encouraged autonomous practice as the expansion and enhancement of nursing roles, based on locally identified need, whilst recognising limitations in one's own practice. Subsequently, new powers of prescribing for nurses (DoH 1989b, 1999b) have gained momentum, providing a much needed professional basis on which to develop nurse-led initiatives even further (see Chapter 29).

Educational

Concomitant to both professional and political influences, educational establishments have taken the opportunity to develop new programmes in preparation for, and in response to, the number of 'new roles' emerging (Gibson 1998).

EXAMPLE OF AN ACNP ROLE

The role of an ACNP was initiated in 1997 by a practice of GPs to enhance the service they provided to their child population. The local community Trust was approached for guidance as to how they should proceed with an initiative to deliver a nurse-led package of primary care to children aged 0–16 years and their families. The vision was to build on the traditions of health visiting whilst utilising the additional nursing skills and expertise of the practitioner in post, a newly qualified Health Visitor (HV) with the Registered Sick Children's Nurse qualification. This role would require enhancement of these specialist skills in order to provide care that met the holistic needs of the child and family presenting with acute minor ailments and chronic illnesses and to facilitate their health awareness through child health promotion and surveillance.

The general practice already had experience and confidence in the Nurse Practitioner concept that originated in America in the early 1960s (Ashburner et al 1997). The GPs were committed to developing a Nurse Practitioner role specialising in child health. Although advanced children's nursing roles in the UK were being developed such as Neonatal Nurse Practitioners (Smith et al 1994), Children's Emergency Nurse Practitioners (Bedford et al 1992, Curry 1994) and condition-specific Children's Nurse Specialists (Jones 1995) there was little UK literature on a role specific to children's nursing within general practice. Therefore the development of this initiative was modeled on the American role of Pediatric Nurse Practitioners (Hamric 1996), a forerunner for their advanced nursing practice (Hoekelman 1998), with the intention of increasing access to primary care for children and their families.

With support from both the GPs and the community Trust the ACNP role developed to provide holistic healthcare through the continuum of health and illness. The role includes:

- assessment and diagnosis, planning care and treatment of undifferentiated acute minor ailments
- child health surveillance to facilitate growth and development

- health education/emotional support for teenage practice population
- health promotion
- coordination/monitoring/support care for children/families with chronic complex health conditions
- advocacy/empowering to retain independence
- assessing/planning/implementing behaviour/parenting management interventions.

The ACNP management of acute minor illness, child health surveillance, chronic complex conditions, teenage health and health promotion and the support of parenting skills are discussed individually.

Acute minor illness

The ACNP is educated and assessed in advanced skills in physical examination and assesses, diagnoses, treats and evaluates care for children who present with acute, undifferentiated, minor ailments independently of medical intervention (Box 30.1).

Box 30.1 Examples of minor ailments treated

▪ Upper respiratory tract infections	Tonsillitis
▪ Ear ache	Conjunctivitis
▪ Eczema	Scabies
▪ Rashes	Impetigo
▪ Constipation	Gastroenteritis
▪ Urinary tract infections	Acute abdomen
▪ Vomiting	Fevers
▪ Minor trauma	Muscle strains

The ACNP independently prescribes from the extended nurse prescriber's formulary. This facilitates a seamless care and treatment experience for the child and family without requiring a GP's authorisation for prescription medicines. When prescription-only medicines are not included in the nurses' extended formulary the ACNP generates the prescription for a GP to sign.

During consultations the ACNP is in a position to educate the child and family on acute minor ailment management, potentially reducing visits to the GP, reducing the need for prescriptions and increasing the independence of the child and family. In the event of a child presenting with a condition unfamiliar to or outside the scope and clinical competence of the ACNP there is always a 'duty' GP on hand to see these children. Here the ACNP will accompany the child and family into the consultation. This further develops the ACNP's assessment and diagnostic skills and facilitates support should any queries or concerns arise from the medical consultation at a later date.

Child health surveillance and health promotion

Child health surveillance and health promotion are within the domain of health visiting for the 0–5-year-old population (DoH 1999a). The ACNP ensures that child health surveillance, developmental screening and health promotion are integral to every aspect of the role. Continuity for the child and family is achieved by the ACNP taking on the physical examination aspect of current child surveillance requirements alongside providing parenting support, health education and a routine health visiting service. For children aged 4–16 years, when concerns arise on aspects of their development, the ACNP can undertake an advanced health and development assessment to ascertain the degree of difficulties. Appropriate timely referrals are made to relevant personnel whilst continuing to support the child and family.

Health education is considered as a continual healthcare need and can be addressed by the ACNP for the 0–5-year-olds and older, empowering children and families to engage in health-enhancing activities through to their teenage years and into early adulthood (see Chapter 13).

Management of chronic and complex conditions

This aspect of the ACNP's workload focuses on patient education toward self-management and monitoring and evaluating the intervention of problems that are predominantly managed in primary care. Conditions may include asthma, epilepsy and food intolerance or allergy.

For children where treatment is initiated and managed by tertiary care services the ACNP acts as a link person between the child's GP and other services involved. In addition the ACNP monitors their condition, growth and development, ensures medication compliance and engages in health education whilst supporting and acting as advocate for the child and family. Acting as a coordinator of care the ACNP ensures continuity of care, effective communication and a well-informed child and family.

Teenage health

The teenage population, aged 13–16 years, are routinely offered health checks at the surgery to include health screening and health education. Specific activities include the provision of sexual health and contraception advice, emergency contraception counselling and prescribing according to the practice protocol. The ACNP can also offer emotional and psychosocial support to teenagers experiencing difficulties with bullying, stress, relationship issues, low self-esteem, etc. Teenagers are encouraged to access these services independently of parents or carers if they wish. Parents (or carers) together with teenagers are encouraged to access the service when there are concerns for the teenager's health and welfare resulting from risk-taking behaviours. Transitional care issues for adolescents experiencing more complex health conditions are addressed through joint consultations. Where adult specialist services are required, liaison and support is given to the young person and their family in order to assist transition to adult services (see Chapter 32).

Parenting and behaviour management

Parents with children experiencing behavioural problems may seek support from their GP or HV. The ACNP can offer advice, help and support on parenting and behaviour management for the 0–4-year-olds as part of routine health visiting activities. For children over the age of 5 years, the ACNP continues to provide advice, help and support following health and psychosocial assessment. Referral to and liaison with the necessary multi-agency teams can be initiated and maintained. Behaviour management care plans are negotiated with the child and family for problems such as sleep difficulties, enuresis and/or encopresis, temper tantrums and/or defiant and risk-taking behaviours and school avoidance.

SERVICE OUTCOMES

The first-phase findings of a research dissertation into the ACNP role described were obtained using focus group interviews (T Malkin, unpublished work, 2001). In these interviews professionals who worked directly with the ACNP or with the same client population, were asked to explore the development of the ACNP role, share their perceptions of how the role could be interpreted as a nurse-led service and highlight potential benefits of having an ACNP in general practice. The themes that emerged are detailed below.

GPs

- Role has the potential to cover an array of health-related issues common to the childhood population.
- This changes what GPs do in relation to their direct input with the practice's childhood population.
- Role allows the GP more time for the ever-growing complexities of adult healthcare needs.

Other nursing professionals

- Awareness of collaboration, communication and coordination between the multi-agency teams involved with children and their families.
- Concerns on the potential for the ACNP role to overlap with others.
- Deskilling of others as the role of the ACNP was seen as all encompassing.
- They would utilise the ACNP as a knowledgeable resource in the future.
- Acknowledge the ACNP as a clinical leader in child health practices.

This phase of the research did not extend to exploring the views of the children and their families. However, the health professionals interviewed expressed their view on how the child and family might benefit from the role (Box 30.2).

Box 30.2 Benefits for the child and family

- Increased access to care at primary care level
- Child- and family-centred care
- Holistic care
- An advocate for the child and family
- Continuity of care
- A coordinated approach to care
- Timely access to support and advice
- A resource with expertise in child health

PROFESSIONAL ISSUES

Training and competence

Advanced nursing practice roles do not evolve by the nurse merely taking on new enhanced clinical skills but by being able to demonstrate autonomous practice, higher-level clinical decision-making skills and clinical leadership in their field of practice (Ludder-Jackson 1995). There also remains disparity in the academic underpinning required to give credibility to such roles, as well as inconsistencies in the nature of care that these roles take on (Gibson 1998). Given the nature and specialist focus of the described ACNP role, the expected level of autonomy and decision-making skills required, the practitioner, local community Trust and GPs considered the nurse should be educated to Masters degree level. The practitioner's prior experience, knowledge and skill base were essential to the developing role together with additional skills in advanced health assessment, physical examination and prescribing. Clinical credibility with medical and nursing colleagues are underpinned by clearly defined practice protocols.

Accountability and liability

Accountability, competency and confidence in practice, within the code of professional practice and the law, are the personal and professional responsibility of the individual nurse (Nursing and Midwifery Council 2002).

Organisational responsibilities

Clinical support in the form of Clinical Supervision and Continuing Professional Development is coordinated between the ACNP, a GP mentor from within the practice and the community Trusts' system for personal review. This is essential for the ACNP to continue to gain new knowledge, develop competence, assume responsibility for their own practice and ensure the protection and safety of children and their families in complex clinical situations (NHS Management Executive 1993).

Future opportunities for the ACNP role

The ACNP as an extension of health visiting is invoking interest as an alternative way forward for meeting the needs of children and their families within General Practice. Anecdotal evidence suggests that the skills and practice of an ACNP can be modelled by primary care nursing services that provide healthcare to children and families, for example Community Children's Nurses (CCNs). ACNPs and CCNs share a philosophy of care that embraces a child- and family-centred and holistic approach to care. Both place an emphasis on the prevention of ill health through health education/promotion activities and supporting and providing nursing care interventions in the event of ill health. They aim to minimise the impact of illness on the child and family in order for them to realise their full health potential. CCNs could expand their role to meet the additional health needs of children and families on their existing case loads (Ludder-Jackson 2000).

CONCLUSION

This chapter outlines a model of advanced nursing practice developed to meet the needs of a child population in a GP practice. Aspects of the role are described to demonstrate the value of this nurse-led initiative for children and their families, health professionals and service providers.

The practical skills of advanced health assessment, physical examination, prescribing and enhanced clinical decision-making skills can be acquired by CCNs to address current issues in access to care. These include reducing hospital admissions and the shortage of medical practitioners (Calman 1993, DoH 2000). The role of the ACNP would appear to challenge the traditional boundaries of nursing and medicine and pave the way towards a new focus for nurse-led services.

REFERENCES

Ashburner L, Birch K, Latimer J & Scrivens E 1997 Nurse Practitioners in Primary Care: The Extent of Practice and Research. Center for Health Planning & Management. Keele University

Bedford H, Jenkins J, Shore C & Kenny P 1992 Use of an East End Children's Accident and Emergency Department for infants. Failure of Primary Health Care? Quality Health Care l(1):29–33

Calman K 1993 Hospital Doctors: Training for the Future. HMSO, London

Curry J 1994 Nurse practitioners in the emergency department, current issues. Journal of Emergency Nursing 6(3):11–14

Department of Health 1989a Working for Patients. HMSO, London

Department of Health 1989b Report of the advisory group on nurse prescribing (Crown Report). HMSO, London

Department of Health 1992 The patients charter. HMSO, London

Department of Health 1997 The new NHS. Modern, Dependable. The Stationery Office, London

Department of Health 1999a Making a Difference. The Stationery Office, London

Department of Health 1999b Review of Prescribing, Supply and Administration of Medicines. Final Report. The Stationery Office, London

Department of Health 2000 The NHS Plan. A Plan for Investment, A Plan for Reform. The Stationery Office, London

Department of Health 2002 Liberating the Talents. Helping Primary Care Trusts and Nurses to Deliver the NHS Plan. The Stationery Office, London

Fulton Y & Philips P 1998 Nurse-led clinics in ambulatory care. In: Glasper E A & Lawson S (eds) Innovations in Ambulatory Care. Macmillan. London

Gibson F 1998 The Development of Advancing Clinical Practice Role within Paediatric Nursing. The Florence Nightingale Foundation, London

Hamric A 1996 A definition of advanced nursing practice. In Hamric A B, Spross J A & Hanson C M (eds) Advanced Nursing Practice: An Integrated Approach. W B Saunders, Philadelphia

Hoekelman R A 1998 Commentary on a program to increase health care for children. The pediatric nurse practitioner program. Pediatrics June Supplement: 245–247

Jones S 1995 The development of the paediatric nurse specialist. British Journal of Nursing 4(1):34–36

Ludder-Jackson P L 1995 Advanced practice nursing – Part 2: Opportunities and challenges for PNPs. Pediatric Nursing 21(1):43–46

Ludder-Jackson P L 2000 Advancing community children's nursing. In: Muir J & Sidey A (eds) Textbook for Community Children's Nursing. Baillière Tindall, Edinburgh, pp 263–271

Muir J & Burnett C 2000 Opportunities for development of nurse-led clinics in community children's nursing. In Muir J & Sidey A (eds) Textbook for Community Children's Nursing. Baillière Tindall, Edinburgh, pp 272–278

National Health Service Management Executive 1993 A Vision for the Future. HMSO, London

Nursing and Midwifery Council (NMC) 2002 Code of Professional Conduct. NMC, London

Smith S, Roch S & Hall M 1994 Neonatal nurse practitioners, delivering further education. Paediatric Nursing 4(2):65–69

UK Central Council for Nursing, Midwifery and Health Visiting (UKCC) 1992 The Scope of Professional Practice. UKCC, London

Chapter 31

Economic evaluation in practice

Caroline Fitzgerald and Tara Davis

KEY ISSUES

- Clarifying the terminology.
- Examining the role of economic evaluation in community children's nursing.
- Considerations for the Community Children's Nurse.

INTRODUCTION

The NHS is undergoing significant change with recent Government initiatives placing particular importance on high-quality care. These include the development of the National Service Framework (the Children's Taskforce), Clinical Governance and the introduction of bodies such as the National Institute for Clinical Excellence. Economic evaluation of health services is an integral part of the Government's quality agenda within the 10-year modernisation initiative (DoH 1998). The concept of clinical effectiveness aims to ensure that services are effective in terms of result and cost. Whilst there will be continuing budgetary restraints, quality is central and clinicians will be required to ensure that the services they provide are appropriate, effective, efficient and economic (DoH 1998).

With the responsibility for commissioning local services now held by Primary Care Trusts (PCTs), Community Children's Nurses (CCNs) will need to be able to demonstrate the effectiveness and efficiency of the services they provide to children, their families and the communities in which they work. This chapter examines the ways in which economic evaluations can inform and influence nursing services for children in the community. Integral to this is the part played by the CCN and some of the issues affecting their role are examined.

CLARIFYING THE TERMINOLOGY

Economic evaluation is the comparative analysis of alternative courses of action in terms of both their costs and the consequences (Drummond et al 1987). Robinson (1993a) describes it as drawing up a balance sheet of the advantages (benefits) and disadvantages (costs) associated with each option so that choices can be made. Economic evaluation (Box 31.1) is only one dimension of the overall evaluation process (Robinson 1993a, Kobelt 2002) and Thomas and Bond (1995) concluded that it is unacceptable to evaluate an intervention without also addressing the cost implications. As such, clinical governance is one way through which organisations can ensure they are providing high-quality, cost-effective care (DoH 1998).

Box 31.1 Glossary of terms commonly used in economic evaluation

- **Costs:** salaries/equipment, etc. and any deleterious effects of a programme
- **Effectiveness:** measure of how successfully or otherwise activities are being undertaken
- **Efficiency:** ensuring best resource is used to provide maximum benefit to client
- **Cost–benefit analysis:** often used to describe all economic evaluations, method in which alternative programmes are compared and costs/benefits valued in monetary terms. Attributing a monetary value to healthcare outcomes is not easy and cost effectiveness analysis is often preferred (Robinson 1993b, Wilson–Barnett & Beech 1994)
- **Cost effectiveness analysis:** employed when costs/consequences of alternative programmes are compared; costs valued in money while common effect measured in natural units (e.g. symptom-free day/ life saved)

ROLE OF ECONOMIC EVALUATION IN COMMUNITY CHILDREN'S NURSING

Effective management should ensure efficiency, quality and accessibility of the service, whilst operating within finite budgetary limits (see Chapter 15 p 180). The allocation of resources needs to be evaluated to ensure that the right service is being provided to the right people at the right cost. Often, services are measured in terms of target numbers, such as number of visits or waiting times. Whilst these may provide some measurable information, they do not fully reflect the volume or complexity of the service, nor are the quality issues addressed (see Chapter 19).

Economic evaluation may be used to assess whether the best use is being made of the resources available, for example when deciding whether to introduce a screening programme or in conjunction with clinical trials. However, the principles of an economic appraisal can be incorporated into an evaluation of a local service or team. Such studies may influence managers in their decisions to continue funding specific projects or they may demonstrate ways in which savings can be made.

New ways of funding community children's nursing services, such as the Diana Teams and those funded by the New Opportunities Fund (NOF), demand that economic evaluation forms part of the overall appraisal process (NOF 2002). The need to demonstrate cost effectiveness alongside other benefits of these pilot projects is vital to ensure that services continue with mainstream funding. Furthermore, demonstrating high-quality, cost-effective community children's nursing services and the dissemination of such information is paramount in developing a theoretical evidence base in an area of nursing which to date has been neglected. As stated by the Health Committee (1997 para 49 p xix): 'We very much regret that no research has ever been conducted into the most cost-effective way of providing the nursing service that children and their carers in the community need.'

Tierney (1993) suggested that tackling the complexities of cost effectiveness research is one of the greatest challenges for nurses. However, these difficulties must be overcome because a lack of data assessing costs and benefits exposes the vulnerability of nurses and nursing in decisions about healthcare financing (International Council of Nurses 1992, Buchan et al 1996) (see Chapters 17 and 19). The difficulties associated with measuring the effectiveness and the outcomes of nursing include distinguishing what exactly it is that nurses do, how this is separated from the input of other disciplines and measuring the success of an intervention that may occur once client contact has ceased (Thomas & Bond 1995, Buchan et al 1996, Lock 1996).

In Bradley's (1997) comprehensive review of community nursing services for children she noted that, while such services offer high-quality care, financial constraints and funding problems may be a threat. It is vital that CCNs demonstrate ways in which their services are beneficial, not only to children and families, as reported in the literature (Bishop et al 1994, Jennings 1994), but also to commissioners of services (Hennessy 1993, Brocklehurst 1996).

In community work, significant time is spent working in areas such as supporting families and their children, health promotion and accident prevention, the impact and long-term effects of which are particularly difficult to demonstrate (Robinson & Hill 1998, Naidoo & Wills 2000). In community children's nursing the psychosocial and other benefits for the child and family are well documented but may be hard to quantify. Financial savings by reducing numbers of hospital beds will not be a reality in the short term (Coast et al 1998, Bagust et al 2002). The establishment of schemes is more likely to increase expenditure initially (While 1991, Royal College of Nursing 1994). Coast et al (1998) compared the mean cost between hospital at home and hospital care and found the hospital at home scheme to be less costly. Although the study focused on elderly patients the authors suggest that the results may be generalised to other hospital at home schemes. Bagust et al (2002) compared the privately borne costs and NHS costs of hospital at home and inpatient care for children with three selected acute conditions. They found that costs to families were reduced but that costs to the NHS were similar. As this was a hospital at home service the limitations of this study include: (i) the specific acute nature of the children's conditions and (ii) it did not include the wide range of both acute and chronic conditions more normally seen by CCNs.

Ways in which community children's nursing services are provided vary widely across the country and the model of hospital at home schemes for children remains few in number (see Chapters 15 and 21). There has been little research evaluating different models of community children's nursing services, either in terms of clinical or cost effectiveness. Eaton (2000) identified the need to evaluate the quality of care delivered, and establish effective models of care provision, in the context of evidence-based healthcare. She discussed the main components important when implementing and evaluating models. A minimum standard for cost effectiveness should be that services are delivered with at least the same cost as hospital services and with high-quality care. It is desirable that services will cost less than hospital services whilst still providing high-quality care (Eaton 2000).

Although the scheme evaluated by While (1991) increased the cost of children's care, because the inpatient bed complement remained unchanged, she was theoretically able to demonstrate cost effectiveness. By calculating the bed nights saved (reported to be 573) and comparing hospital costs with the costs of CCN visits, she proposed that substantial savings could be made. This contrasts with the service evaluated by Jennings (1994), where bed numbers were reduced at the team's inception, thereby reducing costs. A summary of 11 related studies is provided by Whiting et al (2001). Other important benefits, such as child and parent satisfaction and reduced anxiety are well documented (While 1991, Jennings 1994, Bagust et al 2002).

The recent emergence of a primary-care-led NHS and the advent of Children's Trusts, are providing CCNs with opportunities to influence how services are provided. Within this associated financial climate, CCNs may be competing with other services for commissioning. An extensive study of CCN provision found that services are poorly understood and in some cases not welcomed (Procter et al 1998) and it is the responsibility of CCNs and their managers to articulate what it is they do, how much it costs and how effective the service is (see Chapters 16 and 19).

Quality is high on the Government's agenda, and those interventions for which there is good evidence of clinical and cost effectiveness will be promoted (DoH 1998). Demonstrating effectiveness in terms of result and cost will not only help to ensure continued funding of current schemes but act as leverage to set up new schemes. There are still many children in the UK who do not have access to a CCN and the Government has stated that unacceptable variations in services across the country will be addressed (DoH 1997). Undertaking economic appraisals is one way in which CCNs can influence resource allocation and decision making. Whilst complex, there are an increasing number of people with the necessary expertise to help in undertaking such a project (Brocklehurst 1996).

Contributing to financial debates is a further way in which CCNs can impact on decision making. With their unique knowledge and experience they can enhance debates by articulating the quality issues of the services they provide and by representing the viewpoints of children and families they will fulfil client-advocate responsibilities. CCNs must develop budgetary knowledge and skills to meet new challenges associated with the devolvement of budgets, appropriate use of skill mix and the increasing demand for economic evaluation. While commissioners may wish to select the cheaper option, professional arguments in favour of the positive benefits associated with the higher costs could be made.

An appreciation of economic terminology and methodology will enable nurses to recognise whether studies are valid and will increase confidence for participating in debates and for undertaking their own studies. Continuing education opportunities will empower nurses to contribute to this aspect of evaluation (International Council of Nurses 1992, Shamian 1997).

EXAMPLES FROM PRACTICE

Three examples are offered from the author's own previous practice experience:

1. The community children's nursing team demonstrated cost effectiveness by calculating the number of inpatient bed nights saved for children who were discharged early to complete their course of intravenous (IV) antibiotics at home. The one major dimension for the measurement of success, which Drummond et al (1987) suggest is necessary for a cost-effectiveness analysis, is 'bed nights saved'. The cost of the inpatient night was compared with the cost of visits by CCNs. The main motive for community IV treatment should be better care, not simply a reduction in costs (Nathwani & Davey 1996). The provision of the community children's nursing service improved care by facilitating earlier discharge and for some children on long-term medication this enabled a return to school. The conclusion was that the service was cost-effective: there were substantial savings to the hospitals, particularly where children were prescribed once- or twice-daily drugs. In addition the earlier discharge allowed increased bed usage. Clinical effectiveness was demonstrated in terms of both result (early discharge) and cost (savings to hospitals). These findings seem to support those of While (1991). However, because of the influence of local factors upon cost effectiveness, generalisation should be cautionary. The wide variation of visiting costs reported by Jennings (1994) and Whiting et al (2001) illustrate how great local variations can be.

2. CCNs planned to introduce geographical caseloads. There had been no specific division to date but, as the team grew, it was agreed that the change might offer a more efficient service, in terms of reducing travelling time and improving links with primary healthcare teams. Mooney (1992) suggests that cost effectiveness analysis can demonstrate how best to deploy a given budget to meet a particular objective. Whilst the principal aim was not to reduce expenditure, the team's travel budget needed to be used to best effect. The measurements used in the evaluation were:
   - mileage claims
   - travelling times
   - numbers of children visited before and after the change.

     Whilst numbers of children do not encompass quality, they are a measurable indicator and one that was dictated by the purchasers.

A review of the literature to identify previous studies that had examined caseload organisation in community nursing teams revealed little evidence of this type of evaluation. Savings of £50 000 in travelling expenses were cited in one area when nurses began working in defined boundaries (Wilson & Brown 1989). Economic evaluations are specific to a population or location (Edwardson 1992, Muir Gray 1997) and whilst other studies may have been useful they would not necessarily have related to this team. This study did show that the travel budget could be used more effectively as both mileage claims and travelling times were lower. Since less time was spent travelling there was more time available for client contact. The numbers of visits continued to meet contract requirements. Additional effectiveness indicators included an increase in referrals from primary healthcare teams, suggesting improved links and better knowledge of the service, and nurses' knowledge of the local areas improved. The study was limited in that consideration was not given to other organisational styles such as the nurses holding specialist caseloads.

3. The third example is based on anecdotal experience and relates to the provision of continuing care for children with complex needs. This enhanced role of the CCN has been brought about in part by increasing numbers of children with complex and/or technological needs and a greater focus on caring for these children at home (Kirk 1999). For some families the provision of an appropriate package of care may help to promote normality of family functioning, maintain family dynamics and prevent inappropriate hospitalisation used for respite. Care packages may take the form of short breaks away from home and/or care at home, and may be provided by a trained carer or qualified nurse depending on the needs of the child and the views of the parents (Miller 2002, Olsen & Maslin-Prothero 2001). The CCN is required to assess, propose and cost a package of care and negotiate this with health commissioners, social services and education departments. It has been suggested that funding disagreements are common and an additional source of parental stress (Glendinning et al 2001, Kirk 1999). The CCN is able to use professional and clinical skills and examine nursing need and cost of care to obtain and coordinate the most appropriate care package for individual families whilst working with finite resources. This example demonstrates how recommendations made by the CCN can influence budgetary issues and therefore the need to be aware of healthcare economics.

CONCLUSION

Economic evaluation is just one aspect of the evaluation process and one that has not been widely undertaken in relation to nursing services in this country. High quality and cost effectiveness are central to the Government's 'new NHS' (DoH 1997) and nurses will increasingly be required to articulate arguments and proposals in economic as well as professional terms. For community children's nursing to continue to develop and progress, practitioners should include an economic perspective in service evaluations. This will help to ensure that:

- benefits and outcomes are considered in relation to costs
- services are adequately resourced
- economic evaluation is part of the decision-making process when services are being planned and reviewed
- a knowledge base about the value of nursing emerges.

Some of the difficulties include:

- measuring and quantifying nursing outcomes
- generalisability
- financial data may not demonstrate cost effectiveness but the supportive evidence relating to benefits should override this.

Implications for CCNs include:

- requirement of an understanding of the terminology to enable participation in the process
- critical analysis of economic evaluations
- application of the principles to practice
- the need to demonstrate and articulate the effectiveness and efficiency of the quality services being provided through (i) research studies, (ii) service evaluations, (iii) contributions to debates and (iv) participation in decisions about resource allocation.

Given the recommendations that the 'Department of Health should monitor for effectiveness and cost-effectiveness the various local models and structures which currently exist, so that improved advice and guidance can be given to purchasers and providers' (Health Committee 1997 para 49 p xix), it is necessary for CCNs to evaluate the services they are providing and demonstrate clinical effectiveness in terms of both outcomes and cost.

REFERENCES

Bagust A, Haycox A, Sartain S A, Maxwell M J & Todd P 2002 Economic evaluation of an acute paediatric hospital at home clinical trial. Archives of Disease in Childhood 87 (6):489–492

Bishop J, Anderson A & McCulloch J 1994 Hospital-at-home: a critical analysis. Paediatric Nursing 6(6):12–15

Bradley S F 1997 Better late than never? An evaluation of community nursing services for children in the UK. Journal of Clinical Nursing 6:411–418

Brocklehurst N 1996 Selling children's community nursing. Paediatric Nursing 8(9):6–7

Buchan J, Seccombe I & Ball J 1996 Caring Costs Revisited. Institute for Employment Studies, Brighton

Coast J, Richards S H, Peters T J, Gunnell D J, Darlow M & Pounsford J 1998 Hospital at home or acute hospital care? A cost minimisation analysis. British Medical Journal 316:1802–1806

Department of Health 1997 The new NHS. Modern, dependable. The Stationery Office, London

Department of Health 1998 A first class service: quality in the new NHS. The Stationery Office, London

Drummond M F, Stoddart G L & Torrance G W 1987 (reprinted 1995) Methods for the Economic Evaluation of Health Care Programmes. Oxford University Press, Oxford

Eaton N 2000 Children's community nursing service: models of care delivery. A review of the United Kingdom literature. Journal of Advanced Nursing 32(1):49–56

Edwardson S R 1992 Costs and benefits of clinical nurse specialists. Clinical Nurse Specialist 6(3):163–167

Glendinning C, Kirk S, Guiffrida A & Lawton D 2001 Technology-dependent children in the community: definitions, numbers and costs. Child: Care, Health and Development 27(4):321–334

Health Committee 1997 House of Commons Select
Committee. Health services for children and young
people in the community: home and school. Third
report. The Stationery Office, London

Hennessy D 1993 Purchasing community nursing care.
Paediatric Nursing 5(2):10–12

International Council of Nurses (ICN) 1992 Costing
nursing services. Report of the ICN Task Force on
Costing of Nursing Services. ICN, London

Jennings P 1994 Learning through experience: an
evaluation of hospital at home. Journal of Advanced
Nursing 19:905–911

Kirk S 1999 Caring for children with specialized health
care needs in the community: the challenges for
primary care. Health and Social Care in the
Community 7(5):350–357

Kobelt G 2002 Health Economics: An Introduction to
Economic Evaluation. Office of Health Economics,
London

Lock K 1996 The changing organisation of health care:
setting the scene. In: Twinn S, Roberts B & Andrews S
(eds) Community Health Care Nursing: Principles for
Practice. Butterworth Heinemann, Oxford, Ch. 2, p 30

Miller S 2002 Respite care for children who have complex
healthcare needs. Paediatric Nursing 14(5):33–37

Mooney G 1992 Economics, Medicine and Health Care,
2nd edn. Harvester Wheatsheaf, London

Muir Gray J A 1997 Evidence-based Healthcare.
Churchill Livingstone, New York

Naidoo J & Wills J 2000 Health Promotion, 2nd edn.
Baillière Tindall, London

Nathwani D & Davey P 1996 Intravenous antimicrobial
therapy in the community: underused, inadequately
resourced, or irrelevant to health care in Britain?
British Medical Journal 313:1541–1543

New Opportunities Fund (NOF) 2002 Palliative Care for
Children Programme: Guidance notes. NOF, London

Olsen R & Maslin-Prothero P 2001 Dilemmas in the
provision of own-home respite support for
parents of young children with complex health care

needs: evidence from an evaluation. Journal of
Advanced Nursing 34(5):603–610

Procter S, Campbell S, Biott C, Edward S, Redpath N &
Moran M 1998 Preparation for the Developing Role of
the Community Children's Nurse. English National
Board for Nursing, Midwifery and Heath Visiting,
London

Robinson R 1993a Economic evaluation and health care:
what does it mean? British Medical Journal
307:670–673

Robinson R 1993b Cost–benefit analysis. British Medical
Journal 307:924–926

Robinson S & Hill Y 1998 The Health Promoting Nurse.
Journal of Clinical Nursing 7:232–238

Royal College of Nursing (RCN) 1994 Wise Decisions:
Developing Paediatric Home Care Teams. RCN
Paediatric Community Nurses' Forum, London

Shamian J 1997 How nursing contributes towards quality
and cost-effective health care. International Nursing
Review 44(3):79, 84, 90

Thomas L H & Bond S 1995 The effectiveness of
nursing: a review. Journal of Clinical Nursing
4:143–151

Tierney A 1993 Quality, costs and nursing. Journal of
Clinical Nursing 2:123–124

While A E 1991 An evaluation of a paediatric home
care scheme. Journal of Advanced Nursing
16:1413–1421

Whiting M, Greene A & Walker A 2001 Community
Children's Nursing – Delivering on the 'Quality
Agenda'? In: Sines D, Appelby F & Raymond E (eds)
Community Health Care Nursing, 2nd edn. Blackwell
Science, Oxford, p 177

Wilson A & Brown P 1989 Health care units and
neighbourhood nursing. In: Hughes J (ed.) The Future
of Community Health Services. King's Fund Centre,
Primary Health Care Group, London, p 21

Wilson-Barnett J & Beech S 1994 Evaluating the clinical
nurse specialist: a review. International Journal of
Nursing Studies 31(6):561–571

Chapter 32

Transition from children's to adult services

Linda Cancelliere and David Widdas

KEY ISSUES
- The political context and the need for transition.
- Who requires transitional care?
- Programmes to support transition of care.
- The timing of transition.
- Barriers to transition of care.
- Establishing assessment criteria for transitional care.
- The role of the Community Children's Nurse in the process of transition.

INTRODUCTION

Transition is defined as the 'The purposeful, planned movement of adolescents and young adults with chronic physical and medical conditions from a child-centred to adult orientated health care systems' (Blum et al 1993 p 570). The life expectancy of children with chronic, life-limiting or life-threatening conditions has improved significantly and this has been paralleled by the increased availability of community children's nurses (CCNs) (Glendinning et al 1999, Muir & Sidey 2003). This increase in life expectancy, alongside the move from institutional to community-focused and family-centred care, has added to both the recognition and the importance of transitional services (Blum 1995). An unfortunate side effect, arising from the need to transfer care between different services, can be a loss of the skills more associated with children's care. The transfer of young people, particularly those with special health needs, from child to adult services requires specific attention (Health Committee 1997).

Within some specialist services there is a history of transitional care (Viner & Keane 1998, Cuttell 2004). Following recommendations in the DoH document 'Valuing People' (DoH 2001a) learning disability teams are developing transitional services. However, services for children with complex care needs are generally less advanced with transitional care planning due to the complexities of their care (DoH 2001b). Despite examples of good practice, planning for transitional care remains a difficult area in most services (Health Committee 1997).

THE POLITICAL CONTEXT OF THE NEED FOR TRANSITIONAL CARE

There is a growing awareness of the perceived benefits of planned transitional arrangements. However, despite this, the providers of health and social care have yet to achieve the joint policies and procedures required to meet the needs of adolescents with chronic, complex health needs, when transferring from child-centred to adult-oriented healthcare (DoH 1995, Health Committee 1997).

The Government's commitment to the provision of an efficient and seamless health service through multi-agency and multidisciplinary planning, together with an increasing emphasis on empowerment, are key features of current health service policy (DoH 1989, 1991, 1999, 2000, 2001a, 2001b, 2003). Government recommendations acknowledge the lack of recognition of the needs of adolescents within healthcare provision during the transition to adulthood, particularly those with chronic and life-threatening illnesses and disability (DoH 1996, 2003).

The need for key workers and a person-centred approach in transitional planning together with the contribution of the employment facilitators 'Connexions' are highlighted in 'Valuing People' (DoH 2001a). Furthermore, transition is seen as a key theme in the National Service Framework (NSF) and will therefore be considered as a key section within each module of the NSF (DoH 2003). It is anticipated that this will bring a new impetus to the concept of transitional care.

WHO REQUIRES TRANSITIONAL CARE?

It could be said that there are four groups of young people who require planned transitional care and for whom CCNs may be providing or facilitating care. Some young people will span more than one group:

1. Condition specific (cystic fibrosis (CF), diabetes, etc.). For these young people there is a clear transitional pathway to an established adult service but the focus of these services is often very different. In diabetes, children's diabetes nurses have a recommended caseload of 100 families (Paediatric Diabetes Special Interest Group 1998). Anecdotal evidence suggests that within adult services caseloads may exceed 1000 individuals. Diabetes clinics in adult services are overwhelmingly populated by the elderly with a variety of complications from their condition. CCNs at tertiary centres report a lack of involvement in the transition process for children with CF (Cancelliere 2002).
2. Complex care. Transition in complex care is extremely difficult. Young people with a learning disability and complex care needs have no clear referral paths in terms of nursing or medical support. The need for the development of specially commissioned local psychosocial disability teams to coordinate this aspect of care is recognised in 'Bridging the Gaps' (Royal College of Paediatrics and Child Health 2003) (see Chapter 22).

3. Palliative care. Transition and palliative care should be considered together. With an increase in life expectancy, transition is an important part of the care process for some young people. The need for parallel planning is paramount. This should be aimed at following the planned transition of care but also at supporting end-stage care needs if required (Association for Children with Life-threatening or Terminal Conditions and their Families 2001, Royal College of Paediatrics and Child Health 2003) (see Chapter 23).
4. Learning Disabilities. 'Valuing People' has put transition at the forefront of learning disability services (DoH 2001a) (see Chapter 25).

PROGRAMMES TO SUPPORT TRANSITION OF CARE

Viner & Keane (1998) undertook a systematic review of the literature relating to adolescent care within the health service and identified that transitional programmes are particularly poor in areas where no specific adult service exists. This viewpoint is supported by Blum et al (1993) who suggest that adolescents experiencing greater degrees of disability or particularly complex medical conditions are at greater risk of encountering difficulties during transition. They require a formal programme of transition over a longer period. A number of studies identify that where transitional programmes have developed they are largely disease-based or condition-focused programmes, predominantly within CF and diabetes (Viner & Keane 1998, Scal et al 1999, Byron & Madge 2001) (Box 32.1).

Box 32.1 An example of transitional arrangements within a specialist service

Coventry Community Children's Nursing Service
Transitional Programme for Patients with Cystic Fibrosis

- Children's and adult nurses based together
- Families and children know both teams of nurses from diagnosis
- Co-hosted clinics
  (Enter transition September of school year 10 – aged 13–14 years)
- Alternate clinics led by children's and adult nurses
- Care led primarily by adult nurse by year 11
- First adult clinic appointment September of school year 12 with adult nurse, paediatrician and adult CF physician
- Discharged from Community Children's Nursing Service
  (K Thomas, unpublished work, 2000)

THE TIMING OF TRANSITION OF CARE

The need for flexible timing of the transitional process is widely acknowledged (DoH 1991, 1996, Pownceby et al 1996, Viner & Keane 1998). Viner (2001) suggests timing should coincide with developmental readiness and although supporting a target age as being useful, advocates it should not be the sole indicator in identifying readiness to transfer. Blum et al (1993) concluded that transition proceeds at different rates for different individuals and families. In a report on the transition of adolescents with CF, Walshaw (1996) supports the need for flexibility in timing. The American Academy of Pediatrics (1996) states that under 'special circumstances', which include chronic illness and disability, care can be continued within the paediatric setting beyond the age of 21 years where both the provider of children's services and family are in agreement. Conway (1998 p 210) advocates flexibility but states 'keeping patients in a paediatric clinic is tantamount to telling them that their lives will be too short to warrant the bother of moving on'.

The NSF definition of children's services is young people up to 19 years of age (DoH 2003). This definition is now likely to be used in all Government documents, creating an age to base decisions on. Transition from children's services needs to be young-person-centred and planned, have a clear beginning and end but not be a rushed process (Association for Children with Life threatening or Terminal Conditions and their Families 2001). However, a question to be considered is: What is the upper age limit of patients who may receive care from nurses educated on child branch and community children's nursing courses?

BARRIERS TO TRANSITION OF CARE

The reluctance of paediatric professionals to transfer patients, who they have developed close bonds with over many years, is identified by Viner (2001) as the greatest barrier to effective transition. Viner suggests that a lack of trust in the skills and knowledge base of adult services to care for young adults with 'paediatric conditions' also impacts on the reluctance of paediatric professionals to 'let go'. The reluctance of parents to support effective transition is highlighted by Patterson (1999) who identified parental difficulties in 'letting go'. Cancelliere (2002) adds the dimension of disempowerment of young people and their families, by lack of involvement in the process, as a further barrier to effective transition. In addition Patterson (1999) identified 'burnout' (in adolescents and young adults following many years of having to conform to treatments) as a reason for choosing to opt out of the healthcare system.

Viner (2001) suggests that reluctance to lose long-term relationships and fear of the future contribute to adolescent and family resistance to transition. The loss of these relationships may be perceived as a step closer to disease complications or ultimately death and are primary factors influencing adolescent and family resistance. The Association for Children with Life-threatening or Terminal Conditions and their Families (ACT) (2001) summarise the following barriers to transition in palliative care (Box 32.2).

Box 32.2 Barriers to effective transition in palliative care (ACT 2001)

- Families' attachment to children's services
- Paediatrician's reluctance to make the transfer
- Fragmented and impersonal healthcare in adult services
- Poor coordination of services in adult care

- No equivalent adult service available
- Transfer at a time of instability
- Lack of emotional readiness

ESTABLISHING ASSESSMENT CRITERIA FOR TRANSITIONAL CARE

Research by Cancelliere (2002) revealed a wide variation in existing transitional assessment criteria. For example, in a questionnaire to 17 CCNs, five identified age as the only criteria, three identified age and emotional maturity, six identified other criteria including, for example:

- when physicians transfer care
- when they leave school
- if the adolescent requests it
- condition related.

The lack of guidelines to support transition of care was noted by all respondents. The creation of multidisciplinary and multi-agency guidelines would help to steer this process. Blum et al (1993) suggest four key elements for successful transition:

- professional and environmental support
- decision making and developmentally appropriate consent
- family support
- professional sensitivity to the psychosocial issues of disability.

The ACT and the Royal College of Paediatrics and Child Health (RCPCH) guidelines provide suggestions to assist the establishment of criteria (ACT 2001, RCPCH 2003). It is anticipated that the NSF will further advocate clear transitional criteria. This will include that multi-agency and multidisciplinary teams allow for flexibility and choice with the child and family fully engaged in the process. The NSF is also expected to clearly link transition for young people with a disability to the services offered by 'Connexions' (DoH 2003).

THE ROLE OF THE COMMUNITY CHILDREN'S NURSE

The preparation of adolescents for the transition to adult services is considered to be important although problematic. The role of the nurse has been identified as pivotal in the coordination of transitional programmes (Baker & Coe 1993, Betz 1998, Viner & Keane 1998, Patterson 1999). Betz (1998) also supports the need for children's nurses to have appropriate knowledge and skills in the care of adolescents and suggests that nurses are ideally placed to 'bridge the gaps' between child and adult services through their skills of advocacy and communication. In a qualitative study exploring the role of the CCN in caring for children with chronic illness in the community, Carter (2000) identifies skills including facilitating, empowering and enabling as fundamental to the role of the CCN. These skills, which are central to the philosophy of community children's nursing, support the fact that CCNs have a vital role in the transition process. However, Cancelliere (2002) found that 35% of CCNs in her study considered they did not have a role to play in the transition of young people with complex care needs.

CONCLUSION

The publication 'Valuing People' (DoH 2001a) and the children's NSF (DoH 2003) placed transition at the heart of policies underpinning the delivery of care to young people and their families. CCNs have a pivotal role to play within the transition process. This, together with the increasing profile of transitional planning, would suggest that, as part of their advocacy role, they may use their skills and influence to steer and enhance this process. CCNs can influence the formation of local policy and act as key negotiators with the young person and their family. Effective acceptable transition is a key aspect of a young person's care and may be considered a qualitative marker of an effective community children's nursing team. Timely transition of young people to adult services releases staff to provide services to new referrals of children and their families who require experienced child-focused care.

REFERENCES

American Academy of Pediatrics 1996 Transition of care provided for adolescents with special health care needs. Pediatrics 98(6):1203–1206

Association for Children with Life-threatening or Terminal Conditions and their Families (ACT) 2001 Palliative Care for Young People Aged 13–24 Years. ACT, Bristol

Baker K L & Coe L 1993 Growing up with a chronic condition: Transition to young adulthood for the individual with cystic fibrosis. Holistic Nursing Practice 8(1):8–15

Betz C 1998 Adolescent transitions: A nursing concern. Pediatric Nursing 24(1):23–28

Blum R 1995 Transition to adult health care: Setting the stage. Journal of Adolescent Health 17(1):3–5

Blum R, Garell D, Hodgman C H, Jorrissen T W, Okinow N A, Orr D P & Slap G B 1993 Transition from child-centred to adult health care systems for adolescents with chronic conditions. Journal of Adolescent Health 14:570–576

Byron M & Madge S 2001 Transition from paediatric to adult care: Psychological principles. Journal of the Royal Society of Medicine Supplement 40(94):5–7

Cancelliere L 2002 An exploratory study into the experiences of Community Children's Nurses on the transition of adolescents with complex health needs from child centred to adult focused health services. Unpublished dissertation. University College Northampton. Northampton

Carter B 2000 Ways of working: Community Children's Nurses and chronic illness. Journal of Child Health Care 4(2):66–72

Conway S P 1998 Transition from paediatric to adult-orientated care for adolescents with cystic fibrosis. Disability and Rehabilitation 20(6/7):209–216

Cuttell K 2004 Adolescents with diabetes: A Health Action Zone Project. Paediatric Nursing 16(3):32–35

Department of Health 1989 NHS and Community Care Act. The Stationery Office, London

Department of Health 1991 Welfare of Children and Young People in Hospital. HMSO, London

Department of Health 1995 Growing Up and Moving On. Social Services Inspectorate Project, Bristol

Department of Health 1996 Child Health in the Community: A Guide to Good Practice. The Stationery Office, London

Department of Health 1999 Working Together to Safeguard Children. The Stationery Office, London

Department of Health 2000 The NHS Plan. The Stationery Office, London

Department of Health 2001a Valuing People: A new strategy for learning disability for the 21st century. The Stationery Office, London

Department of Health 2001b The Expert Patient: A new approach to chronic disease management for the 21st century. The Stationery Office, London

Department of Health 2003 Getting The Right Start: The National Service Framework for Children, Young People and Maternity Services – Emerging Findings. The Stationery Office, London

Glendinning C, Kirk S, Guiffrida A & Lawton D 1999 The Community Based Care of Technology-dependent Children in the UK: Definitions, Numbers, and Costs. National Primary Care Research and Development Centre, Manchester

Health Committee 1997 Health Services for Children and Young People in the Community: Home and School. The Stationery Office, London

Muir J & Sidey A 2003 Community children's nursing. In: Watkins D, Edwards J & Gastrell P (eds) Community Health Nursing. Baillière Tindall, Edinburgh, pp 271–280

Paediatric Diabetes Special Interest Group 1998 The Role and Qualifications of the Nurse Specializing in Paediatric Diabetes. Royal College of Nursing, London

Patterson D 1999 Adolescent Health Transitions: Focus Group Study of teens and young adults with special health care needs. Family and Community Health 22(2): 43–58

Pownceby J, Ratcliffe D, Abbott J & Kent P 1996 The Coming of Age Project. A study of the transition from paediatric to adult care and treatment adherence amongst young people with Cystic Fibrosis. Cystic Fibrosis Trust. Kent

Royal College of Paediatrics and Child Health (RCPCH) 2003 Bridging the Gaps: Health Care for Adolescents. RCPCH, London

Scal P, Evans T, Blozis S, Okinow N & Blum R 1999 Trends in transition from pediatric to adult health care services for young adults with chronic conditions. Journal of Adolescent Health 24(4):259–264

Viner R 2001 Barriers and good practice in transition from paediatric to adult care. Journal of the Royal Society of Medicine 94 Supplement 40:2–4

Viner R & Keane M 1998 Youth Matters. Caring for Children in the Health Service. Action for Sick Children, London

Walshaw M J 1996 The transfer of adolescents with cystic fibrosis to an adult clinic. Paediatric Respiratory Medicine 2(4):16–18

Chapter 33

Launching further research in community children's nursing

Steve Campbell and Susan Procter

KEY ISSUES

- The current research foundation in community children's nursing.
- Analysis of specific research studies and their relative findings.
- Indications for future research opportunities in community children's nursing.

INTRODUCTION

Research into community children's nursing is a relatively new phenomenon. The research that has been undertaken has tended not to include the children themselves. This is a challenge that all children's nursing researchers need to take on if research into the practice of community children's nursing is to develop: balancing the needs of children with those of their primary carer(s). Broome (1998 p 305) commented:

'Investigators who study children must assemble a team of investigators who are experts in child development and the study of children, who are familiar with methodological limitations of some methods with children, and who know how to protect children from undue burden. Society has much to gain from new research conducted with children.'

Children's nursing research in the UK has developed along family-centred lines. This tends to mean the involvement of parents and prime carers; however, future studies need to be balanced in favour of a children's focus. Such approaches are well supported by the NHS drive for greater patient involvement and implicit within the National Service Frameworks for children.

The content of this chapter is influenced by a nationally funded, English National Board for Nursing, Midwifery and Health Visiting (ENB) research study carried out between 1997 and 1998, of which the two authors were the principal investigators (Procter et al 1998a, 1998b, 1999). While there has been considerable development in the number of community children's nursing services since this report, the authors believe the findings to be enduring. Despite the contemporary nature of the study, the authors are aware that the study would have been enhanced by the greater involvement of children as primary sources of evidence.

The themes that were evident, and continue to be the source of inspiration for further research, are 'Burden of care', 'Guiding principles of care' and 'Forms of service'. These themes are presented as the structure to this chapter. To provide some clarity and order to these themes, a brief description of the research study (Procter et al 1998a, 1998b, 1999) will be presented.

BRIEF OUTLINE OF THE ENB RESEARCH STUDY

The study was designed to elicit a training needs analysis for Community Children's Nurses (CCNs) based on an analysis of the needs of families caring for sick children at home. The research used a variety of methods to:

- Map existing service provision nationally (England).
- Select six sites providing community children's nursing services (these were purposively sampled from all available NHS Trusts on the basis of a series of variables identified by an expert group) and undertake interviews with CCNs, their managers and professional colleagues.
- Undertake interviews with families receiving care from each of the services used in the research.
- Conduct three focus groups: a multiprofessional group, a group of nurse educationalists providing courses for CCNs and a group of representatives from children's charities with an interest in sick children being cared for at home (Procter et al 1998b).

The data were analysed qualitatively. Themes relating to service provision from a management, organisational and practitioner perspective were derived from the interviews with professional staff. The data from families drew on a theoretical analysis of need within a framework of health promotion and disease prevention. These were the families of a sample of children who could be characterised as largely having problems associated with chronic illness. A process model for service and curriculum development was produced, centred on a set of guiding principles and based on an analysis of the needs of families caring for sick children at home (Procter et al 1998b). The process of this research and outcomes of the study left the authors with a number of key issues that remain largely unresolved nationally and need to be the focus of further research.

BURDEN OF CARE

In reading the transcripts of the interviews with parents, the vast majority being mothers of chronically ill children, there was an impression of the enormous burden of care that parents and, in particular, mothers were obliged to take on. This burden was tempered, if not balanced, by the pride these parents took in being able to care for their child and the improvements they saw in their child. The obligation that these parents feel to care for their child at home is natural, but we are not yet clear as to how far we (or their sick children) can or should push parents into providing this care at home. The resources of the parents and the capacity of that family to care for the child are currently assessed by the multidisciplinary team involved. However, this assessment may be influenced by two conflicting perspectives: whilst getting the child home is philosophically the right thing to do, it also saves hospital funds. Such pressures on acute hospital beds will increase, making decisions about discharge even more important. The multidisciplinary team assessment tends to focus on the child and the prime carer(s) rather than the total family, because those involved are most aware and most specifically concerned with the dynamic of the relationship between these two. There is a need to examine the evidence and research base on which children, particularly those with complex needs, are discharged into the care of their family, with or without the support of a CCN. The current approach to assessing the family would seem, in the main, to be too narrow. This approach fails to draw on the potential of the whole family, their ability to problem solve and utilise their full resources.

The CCN appears to be in a key position to assess the needs of the whole family that takes on the care of the sick child at home. This is perhaps best exemplified by the position of many mothers, who find themselves providing the majority of the care to the chronically ill child. Baldwin and Twigg (1991) discuss the notion of delegating care to families, but caution that this should not prevent them leading 'relatively ordinary lives'. Systematic strategies for CCNs to help the members of families to lead relatively ordinary lives have not been explored to any great extent in practice, let alone through research.

The potential use of McCubbin and McCubbin's (1993) model of family resiliency has great potential as a focus for helping CCNs to find these new ways of working. The model can be regarded as outlining the process by which families adjust and adapt to illness. By allowing objectification of a family's collective reaction to a child's illness, the model affords the CCN the opportunity to find ways of intervening in the process of adaptation, so that there is greater opportunity for all members of the family to lead relatively ordinary lives. It has been commented that such a role would be better carried out by a social worker rather than a CCN, the justification being the social basis of this intervention and the social worker's potential knowledge of family therapy. However, such an approach is not family therapy and when challenging a focus group of special interest groups (Procter et al 1998a, 1999) with this proposition, the group was unanimous that this role needed to be carried out by CCNs because it was they who had the knowledge and credibility with the family. Such an approach would form an exciting action research project (Whyte et al 1998). Action research has been grasped as a methodology, although not applied to this arena, Livsey (2003) has used this approach to explore the development of a community children's nursing service.

GUIDING PRINCIPLES OF CARE

Procter et al (1998a, 1998b) suggested 17 guiding principles for community children's nursing practice (Box 33.1).

Box 33.1 Guiding principles of community children's nursing practice (Procter et al 1998a, 1998b)

1. Promoting family-centred care rather than child-centred care
2. Maintaining/improving the quality of life of the family, rather than focusing on medical needs
3. Minimising stressful events rather than giving routinised care
4. Fostering family empowerment rather than learned helplessness/dependency on professionals' problem-solving abilities
5. Having an approach of partnership rather than the imposition of professional expertise
6. Appreciating the complexity of a problem rather than oversimplifying it
7. Solving/re-framing problems rather than avoiding them
8. Recognising boundaries of own expertise and knowing where to turn for appropriate help rather than trying to solve all the problems yourself
9. Establishing credibility with paediatric and primary healthcare colleagues through working together openly rather than having an insular approach
10. Having a flexible/organic/responsive role, rather than a formally directed set of functions
11. Having knowledge gained through experience rather than procedures
12. Having the knowledge to anticipate/plan for future directions in the care needs of the child rather than reacting to crisis
13. Being available (light touch) for the family when the family wants it rather than when it is most convenient to services
14. Promoting the health of families rather than focusing solely on tertiary interventions
15. Lightening the burden through manner of approach, rather than getting caught up in the anxieties of the situation/reinforcing the burden
16. Enabling children and families to lead ordinary lives, rather than this being regarded as secondary to biomedical interventions
17. Listening/discovering rather than imposing ready-made solutions from elsewhere

---

Many of these principles are fundamental to the nature of good children's nursing in any setting, including hospital. Therefore, there is a need to identify those principles that are peculiar to the practice of a CCN and those that have been built up through practice in other fields of children's nursing, or even from nursing in general. Further work needs to be done to establish whether these 17 principles are exhaustive (i.e. whether there are further principles). This is especially pertinent, since the majority of the sample in this study were children with a chronic illness (Procter et al 1998a, 1998b). The nursing in the community of children with an acute illness might well elicit different guiding principles and is an area yet to be studied (see Chapter 21). Further to this, there would appear to be relationships between some of these 17 principles. This raises the issue of whether there is a need for *all* of these principles, or whether some could be conflated. Such a study could be carried out by identifying the major theme areas underlying these principles and grouping them together.

Given that these principles were derived from interviews with the families involved in the study (Procter et al 1998a, 1998b, 1999), it would be possible to construct some form of evaluation tool based upon the ways that families with a chronically ill child would like CCNs to behave. As an evaluative instrument, such as a linear analogue (Burns 1979, Cella & Perry 1986), this could then be completed by the families. Such an evaluation tool would be useful for many community children's nursing services. In the process of the ENB study, many managers of community children's nursing services indicated that they were struggling to provide data to support their practice. Specialist services, such as paediatric oncology, may be able to provide data such as morbidity and mortality statistics to justify their practice. However, generalist community children's nursing practice may be concerned much more with the quality of life of the child and family, but these issues are more challenging to evaluate. Assessing the extent to which each family believes their CCN to have worked to the principles may well help to provide some meaningful data for managers of these services.

FORMS OF SERVICE

Since the publication of 'Wise decisions' (Royal College of Nursing 1994), there has been a preoccupation with the different models of community children's nursing services based upon need. More recently, Eaton and Thomas (1998) and Whiting (Chapter 2) characterised models of service provision with clear relationships between each. It may be possible, with further analysis, to identify a continuum of their characteristics and to also identify the different forms of service, with these models as important areas of activity on that continuum.

CCNs will be required now and in the future to be sure of where their practice needs to be placed; further work should be undertaken to establish the nature and form of this need. In particular, this work should be influenced by key authors in this area, such as Bradshaw (1972) and his form of need: normative, relative, felt and expressed (see Chapter 17). There are challenging questions to be answered with respect to how it is possible to articulate a notion of need in relation to a family.

The nature of 'good' community children's nursing services is linked to the guiding principles laid out in Box 33.1. Is this a function of the people involved in the service, or is it derived from the nature of the form of the service? Eaton and Thomas (1998) have identified evaluative criteria derived from quality management theoretical material. These criteria have a relationship with the guiding principles, although they focus on the service itself. The criteria identified by Eaton and Thomas (1998) assist in answering important questions about what part of the organisation of the service lends itself to promotion of this 'good' community children's nursing service. However, if the success of a service is derived from the people concerned, from where did they gain these qualities? Were they innate, or taught to them in practice or in their nurse training, or learned in other forms of practice or from role models? All of these questions represent lines of enquiry in the practice of a CCN.

CONCLUSION

In this chapter it has been possible only to hint at aspects of the potential for research building on the currently limited foundations available. These foundations are strong, but need to be developed and to be part of a balance of family-focused and child-focused research.

REFERENCES

Baldwin S & Twigg J 1991 Women and community care – reflections on debate. In: Maclean M & Groves D (eds) Women's Issues in Social Policy. Routledge, London, pp 117–135

Bradshaw J 1972 The concept of social need. New Society 30:640–643

Broome M E 1998 Researching the world of children. Nursing Research 47(6):305–306

Burns R E 1979 The use of visual analogue mood and alert scales in diagnosing hospitalised affective psychosis. Psychological Medicine 9:155–164

Cella D F & Perry S W 1986 Reliability and validity of three visual analogue mood scales. Psychological Reports 59:827–830

Eaton N & Thomas P 1998 Community children's nursing: an evaluative framework. Journal of Child Health Care 2(4):170–173

Livsey P 2003 Contradictions and Confusions in the Provision of Community Children's Nursing Services. PhD Thesis, Lancaster University

McCubbin M A & McCubbin H I 1993 Families coping with illness: the resiliency model of family stress, adjustment and adaptation. In: Danielson C B, Hamel-Bissell B & Winstead-Fry P (eds) Families, Health and Illness. Mosby, St Louis

Procter S, Biott C, Campbell S, Edward S, Redpath N & Moran M 1998a Preparation for the Developing Role of the Community Children's Nurse. English National Board for Nursing, Midwifery and Health Visiting, London

Procter S, Biott C, Campbell S, Edward S, Redpath N & Moran M 1998b Preparation for the Developing Role of the Community Children's Nurse. Research Highlights, no. 32. English National Board for Nursing, Midwifery and Health Visiting, London

Procter S, Biott C, Campbell S, Edward S, Redpath N & Moran M 1999 Preparation for the Developing Role of the Community Children's Nurse. Researching Professional Education: Research Report Series, no. 11. English National Board for Nursing, Midwifery and Health Visiting, London

Royal College of Nursing (RCN) 1994 Wise Decisions. Developing Paediatric Home Care Teams. RCN Paediatric Community Nurses Forum, London

Whyte D, Barton M E, Lamb A et al 1998 Clinical effectiveness in community children's nursing. Clinical Effectiveness in Nursing 2: 139–144

Conclusion

Anna Sidey and David Widdas

Community children's nursing has a relatively short history compared with nursing as a whole. The enormous societal changes since the Industrial Revolution have had a profound influence on how we practice and develop nursing services. In Chapter 1 we read that in 1095 the monks were delivering community-based care in a self directed manner. This chapter describes the development of nursing towards the end of the following thousand years, a time that saw alongside the industrial revolution the rise of the medical profession, subservience of nurses and a concentration on the secondary model of care. The first challenges to this model of care for children and their families came from Dr West at Great Ormond Street in the 1880s. The scene was then set for one of the slowest revolutions in healthcare history! One hundred years later only 24 services, most staffed by only one or two Community Children's Nurses (CCNs), existed (Chapter 2).

Recent history offers some answers to the slow pace of this revolution. CCNs based in the community and offering nurse-led services challenged the dominance of secondary care and the medical profession. The Community Children's Nursing Forum of the Royal College of Nursing, established in 1988, set about revolutionising the pace of reform. The contributions of the early 'heroes' of the forum, as described in Chapters 2, 8 and 10 contributed to the publication of numerous documents to influence and support practice, service development and political thought and direction. CCNs now have opportunities unparalleled in the first 100 years of their development.

Are these opportunities being fully realised? Two waves of new (time-limited) funding have become available with the Diana and the New Opportunity Fund (NOF) monies. In addition Continuing Care funding is supporting some children with complex care needs (Chapter 22) and more acutely ill children are cared for at home (Chapter 21). These developments are supported by the increasing number of nurse prescribers (Chapter 29), and new roles such as Nurse Consultants (Chapter 16) and Nurse Practitioners (Chapter 30). Community children's nursing services are increasingly multiprofessional and skill mixed. However, at the time of writing many children, young people and their families do not have access to a CCN despite the number of services listed in the latest directory of CCNs and figures for the percentage of the country covered by services.

Whiting (Chapter 2) identifies a core group of children visited by CCNs but recent developments have focused on life-limited children and children who fit the tight criteria for Continuing Care. A new way of calculating service coverage is required.

The time-limited nature of Diana and NOF funding is a major issue for commissioners in Primary Care Trusts. The evidence base for commissioning has to some extent been improved by the Diana team evaluations but no common evaluation was undertaken. A meter study is now required to combine these evaluations. The Children's National Service Framework (NSF) team, as part of its remit, is evaluating the existing evidence on the effectiveness of community children's nursing.

The development of community children's nursing has resulted in wide variations in service provision. These variations could be seen as local responses to local needs or as an example of the so-called postcode lottery. The lack of a corporate identity (Chapter 10) has contributed to discrepancies in provision that may exist even within the same county. Modern families are highly mobile and for families with children with complex conditions, availability and acceptance criteria of the local community children's nursing team is a consideration when moving home or changing employment or lifestyle.

Nursing's history is characterised by divided movement and this division has consistently undermined the influence of nursing (Chapter 1). The power of CCNs working together was demonstrated in 1997 by their effect on the House of Commons select committee report (Chapter 2). However will the lack of a corporate strategy and shared national identity ultimately divide CCNs? The degree course provides a bedrock to our shared identity but do all teams aspire to second their staff to these courses? Are placements always appropriately negotiated and are CCNs taught by CCNs (p 111)?

Some teams are led and/or managed by nurses with either no community qualification and/or no children's nursing qualification. Anecdotal evidence suggests a worrying number of CCNs themselves feel without local, regional and national leadership, especially in services not connected to successful urban children's centres. Some services are observed to be reinventing 'wheels' invented by their predecessors as they attempt to fill a leadership vacuum. Nationally, 20 years ago a small number of individual CCNs supported and guided each other's innovative practice. Today CCNs still feel the need to do the same.

Many services suffer from the shortage of effective CCN managers able to appropriately lead services through the maze of secure service provision and development, clinical management and the world of commissioners and their employing trust's adjusting structures. More local role models, with robust backgrounds in practice, education, and management, need to be 'grown' from within the profession to contribute to the essential growth of a national strategy and corporate identity. The passion that may guide practice must be supported by sophisticated information, an ability to deliver it in the 'language' of the new NHS and the leadership to do so. The supervision of the practice of children's nurses providing and facilitating care in community settings is less rigorous in some areas than others and contributes to concerns over the essential enabling and empowering nature of practice (see Introduction and p 135).

The dream of 100% national service coverage is nearer but a national holistic community children's nursing service remains a distant vision. The NSF offers another opportunity for community children's nursing to develop. The focus of the NSF, on a clear evidence base, must be utilised by CCNs to create a national service module to ensure a truly equitable national service.

'There can be no keener revelation of a society's soul than the way in which it treats its children'

(Nelson Mandela)

Chapter-linked websites

CHAPTER 24
www.mentalhealth.org.uk *Mental Health Foundation*
www.youngminds.org.uk *Mental health for young people, parents and professionals*
www.focusproject.org.uk *Focus, an organisation which aims to promote effective practice in child and adolescent mental health services*
www.ru-ok.com *Interactive website to promote mental well-being for teenagers*
www.rethink.org/at-ease *Mental health resource for young people under stress or worried about their thoughts and feelings*

CHAPTER 25
www.APLD@apld.freeserve.co.uk *Association of Practitioners in Learning Disabilities*
www.Bild@bild.demon.co.uk *British Institute for Learning Disability (BILD)*
www.dh.gov.uk/vpst *Valuing People support team*
www.dh.gov.uk/learningdisabilities/ *Learning disabilities site at DoH*

CHAPTER 26
www.carersonline.org.uk *Carers UK*
www.ycrg.org.uk *Young Carers Research Group*
www.bubblycrew.org.uk *Hammersmith and Fulham Young Carers*
www.disabledparentsnetwork.org.uk *The Disabled Parents Network*
www.youngminds.org.uk *Young Minds*
www.youngcarers.net

CHAPTER 28
www.aor.org.uk *Association of Reflexologists*
www.acupuncture.org.uk *British Acupuncture Council*
www.bhma.org *British Holistic Medical Association*
www.icmedicine.co.uk *Institute for Complementary Medicine*
www.IFPAroma.org *International Federation of Professional Aromatherapists*
www.rccm.org.uk *Research Council for Complementary Medicine*
www.homeopathy-soh.org *Society of Homeopaths*
www.miami.edu/touch-research *Touch Research Institute*

CHAPTER 29
www.dh.gov.uk/PolicyAndGuidance/MedicinesPharmacyAndIndustry/Prescriptions/NursingPrescribing *Policy on nurse prescribing, lists products formulary for extended prescribers, details of training course*
www.npc.co.uk *National Prescribing Centre, competency framework*
www.nurse-prescriber.co.uk/ *List of recently published articles*

CHAPTER 31
www.ohe.org *Office of Health Economics providing independent research, advisory and consultancy service*
www.healtheconomics.com

Generic websites

www.act.org.uk *Association for Children with Life-threatening or Terminal Conditions and their Families*

www.actionforsickchildren.org *offers standards/guidance/reports/training packs on provision of health services for children/young people*

www.BACCH.org.uk *British Association for Community Child Health*

www.barnardos.org.uk

www.childrenssociety.org.uk *The Children's Society*

www.dh.gov.uk *provides access to all reports/circulars, most documents available in PDF format*

www.dh.gov.uk/bristolinquiryresponse.htm *recommendations from Bristol Enquiry and DoH responses*

www.dh.gov.uk/childrenstaskforce

www.dh.gov.uk/childrenstrust/index.htm *frequently asked questions about Children's Trusts*

www.dh.gov.uk/nsf/children *children's NSF, allows users to leave comments*

www.hda-online.org.uk *Health Development Agency*

www.healthaction.nhs.uk *information on Health Needs Assessment and profiling*

www.healthy.net *Health World Online*

www.hfht.org/chiq/ *Centre for Health Information Quality*

www.hse.gov.uk *Health and Safety Executive*

www.hsj.macmillan.com *Health Services Journal, free access to strategic/managerial information on NHS*

www.integratedcarenetwork.gov.uk *Integrated Care Network*

www.jrf.org.uk *Joseph Rowntree Trust, publishes research on children/families/disability/support need*

www.mencap.org.uk

www.ncb.org.uk/cdc *Council for Disabled Children*

www.ndt.org.uk *National Development Team*

www.nelh.nhs.uk/childhealth *National Electronic Library for Child Health*

www.nmap.ac.uk *UK resources for nurses/midwives/allied professionals*

www.rcn.org.uk/resources/clinicalleadership *RCN Clinical Leadership*

www.rcpch.ac.uk *Royal College of Paediatrics and Child Health*

www.statistics.gov.uk/ *Office for National Statistics*

www.through-the-maze.org.uk/pages/ContactAFamily *support for people with learning disabilities/families/carers*

www.who.int/en/ *World Health Organisation*

www.wiredforhealth.gov.uk

www.york.ac.uk/inst/spru/ccnuk.htm *Care Co-ordination Network UK promoting care co-ordination/key working for children with disabilities and their families*

Chapter-linked further reading

CHAPTER 5   Crawshaw P, Bunton R & Gillen K 2003 Health Action Zones and the problem of community. Health and Social Care 11(1):36–44
Uses findings of ongoing study into zone in north east of England to consider community involvement in practice

Harris M & Rochester C 2001 Voluntary organisations and social policy in Britain. Palgrave, Basingstoke
Analyses numerous/complex ways that formulation and implementation of social policy is dependent on contributions of voluntary sector

Kendall J & Knapp M 1996 The voluntary sector in the UK. Manchester University Press
Provides first ever comprehensive, consolidated/detailed account of scope of UK voluntary sector and traces sector's historical development

Wyatt M 2002 Partnership in Health and Social Care. Policy and Politics 30(2):167–182
Implications of Government guidance in the 1990s in England, particular reference to voluntary organizations

CHAPTER 7   Department for Education and Employment 1999 The Special Educational Needs Code of Practice. The Stationery Office, London
Sets out current arrangements for identification/assessment of special educational needs, including contribution of community child health and nursing services to assessment/reviews

Department for Education and Skills (DfES) 2002 Accessible Schools: planning to increase access to schools for disabled pupils. DfES Publications, Nottingham
Explains new planning duties for schools and gives extensive set of references/ useful organisations

Department for Education and Skills 2002 Inclusive Schooling: Children with special educational needs. DfES Publications, Nottingham
Guidance sets out Government's statutory framework for inclusion and summarises a wide range of legislation that protects interests of children with special educational needs

Disability Rights Commission 2002 Code of Practice for Schools. Disability Rights Commission, London
Code of Practice, sets out duties for schools/LEAs associated services under Disability Discrimination Act 1995 Part 4. Contains practical advice/examples of education and health services working together/extensive references to other guidance/Disability Rights Commission's free Help-Line/Casework Service

CHAPTER 11

Morse J 1991 Negotiating commitment and involvement in the nurse–patient relationship. Journal of Advanced Nursing 16:455–468
Uses grounded theory methodology to explore relationship between nurse/patient

CHAPTER 12

Dimond B 1996 The legal aspects of child health care. Mosby, London

Dimond B 1996 The right to die, euthanasia and advanced directives. In: Greaves D & Upton H (eds) Philosophical problems in health care. Avebury, London
Sets out law relating to letting die/killing

Dimond B 1997 Legal aspects of care in the community. Macmillan, London

Dimond B 2004 The legal aspects of nursing. 4th ed. Pearson Education, Harlow, Essex
Overview of law relating to nursing, relevant to the healthcare of the child, specifically considers practical aspects of child care in the community

Dimond B 2002 The Legal Aspects of Pain Management. Quay Publications, Dinton, Wiltshire
Looks at legal issues arising in palliative care/pain management, considers issues relating to chronically sick/dying children

Dimond B 2003 The Legal Aspects of Consent. Quay Publications, Dinton, Wiltshire
Considers legal issues arising across wide field of topics where consent arises, including research/life saving treatment/rights of the child and young person in comparison with the rights/responsibilities of parents

CHAPTER 13

Downie R S, Tannahill C & Tannahill A 2002 Health promotion: models and values. 2nd edn. Oxford University Press, Oxford
Comprehensive overview of key concepts surrounding health promotion

Ewles L & Simnett I 1995 Promoting health. A practical guide. 3rd edn. Scutari Press, London
Guide for professionals working as health promoters

Naidoo J & Wills J 2000 Health promotion. Foundations for practice. 2nd edn. Baillière Tindall, London
Comprehensive text, provides valuable insight into multifaceted perspectives of health promotion

CHAPTER 14

Dwivedi K N & Varma V P 1996 Meeting the needs of ethnic minority children. Jessica Kingsley, London
Addresses social/health care of children from minority ethnic families in UK, particular focus on meeting psychological needs

Helman C G 2000 Culture, health and illness. 4th edn. Butterworth–Heinemann, London
Medical anthropology text, well organized into chapters that enable reader to dip in. Little information on children but useful for insight into culture of medical care

Prout A 1996 Families, cultural bias and health promotion implications of an ethnographic study. Health Education Authority, London
Ethnographic study examining impact of culture on health promotion in the family, an insight into the complexities of how families make decisions about health, children's own contribution

Slater M 1993 Health for all our children: achieving appropriate health care for black and ethnic minority children and their family. Action for Sick Children, London
Report of study reviewing experiences of minority ethnic families within health service, provides examples of good practice/training package

CHAPTER 19

Needham J 1997 Accuracy in Workload measurement: a fact or fallacy? Journal of Nursing Management 5(2):83–87
Written by children's nurse, examines accuracy of workload measurement systems, advocates using patient dependency as an assessment tool

Roberts W & Ross R 1996 Make it so: leadership lessons from Star Trek: The Next Generation. Pocket Books, New York
Excellent source of illustrations of good leadership qualities, highlights importance of keeping logs and records, notes 'Apathy, laziness, distraction, and interference can all lead to a self inflicted workplace crisis created by the failure to do what needs to be done within acceptable time limits, or according to established standards'!

CHAPTER 20

Thompson C & Dowding D (eds) 2002 Clinical decision making and judgement in nursing. Churchill Livingstone, Edinburgh
Overview of research/practical experience of implementing decision making in practice with links to information management, clinical governance and autonomous nursing roles

Thompson D & Wright K 2003 Developing a Unified Patient Record: A Practical Guide. Radcliffe Medical Press, Oxford
Summarises drivers for integrated, multi-professional record keeping, provides examples of unified records, approaches to changing practice in record keeping

CHAPTER 22

National Health Service Executive 1998 Evaluation of the pilot project programme for children with life threatening illnesses. The Stationery Office, London
Provides examples of good practice in meeting the needs of sick children in the community, contains practical examples including eligibility criteria/training protocols for carers

National Primary Care Research and Development Centre (NPCRDC) 1999 Supporting Parents Caring for a Technology Dependent Child NPCRDC, Manchester
Provides information on numbers/types of children who are technology dependent at home/recommendations for planning care

Servian R, Jones V, Lenehan C & Spires S 1998 Towards a healthy future. Shared Care Network, London
Provides examples of guidelines/training packages, useful definitions for agreeing local policies

CHAPTER 23

PaedPalLit. Association for Children with Life-threatening or Terminal Conditions and their Families, Bristol
Quarterly literature search for those working with children with life-limiting conditions

Twycross A, Moriarty A & Betts T 1998 Paediatric Pain Management. Radcliffe Medical Press, Oxford

CHAPTER 24

Edwards E & Davis H 1997 Counselling children with chronic medical conditions. BPS Books, Leicester
Important book for all healthcare workers in contact with children, includes detailed information about practical skills to promote supportive/facilitative communication

Sharman W 1997 Children and adolescents with mental health problems. Baillière Tindall, London
Excellent introduction to mental health difficulties experienced by children/ young people from a nursing perspective

CHAPTER 25

Abbot D, Morris J & Ward L 2000 Disabled Children and Residential Schools: a Study of Local Authority Policy and Practice. Norah Fry Centre
Looks at practice of local authorities and placement of young disabled adults in residential schools

Brown H 2000 Abuse and Protection issues, Centre for Applied Social and Psychological Development. Christ Church University Press, Canterbury
Insight into issues surrounding abuse/protection in children/adults with learning disability

Department of Health 2002 Action for Health Action Plans and Health Facilitation. Good Practice Guidance on Implementation for Learning Disability Partnership Boards. The Stationery Office, London
Guide on how/why people with learning disabilities should be offered health action plans

CHAPTER 26   Department of Health 1999 Caring about carers: a national strategy for carers. The Stationery Office, London
Ch. 8 summarises situation for young carers, endorses Government's belief in multi-agency work

McClure L 2001 School-age caregivers: Perceptions of school nurses working in central England. Journal of School Nursing 17(2)
Identifies school nurses' perceptions of young carers encountered, could be replicated to discover CCN's perceptions of young carers they know

Tucker S & Taturn C 1999 On small shoulders. The Children's Society, London
Research initiated by OU and Children's Society examines some long-term effects of being a young carer

CHAPTER 27   McMahon L 1992 The Handbook of Play Therapy. Routledge, London
Comprehensive introduction to theory/practice, provides practical guide to basic skills necessary to begin tapping healing potential of play

CHAPTER 28   Buckle J 2003 Clinical aromatherapy. Churchill Livingstone, Edinburgh
Evidence based, examines key facts/issues in aromatherapy practice, applies them within a variety of contexts, highlights how aromatherapy can enhance clinical care

Mantle F 2004 Complementary and alternative medicine in child and adolescent care. Butterworth-Heinemann, Edinburgh

Null G 1997 The clinician's handbook of natural healing: the first comprehensive guide to scientific review studies of natural supplements and their proven treatment values. Kensington Books, New York

Pietroni P & Pietroni C 1996 Innovation in community care and primary health. The Marylebone Experiment. Churchill Livingstone, Edinburgh
Describes benefits (and pitfalls) of integrating complementary therapies/mainstream primary care

Price S & Price L 1999 Aromatherapy for health professionals. 2nd edn. Churchill Livingstone, Edinburgh

Rankin-Box D (ed.) 2001 The nurses' handbook of complementary therapies. 2nd edn. Churchill Livingstone, Edinburgh

Rankin-Box D 2002 Clinical reflexology: a guide for health professionals. Churchill Livingstone, Edinburgh

CHAPTER 31

Kernick D (ed.) 2002 Getting Health Economics into Practice. Radcliffe Medical Press, Oxford
Illustrates practical help that concept/principles of health economics can offer, addresses gap between health economic theory/realities of the healthcare environment, highlights practical value of health economics

Kobelt G 2002 Health Economics: an introduction to economic evaluation. 2nd edn. Office of Health Economics, London
Provides accessible/practical introduction to principles behind economic analysis, step by step guide to methods used when undertaking economic evaluations of healthcare interventions

Morris S 1997 Health Economics for Nurses: an Introductory Guide. Prentice-Hall, Essex
Offers account of economic relevant concepts, aims to explain economic theory underlying healthcare policy in the NHS, examines economic techniques to improve understanding of cost effectiveness

Royal College of Nursing 1998 Marketing community and specialist nursing services – an RCN guide. Royal College of Nursing, London
Contains useful information/case examples on marketing/analysing services/demonstrating cost effectiveness of nursing

CHAPTER 32

Association for Children with Life-threatening or Terminal Conditions and their Families (ACT) 2001 Palliative Care for Young People Aged 13–24 Years. ACT, Bristol
Seminal publication, provides essential overview of identified key issues for young people with palliative care needs, contains specific chapter dedicated to transition

Soanes C & Timmons S 2004 Improving Transition: a qualitative study examining the attitudes of young people with chronic illness transferring to adult care. Journal of Child Health Care 8(2):102–112

Generic further reading

Antrobus S 1998 Political leadership in nursing. Nursing Management 5(4):26–28
Describes political leadership in nursing/expresses view that nurses require appropriate knowledge to influence policy and practise effectively

Antrobus S & Kitson A 1999 Nursing leadership: influencing and shaping health policy and nursing practice. Journal of Advanced Nursing 29(3):746–753
Considers sociopolitical factors that have impact on nursing leadership

Association for the Care of Children with Life-threatening or Terminal Conditions and their Families (ACT) 2003 Voices for Change. ACT, Bristol
Explores current perceptions of parents/professionals on accessibility/delivery of services

Association for the Care of Children with Life-threatening or Terminal Conditions and their Families (ACT) & Royal College of Paediatrics and Child Health 2003 A guide to the development of children's palliative care services. 2nd edn. ACT, Bristol
Overview of measures to help families/professionals meet emotional/therapeutic/spiritual/psychological needs of children

Association for the Care of Children with Life-threatening or Terminal Conditions and their Families (ACT) 2004 Information Pack for Families. ACT, Bristol
Information for families on support available

British Medical Association 2001 Consent, Rights and Choices in Health Care for Children and Young People. British Medical Journal Books, London
Account of issues in decision making

Burr S 1998 Making waves. Nursing Management 5(6):8–11
The potential of HoC Health Select Committee as powerful mechanism to influence healthcare policy is explored, specific reference to Inquiry into Services for Children/Young People

Cunningham G & Kitson A 2000 An evaluation of the RCN's clinical leadership development programme – part 1. Nursing Standard 15(12):34–37

Dale N 1996 Working with Families of Children with Special Needs: Partnership and Practice. Routledge, London
Exploration of relationship between family/professional, considers issues such as consent/confidentiality/breaking news of diagnosis

Department for Education and Skills (DfES) 2003 Every Child Matters. DfES Publications Unit, Nottingham
Government's Green Paper sets out radical plans to reform children's services

Department of Health and Department for Education and Skills (DfES) 2003 Together from the start: practical guidance for professionals working with young disabled children and their families birth to three. DfES Publications Unit, Nottingham
Government's guidance for professionals working with young disabled children and their families

Department for Education and Skills (DfES) 2004 The SEN Action Programme. DfES, Nottingham
Sets out new agenda for children with disabilities and special educational needs

Department of Health 1998 Government response to the reports of the Health Committee on health services for children and young people. The Stationery Office, London
Two publications offering invaluable information on policy/practice/developing community children's nursing services

Department of Health 2004 The Chief Nursing Officer's review of nursing, midwifery and health visiting contribution to vulnerable children and young people. The Stationery Office, London
Sets out changes needed to improve health and well-being

Department of Health (DoH) & Department for Education and Skills 2004 National Service Framework for Children, Young People and Maternity Services. DoH, London

Eaton N & Thomas P 1998 Community children's nursing: an evaluative framework. Journal of Child Health Care 2(4):170–173
Explores components of comprehensive evaluation which considers views/perspectives of key stakeholders in a community children's nursing service

English National Board for Nursing, Midwifery and Health Visiting (ENB) & Department of Health 1999 Sharing the care. Resource pack to support Diana, Princess of Wales Community Children's Nursing Teams. ENB, London
Guidance for establishing community nursing teams specialising in care of children with life limiting/threatening illness

Health Committee 1997 The House of Commons Health Select Committee. Health services for children and young people in the community: home and school. Third Report. The Stationery Office, London

Lenehan C & Carlin J 2003 The Risk Management Handbook. National Children's Bureau, London
Practical guidance on the management of risk

Lenehan C, Morrison J & Stanley J 2004 The dignity of risk. Council for Disabled Children, London
Provides examples of/advice on risk management strategies

Procter S, Biott C, Cambell S, Edward S, Redpath N & Moran M 1998 Preparation for the role of the community children's nurse. English National Board for Nursing and Midwifery, London
Comprehensive study/process model for service/curriculum development centred on set of guiding principles based on analysis of needs of families caring for sick children at home (see Chapter 33)

Rosina R, Starling J, Nunn K et al 2002 Telenursing: Clinical Nurse Consultancy For Rural Paediatric Nurses. Journal of Telemedicine and Telecare. 8 Suppl 3:S3:48–49
Reports a project using technology to link ward nurses/local community teams to enhance nursing care of young people psychological/physical health problems

Royal College of Nursing 2000 Children's Community Nursing. Promoting effective teamworking for children and their families. RCN, London
Guide to planning/auditing community children's nursing services

Royal College of Nursing 2002 Community Children's Nursing. RCN, London
Information for Primary Care organisations/Strategic Health Authorities/ professionals working with children

Royal College of Nursing Publishing Company. 'Paediatric Nursing' and 'Primary Health Care', London
Journals address current issues/dilemmas in children's and community nursing

Russell P 1998 Having a say? Partnership in decision-making with disabled children. National Children's Bureau, London
Looks at positive partnerships between range of healthcare/other professionals/ children/young people with disabilities and special healthcare need/gives practical examples of involving children (and families) in decision making/treatment

Servian R, Jones V & Lenehan C 1998 Towards a healthy future: multi-agency working in the management of invasive and life-saving procedures for children in family based services. Norah Fry Research Centre, Bristol
Advice on management of children with complex health care needs in the community

Sines D, Appelby F & Raymond E 2001 (eds) Community Health Care Nursing. 2nd edn. Blackwell Sciences, Oxford
General community nursing textbook, considers key issues for the introduction and implementation of infrastructure for health care nursing/quality of service delivery in community children's nursing

The Audit Commission 2003 'Let me be me'. Online. Available: www. auditcommission.gov. uk/disabledchildren/downloads/handbook.pdf
Handbook for managers/staff working with disabled children/families, draws on experiences of a large interview sample, aims to be tool to integrate services provided by staff from different agencies, includes service planning/workforce/ inclusion in everyday life/transition to adult services

Townsley R, Abbot D & Watson W 2003 Making a difference? The Policy Press, York
Findings from research by Family Fund/Norah Fry into multi-agency services which provide effective and focused multi-agency support to families with children with disabilities/complex health needs

Watkins D, Edwards J & Gastrell P (eds) 2003 Community Health Nursing – Frameworks for practice 2nd edn. Baillière Tindall, London
Key text for students of community nursing, identifies current pressures for change, public health agenda, family as a framework for practice, psychological/sociological perspectives, shifting boundaries of community practice, specific chapter for CCNs providing comprehensive summary of speciality

Whiting M, Greene A & Walker A 2001 Community Children's Nursing – Delivering on the 'Quality Agenda'. In: Sines D, Appleby F & Raymond E (eds) Community Healthcare Nursing. 2nd edn. London: Blackwell Science. Ch 11
Systematic examination of range of strategies utilised to demonstrate attainment of 'quality' in community children's nursing

Whyte D A 1997 Explorations in family nursing. Routledge, London
Examines a systemic approach to nursing care which can be applied widely in both hospital and community settings

Index

Page numbers suffixed by 'f' refer to figures; those with 't' refer to tables; those with 'b' refer to boxed material.

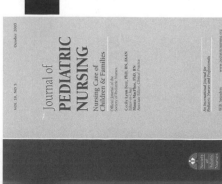